T0226552

Endocrine Surgery

Editor

PETER J. MAZZAGLIA

SURGICAL CLINICS
OF NORTH AMERICA

www.surgical.theclinics.com

Consulting Editor
RONALD F. MARTIN

June 2014 • Volume 94 • Number 3

ELSEVIER

1600 John F. Kennedy Boulevard • Suite 1800 • Philadelphia, Pennsylvania, 19103-2899

http://www.surgical.theclinics.com

SURGICAL CLINICS OF NORTH AMERICA Volume 94, Number 3
June 2014 ISSN 0039–6109, ISBN-13: 978-0-323-29933-6

Editor: John Vassallo, j.vassallo@elsevier.com

Developmental Editor: Yonah Korngold

Surgical Clinics of North America (ISSN 0039–6109) is published bimonthly by Elsevier Inc., 360 Park Avenue South, New York, NY 10010-1710. Months of publication are February, April, June, August, October, and December. Business and Editorial Offices: 1600 John F. Kennedy Blvd., Suite 1800, Philadelphia, PA 19103-2899. Periodicals postage paid at New York, NY and additional mailing offices. Subscription prices are $370.00 per year for US individuals, $627.00 per year for US institutions, $180.00 per year for US students and residents, $455.00 per year for Canadian individuals, $793.00 per year for Canadian institutions, $510.00 for international individuals, $793.00 per year for international institutions and $250.00 per year for Canadian and foreign students/residents. To receive student/resident rate, orders must be accompanied by name of affiliated institution, date of term, and the *signature* of program/residency coordinator on institution letterhead. Orders will be billed at individual rate until proof of status is received. Foreign air speed delivery is included in all *Clinics* subscription prices. All prices are subject to change without notice. POSTMASTER: Send address changes to *Surgical Clinics*, Elsevier Health Sciences Division, Subscription Customer Service, 3251 Riverport Lane, Maryland Heights, MO 63043. **Customer Service (orders, claims, online, change of address): Telephone: 1-800-654-2452 (U.S. and Canada); 314-447-8871 (outside U.S. and Canada). Fax: 314-447-8029. E-mail: journalscustomerservice-usa@elsevier.com (for print support); journalsonline support-usa@elsevier.com (for online support).**

Reprints. For copies of 100 or more, of articles in this publication, please contact the Commercial Reprints Department, Elsevier Inc., 360 Park Avenue South, New York, New York 10010-1710. Tel. 212-633-3874, Fax: 212-633-3820, E-mail: reprints@elsevier.com.

The Surgical Clinics of North America is also published in Spanish by McGraw-Hill Interamericana Editores S.A., P.O. Box 5-237 06500 Mexico D.F. Mexico; and in Portuguese by Interlivros Edicoes Ltda., Rua Comandante Coelho 1085, CEP 21250, Rio de Janeiro, Brazil; and in Greek by Paschalidis Medical Publications, Athens Greece.

The Surgical Clinics of North America is covered in *MEDLINE/PubMed (Index Medicus)*, *EMBASE/Excerpta Medica*, *Current Contents/Clinical Medicine*, *Current Contents/Life Sciences*, *Science Citation Index*, and *ISI/BIOMED*.

Printed in the United States of America.

Contributors

CONSULTING EDITOR

RONALD F. MARTIN, MD, FACS
Staff Surgeon, Department of Surgery, Marshfield Clinic, Marshfield, Wisconsin; Clinical Associate Professor, University of Wisconsin School of Medicine and Public Health, Madison, Wisconsin; Colonel, Medical Corps, United States Army Reserve

EDITOR

PETER J. MAZZAGLIA, MD, FACS
Associate Professor, Department of General Surgery, Rhode Island Hospital, The Warren Alpert School of Medicine, Brown University, Providence, Rhode Island

AUTHORS

EREN BERBER, MD
Section of Endocrine Surgery, Endocrinology and Metabolism Institute, Cleveland Clinic Foundation, Cleveland, Ohio

TOBIAS CARLING, MD, PhD
Section of Endocrine Surgery, Department of Surgery; Yale Endocrine Neoplasia Laboratory, Yale University School of Medicine, New Haven, Connecticut

DENISE CARNEIRO-PLA, MD, FACS
Associate Professor of Surgery, Division of Oncologic and Endocrine Surgery, Medical University of South Carolina, Charleston, South Carolina

JOHN A. CHABOT, MD
David V. Habif Professor of Clinical Surgery; Chief, Division of GI/Endocrine Surgery, Columbia University, New York, New York

RYAZ CHAGPAR, MD, MSc
Section of Endocrine Surgery, Endocrinology and Metabolism Institute, Cleveland Clinic Foundation, Cleveland, Ohio

DINA ELARAJ, MD
Assistant Professor, Section of Endocrine Surgery, Department of Surgery, Feinberg School of Medicine, Northwestern University, Chicago, Illinois

ADRIAN M. HARVEY, MD, MEd, MSc, FRCSC, FACS
Clinical Assistant Professor, Section of General Surgery and Surgical Oncology, Department of Surgery, Faculty of Medicine, Foothills Medical Center, University of Calgary, Calgary, Alberta, Canada

JOHN W. KUNSTMAN, MD
Department of Surgery, Yale University School of Medicine, New Haven, Connecticut

JENNIFER H. KUO, MD
Endocrine Surgery Fellow, Division of GI/Endocrine Surgery, Columbia University, New York, New York

JAMES A. LEE, MD
Director, COACH Education; Assistant Professor of Surgery; Chief, Endocrine Surgery; Co-Director, Adrenal Center; Co-Director, New York Thyroid/Parathyroid Center; Associate Medical Director, Simulation Center, Columbia University, New York, New York

AARTI MATHUR, MD
Endocrine Surgery Fellow, Department of Surgery, Johns Hopkins University School of Medicine, Baltimore, Maryland

PETER J. MAZZAGLIA, MD, FACS
Associate Professor, Department of General Surgery, Rhode Island Hospital, The Warren Alpert School of Medicine, Brown University, Providence, Rhode Island

CHRISTOPHER R. MCHENRY, MD
Professor of Surgery; Vice Chairman, Department of Surgery, MetroHealth Medical Center, Case Western Reserve University School of Medicine, Cleveland, Ohio

MIRA MILAS, MD, FACS
Department of Surgery, Knight Cancer Institute, Oregon Health and Science University, Portland, Oregon

RICHARD B. NOTO, MD
Professor of Diagnostic Imaging (Clinical), Department of Diagnostic Imaging, Rhode Island Hospital, The Warren Alpert Medical School of Brown University, Providence, Rhode Island

MATTHEW T. OLSON, MD
Assistant Professor, Department of Pathology, Johns Hopkins University School of Medicine, Baltimore, Maryland

SAREH PARANGI, MD
Unit of Endocrine Surgery, Massachusetts General Hospital, Harvard Medical School, Boston, Massachusetts

UMA RAJHBEHARRYSINGH, MD
Department of Surgery, Oregon Health and Science University, Portland, Oregon

ALLAN E. SIPERSTEIN, MD
Section of Endocrine Surgery, Endocrinology and Metabolism Institute, Cleveland Clinic Foundation, Cleveland, Ohio

CARMEN C. SOLORZANO, MD, FACS
Professor of Surgery and Director of Endocrine Surgery, Division of Surgical Oncology and Endocrine Surgery, Vanderbilt University Medical Center, Nashville, Tennessee

LEE F. STARKER, MD, PhD
Department of Surgery, Yale University School of Medicine, New Haven, Connecticut

JONAH J. STULBERG, MD, PhD, MPH
Department of Surgery, University Hospitals, Case Medical Center, Cleveland, Ohio

CORD STURGEON, MD, MS, FACS

Director of Endocrine Surgery, Section of Endocrine Surgery; Associate Professor, Department of Surgery, Feinberg School of Medicine, Northwestern University, Chicago, Illinois

HYUNSUK SUH, MD

Endocrine Surgery Fellow, Department of General Surgery, Massachusetts General Hospital, Boston, Massachusetts

MATTHEW TAYLOR, MD

Division of Hematology & Medical Oncology, Knight Cancer Institute, Oregon Health and Science University, Portland, Oregon

SCOTT WILHELM, MD, FACS

Section Head, Endocrine Surgery; Associate Professor, Department of Surgery, University Hospitals Case Medical Center, Cleveland, Ohio

DON C. YOO, MD

Associate Professor of Diagnostic Imaging (Clinical), Department of Diagnostic Imaging, Rhode Island Hospital, The Warren Alpert Medical School of Brown University, Providence, Rhode Island

MARTHA A. ZEIGER, MD, FACS, FACE

Professor of Surgery, Oncology, Cellular and Molecular Medicine; Chief of Endocrine Surgery; Associate Vice Chair of Faculty Development; Associate Dean of Postdoctoral Affairs, Department of Surgery, Johns Hopkins University School of Medicine, Baltimore, Maryland

Contents

Thyroid nodules are an extremely common endocrine disorder with a generally accepted prevalence of around 4% to 7%. Incidental thyroid nodules are typically nonpalpable thyroid nodules found during radiographic evaluation for a non-thyroid-related issue (eg, computed tomographic scan, positron emission tomography scan, carotid duplex). Incidental thyroid nodules are contributing to but are not the sole reason for the rising incidence of thyroid cancer in the Unites States and other developed nations.

Follicular lesions of the thyroid encompass a wide spectrum of diseases with clinicopathologic overlap, including benign follicular adenoma, malignant follicular carcinoma, and follicular variant of papillary cancer. This review addresses the clinical presentation, preoperative diagnosis in the era of molecular markers, pathologic diagnosis, treatment, and prognosis of follicular lesions, taking into account the frequent controversy about definitive histologic diagnoses.

Thyroid nodules are common, with increasing incidence, but only 5% to 15% of nodules are malignant. Genetic markers should only be used as an ancillary diagnostic tool for indeterminate thyroid nodules. Veracyte Afirma may improve the diagnostic accuracy for a subset of indeterminate cytologic diagnosis. Overall clinical, imaging, and cytopathologic evaluation in addition to patient preference should guide the management of indeterminate nodules. Further multicentered and independent validation studies are needed in order to prove the efficacy of commercially available genetic markers.

Prophylactic central compartment neck dissection (pCCND) is a CCND in patients with thyroid cancer who have no clinical, sonographic, or intraoperative evidence of abnormal lymph nodes. Whether pCCND should be

rate between focused parathyroidectomy and bilateral exploration. Costs of the two techniques differ depending on the preoperative and intraoperative localization used, speed of the operation, ability to discharge the patient on the same day as the operation, cure rate, and complications. It may be less costly and more effective to use a policy of routine 4-gland exploration without the use of preoperative or intraoperative localization studies. The potential economic impact and the expected outcome of the various strategies should be formally evaluated.

Refinements in both diagnostic criteria and surgical techniques, as well as the increasing use and study of novel multimodality therapies for ACC, have provided advances in the treatment of these patients, and renewed hope for meaningful improvements in patient outcomes.

Jennifer H. Kuo, James A. Lee, and John A. Chabot

Pancreatic neuroendocrine tumors are a group of rare, heterogeneous neoplasms that have been increasing in incidence the past few decades largely because of the diagnosis of pancreatic incidentalomas on cross-sectional imaging. Although these tumors are classically associated with clinical syndromes that result from excess secretion of particular hormones, most pancreatic neuroendocrine tumors are nonfunctional tumors presenting with symptoms secondary to mass effect, metastatic disease, or as incidental findings. This article reviews the diagnostic algorithm, surgical management, and available systemic therapies for nonfunctional pancreatic neuroendocrine tumors.

SURGICAL CLINICS
OF NORTH AMERICA

DOWNLOAD
Free App!

Review Articles
THE CLINICS

NOW AVAILABLE FOR YOUR iPhone and iPad

Foreword

Endocrine Surgery

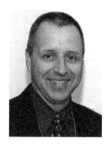

Ronald F. Martin, MD, FACS
Consulting Editor

By the time this issue of the *Surgical Clinics of North America* is distributed, we will be approaching the end of another academic year and the beginning of a new one. The start of a new academic year is more than just a calendar event; it is an opportunity to reassess what we surgeons do and why—at least if you are a program director.

One of the more frustrating aspects of being a program director is the Sisyphean nature of the job as the boulder of educating residents seems to roll back down the mountain every year. It appears as if we just keep repeating ourselves while covering familiar ground year after year. Of course, the perception is false for two fundamental reasons: it is always a new group of residents for whom it is not repetition and we don't really cover the same ground. Those who have completed their training move on to new adventures and those left behind look at things through slightly different lenses each day. Also, while one never steps in the same river twice, as the proverb goes, you get wet every time you step in a river.

Some things are fairly consistent year after year though. Invariably one of our new residents will refer to a patient's operation as a "surgery" and that will cause me to remind them that surgery is a way of life, a state of mind, and a discipline—occasionally a passion. I will also tell them operations are procedures performed by surgeons in operating rooms and ramble on as I sometimes do. As I have stated before, if one looks up the definition of "Surgery," one will find my new resident was well within her rights to use the term as she did. Nonetheless, I will remain undaunted by facts in my reticence to acquiesce to low-grade terminology. In this instance, I stand my ground for one reason: I need the resident to understand that surgery is only to a very minor degree about operating. Our discipline is about everything in regard to the care of the patient and operating is but one of the tools we use to make our communities better and safer places to live.

I can think of few better topics than Endocrine Surgery to illustrate this point. As one reads through the outstanding articles in this issue by Dr Mazzaglia and his colleagues, one will quickly discern that much of what we focus on in the care of patients with

Surg Clin N Am 94 (2014) xiii–xiv
http://dx.doi.org/10.1016/j.suc.2014.04.002
0039-6109/14/$ – see front matter © 2014 Published by Elsevier Inc.

endocrine disorders involves almost anything but the operative considerations. That, by no means, diminishes the value and importance of excellent operative skills being essential to the endocrine surgeon. However, to be effective as a surgeon who manages patients with endocrine disorders, one must have a clear and detailed grasp of the biochemical, genetic, and physiologic aspects of endocrine disease as well as an excellent understanding of the imaging techniques used and their scientific basis.

Occasionally distance and time are required to achieve perspective on change. If one reviews past issues of our series on endocrine surgery, the evolution of discourse from operative management to comprehensive understanding is clear. Endocrine surgery may well be a bellwether to us all that our role will be to expand our comprehensive management of the patient while rapidly decreasing the degree of invasion and operative management to whatever degree possible. I encourage the reader to study these articles well and I thank Dr Mazzaglia and his colleagues for an excellent contribution to this series.

Ronald F. Martin, MD, FACS
Department of Surgery
Marshfield Clinic
1000 North Oak Avenue
Marshfield, WI 54449, USA

E-mail address:
martin.ronald@marshfieldclinic.org

Preface

Endocrine Surgery

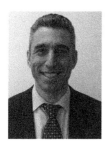

Peter J. Mazzaglia, MD, FACS
Editor

The field of endocrine surgery continues to witness scientific and technical advances that are reshaping the ways that we take care of patients with thyroid, parathyroid, adrenal, and pancreatic neoplasms. Endocrine surgeons and their colleagues in endocrinology and radiology are actively studying better ways to diagnose and manage many disease processes. This issue of the *Surgical Clinics of North America* aims to cover areas within endocrine surgery that are actively being transformed by our research efforts. It also addresses the necessity of dealing with increased recognition of disease at a time of shrinking health care dollars.

The growing number of incidentally detected thyroid neoplasms has led to more investigation of their prognostic significance, and a need to determine what should be the impact on nationally recognized guidelines. Evolving concepts and understandings of thyroid cancer biology are influencing recommendations about when to perform lymph node dissections, and which patients benefit from radioiodine ablation. Exciting research into genetic markers is changing the way we approach some thyroid nodules and malignancies.

Despite everything that's been written about hyperparathyroidism, debate over its management continues. Controversy exists over the best localizing studies, and which preoperative strategy is most cost-effective. There is still lively debate about the best operative approach, and the door is far from closed on four-gland exploration.

Due to the current high volume of cross-sectional imaging studies of the chest and abdomen, adrenal incidentalomas are increasingly recognized. While determining which are functional is relatively straightforward, there are complex management decisions required for patients with subclinical Cushing syndrome and hyperaldosteronism. For the nonfunctioning adrenal neoplasms, determining malignant potential is paramount to proper management. Radiographic characterization is playing a larger role in this process. Once adrenocortical cancer is recognized, judicious, timely treatment administered by a team of surgeons, endocrinologists, and oncologists is necessary.

Surg Clin N Am 94 (2014) xv–xvi
http://dx.doi.org/10.1016/j.suc.2014.04.001
0039-6109/14/$ – see front matter © 2014 Elsevier Inc. All rights reserved.

surgical.theclinics.com

Finally, just as with adrenal neoplasms, more and more frequently we are faced with the incidental pancreatic neuroendocrine tumor. Understanding its differential diagnosis and possible manifestations is essential to the management of these multiple diseases.

The authors who contributed to this issue represent present and future leaders in the fields of endocrine surgery, endocrinology, radiology, and oncology. Their comprehensive reviews on these timely topics will be helpful references for surgeons, endocrinologists, and all other practitioners providing care for patients with endocrine neoplasms.

Peter J. Mazzaglia, MD, FACS
Department of General Surgery
The Warren Alpert School of Medicine
Brown University
593 Eddy Street, APC 4
Providence, RI 02905, USA

E-mail address:
peterjmazzaglia@gmail.com

Evaluation of Thyroid Incidentaloma

Scott Wilhelm, MD

KEYWORDS

- Incidental thyroid nodule • Thyroid cancer • Ultrasound
- Fine needle aspiration biopsy

KEY POINTS

- Incidental thyroid nodules are typically nonpalpable thyroid nodules found during radiographic evaluation for a non-thyroid-related issue (eg, computed tomographic scan, positron emission tomography [PET] scan, carotid duplex).
- The prevalence of thyroid incidentalomas ranges from 1.6% to 67% based on the radiographic modality of detection.
- The overall risk of malignancy in the incidental thyroid nodule is approximately 15%, but ranges from 4% to 50% based on the mechanism of identification and other nodule characteristics.
- Incidental thyroid nodules should be referred to an endocrine specialist (endocrine surgeon, endocrinologist, otolaryngologist, or a general surgeon comfortable with thyroid surgery) for proper evaluation.
- Solid thyroid nodules more than 1 cm in size should undergo ultrasound-guided fine-needle aspiration biopsy according to American Thyroid Association guidelines. PET scan and nodules, or nodules less than 1 cm with worrisome ultrasonographic features, should also be "considered for biopsy" because of higher concern for cancer.
- Incidental thyroid nodules are contributing to but are not the sole reason for the rising incidence of thyroid cancer in the Unites States and other developed nations.

INTRODUCTION

Thyroid nodules are an extremely common endocrine disorder with a generally accepted prevalence of around 4% to 7%. The Framingham study,[1] completed in 1968, demonstrated an overall prevalence of thyroid nodules in the general population of 4.2% (women 6.4%, men 1.5%). The Whickham survey[2] completed in England in 1977 had a similar overall prevalence of 3.7%. A more contemporary study[3] still quotes a prevalence of 3% to 6%. Thus, based on US population data in 2012, up to 12 to 21 million adults may harbor a thyroid nodule. All of these studies are based

Department of Surgery, University Hospitals Case Medical Center, 11100 Euclid Avenue, Cleveland, OH 44118, USA
E-mail address: Scott.Wilhelm@UHhospitals.org

Surg Clin N Am 94 (2014) 485–497
http://dx.doi.org/10.1016/j.suc.2014.02.004
0039-6109/14/$ – see front matter © 2014 Elsevier Inc. All rights reserved.

on nodules that are considered "palpable." However, true prevalence of thyroid nodules based on autopsy data can be much higher, ranging from 10% to 60%. The Mayo Clinic study[4] in 1955 (821 consecutive autopsies) demonstrated that up to 50% of patients who underwent autopsy with no history of thyroid disease could be found to have incidental nodular thyroid disease. Modern prevalence studies based on standard radiographic analysis with neck ultrasound (U/S) concur with autopsy data that up to 42% to 67% of patients who undergo neck U/S can be found to have a nonpalpable, incidental thyroid nodule.[5,6]

A thyroid incidentaloma can be defined as an unsuspected thyroid nodule found on a diagnostic radiographic examination performed for a reason other than "thyroid disease." Most of these are nonpalpable, but once known may actually be palpable. Because these nonpalpable thyroid nodules can occur in up to 30% to 50% Americans, some endocrinologists have termed the incidental thyroid lesion as a modern day epidemic.[7] Based on US population data from 2012, up to 93 to 156 million people may actually harbor a nonpalpable, incidental thyroid nodule. Therefore, it is important to determine guidelines for the appropriate identification and risk stratification of these nodules to determine adequately which nodules need further examination, biopsy, and surgical evaluation. It is also important to recognize the risk of malignancy in the incidental thyroid nodule and how it varies based on mechanism of identification and radiographic characteristics. Finally, this article puts into perspective the contribution of the incidental thyroid nodule to the rising incidence of thyroid cancer.

DETECTION OF INCIDENTAL THYROID NODULES

Incidental thyroid nodules can be found during multiple different radiographic evaluations, including computed tomographic (CT) scan, positron emission tomography (PET) scan, carotid duplex, and neck U/S. Other less common modalities would include chest radiograph, magnetic resonance imaging, and nuclear medicine tests, such as octreotide or sestamibi scanning. The following case presentations highlight the most common modalities where incidental thyroid nodules are detected.

CT SCAN DETECTION OF INCIDENTAL THYROID NODULES
Case Presentation

A 55-year-old white woman who had a history of surgically resected stage III rectal cancer underwent an annual surveillance CT scan of the chest, abdomen, and pelvis. Upper cuts of the chest revealed what the radiologists described as a "1.5-cm hypodense mass in the right thyroid lobe with smooth borders... likely benign" (**Fig. 1A**). The patient was then referred for further evaluation. The patient had no prior history of nodular thyroid disease, and she was clinically euthyroid with a thyroid-stimulating hormone (TSH) count of 0.53. She had received radiation treatment to her rectal cancer, but had no history of head, neck, or chest or radiation exposure. There was no family history of thyroid cancer. On detailed physical examination by a dedicated endocrine surgeon, the lesion was palpable and mobile. A dedicated history and physical examination may reveal risk factors for thyroid cancer (**Box 1**).

An office-based U/S demonstrated a 1.7 × 1.2-cm right thyroid nodule, which had worrisome ultrasonographic features, including hypoechoic appearance compared with surrounding thyroid tissue and irregular borders with evidence of localized invasion into the overlying strap musculature and into surrounding thyroid parenchyma (see **Fig. 1B**). Based on this, a U/S-guided fine-needle aspiration biopsy (FNABx) of the mass was performed. Cytology demonstrated evidence of papillary thyroid carcinoma. Therefore, the patient underwent total thyroidectomy. At the time of the operation, the

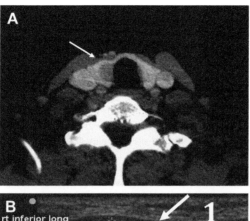

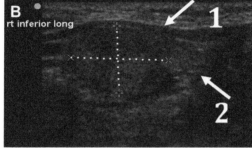

Fig. 1. (*A*) A CT scan demonstrating a 1.5-cm incidentally discovered right thyroid mass (*arrow*). This scan was read as "benign-appearing." (*B*) Office-based thyroid U/S of the same lesion demonstrates a 1.7-cm heterogeneous mass with irregular borders showing local invasion into the overlying sternothyroid musculature (*arrow 1*) and invasion into surrounding thyroid parenchyma (*arrow 2*), highly suspicious for malignancy.

tumor demonstrated local invasion into the overlying sternothyroid musculature (consistent with preoperative U/S) and was resected en bloc with the tumor.

CT scan is a common mechanism for the discovery of incidental thyroid nodules. According to prior studies, 16% of cervical or thoracic CT scans will yield a diagnosis of an incidental thyroid nodule.[8,9] However, although CT scans are good at detecting thyroid nodules, they have several pitfalls. First, CT can often underestimate the size of nodules.[10] The author's group has previously published a correlational analysis study[11] comparing CT and U/S measurements of thyroid nodules to final pathologic nodule size after surgical resection. CT scan had a Pearson correlation r^2 factor of

---

Box 1
Risk factors for thyroid cancer based on history and physical examination

- Prior personal history of thyroid cancer
- Family history of thyroid cancer, including papillary and medullary thyroid cancer (multiple endocrine neoplasia syndrome, type IIA and IIB)
- History of head and neck or upper chest radiation exposure
- Fixed palpable mass in the thyroid gland
- Palpable cervical lymphadenopathy in a patient with a thyroid nodule
- Hoarseness of the voice (representing invasion of the recurrent laryngeal nerve.)

0.83 with a P value of .005 to thyroid nodules at final pathology. However, U/S was consistently more accurate with a Pearson correlation r^2 of 0.90 with a P value of .0001. Correctly determining the size of the nodule is an important first step in determining which nodules need further evaluation. If American Thyroid Association guidelines[12] are to be adhered to to biopsy nodules without worrisome ultrasonographic features greater than 1 cm in size, these nodules must be reliably measured.

CT may also overestimate or underestimate the number of thyroid nodules. In a 3-year study (1998–2001), Shetty and colleagues[13] examined all cervical and thoracic CT scans performed at the Massachusetts General Hospital in Boston. They identified 230 patients with a CT-based thyroid abnormality that subsequently underwent thyroid U/S. They found that CT scan findings agreed with U/S for lesion size only 53% of the time; CT identified the dominant nodule but missed multinodularity 30% of the time and had a false positive identification of a thyroid nodule 4.3% of the time. Another recent review of thyroid incidentalomas by Jin and colleagues[14] described other limitations of CT, including "CT scans of the chest often do not image the entire thyroid gland" (thus a false negative for nodules may occur), routine CT cuts of 3 to 5 mm may miss lesions, and, during chest CT, "the patient's arms are positioned over the head, which often results in beam hardening artifacts in the thyroid." Nonetheless, CT is the most likely radiographic test to detect incidental thyroid nodules.

In regard to CT's ability to detect malignancy in a thyroid nodule, Shetty and colleagues[13] found that the overall risk of malignancy based on CT identification of an incidental nodule was 3.9% to 11.3%. (This is similar to the risk of malignancy in a palpable thyroid nodule that is generally quoted at 5%.) When they looked for any risk factors (found by CT scan) that accurately predicted a malignant outcome, the only finding was that malignant nodules were significantly larger (mean 2.79 cm) than benign nodules (mean 2.16 cm) (P value .03). They also looked at the CT presence of microcalcifications in the nodule. It is well accepted that "ultrasonographically" detected microcalcifications are a worrisome finding that increases the likelihood of malignancy at the time of FNABx. A recent study[15] of almost 1500 patients with greater than 2000 thyroid nodules found that the sensitivity of "ultrasonographically" discovered microcalcifications for predicting a final pathologic diagnosis of malignancy was 49.6% with a specificity of 93.6%. However, CT scan identification of calcifications does not correlate to a final diagnosis of thyroid cancer with a P value of .72.[13] Finally, unlike incidental adrenal nodules, there are no reliable data on absolute Hounsfield Units of an incidental thyroid nodule that correlate to an increased risk of thyroid cancer.[14]

Therefore, although CT is a common mechanism for detecting incidental thyroid nodules, it is quite limited, by itself, in measuring nodule size accurately, predicting the correct number of thyroid nodules, or assessing for the risk of malignancy. Therefore, it is currently recommended that incidental thyroid nodules discovered on CT scan should undergo a dedicated thyroid U/S and referral to an endocrine specialist (endocrine surgeon, endocrinologist, ENT, or general surgeons with high volume practices of thyroid disease) to determine the next step in nodule evaluation.

Finally, CT scan plays a role in the evaluation of thyroid disease, but should not be used as a "screening tool" for thyroid nodules for many of the reasons listed above. The role of CT scan in thyroid disease is generally confined to (1) evaluation of the extent of substernal goiters for surgical planning (need for sternotomy, intubation risks); (2) assessment of large thyroid cancers suspicious for local invasion into trachea, great vessels, and others, that again may alter surgical planning or extent of resection; (3) staging of thyroid cancer, looking for metastatic disease; and (4) follow-up evaluation of the thyroid bed or lymph nodes after thyroidectomy for cancer (may be used as an adjunct to neck U/S).

> **Key points for CT scan detected incidental thyroid nodules**
>
> - 16% of all cervical and thoracic CT scans will identify an incidental thyroid nodule.
> - CT scans do not reliably predict the correct size or number of thyroid nodules.
> - The risk of malignancy in an incidentally discovered thyroid nodule (found by CT) is 3.9% to 11.3%.
> - Incidental thyroid nodules found on CT scan should undergo a dedicated thyroid U/S and referral to an Endocrine specialist.

PET SCAN DETECTION OF INCIDENTAL THYROID NODULES
Case Presentation

The patient is a 59-year-old woman who recently underwent hysterectomy for endometrial cancer. A staging PET scan was ordered after her recovery that showed no residual disease in the pelvis but intense uptake with a solitary focus in the right thyroid lobe (**Fig. 2**). The patient had no history of nodular thyroid disease and was biochemically euthyroid with a TSH of 2.3 and a negative anti-thyroid peroxidase (anti-TPO) antibody effectively ruling out Hashimoto thyroiditis. There was no family history of thyroid cancer. She denied history of head, neck, or chest radiation exposure. On physical examination, the nodule was somewhat palpable in the right thyroid lobe. She underwent an office-based thyroid U/S demonstrating a 1.5-cm nodule in the right thyroid lobe as well as a 1.5-cm nodule in the left lobe (nonpalpable and not PET avid) and other subcentimeter nodules scattered throughout the thyroid. The right-sided nodule had irregular borders and microcalcifications suspicious for malignancy. FNABx was performed and yielded a cytologic diagnosis of papillary thyroid carcinoma. The patient underwent a total thyroidectomy. Final pathology demonstrated a 1.5-cm, papillary thyroid carcinoma in the right thyroid lobe. The left-sided nodule was benign.

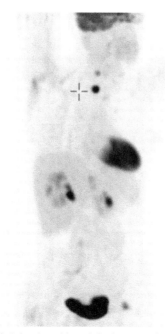

Fig. 2. Patient with PET and right thyroid nodule (seen to the right of the cross-hairs).

PET scans are commonly performed as cancer surveillance and staging tools. Thus, the finding of an incidental thyroid nodule can be a source of stress for patients already diagnosed with another primary malignancy. Fluorodeoxyglucose or FDG-PET relies on the principle that tissue with a high metabolic demand (cancer, inflammation, infection) will uptake more of the tracer. PET scan uptake patterns for thyroid disease generally come in 2 forms. The first form is diffuse uptake throughout the thyroid gland. This uptake is generally representative of thyroiditis or Graves disease. As such, this pattern generally indicates benign disease of the thyroid. The second pattern of uptake is that of a solitary focus that corresponds to a nodule in the thyroid and raises suspicion for malignancy.

Although the prevalence of incidental thyroid nodules found on CT scan is 16% as outlined above, the prevalence of thyroid nodules discovered on PET scan is much lower. A large meta-analysis[16] recently reviewed 22 articles pertaining to PET and thyroid nodules. Of more than 125,000 patients who underwent FDG-PET for varying indications, only 1.6% had a thyroid incidentaloma discovered. Despite the lower overall incidence of thyroid nodules found during PET scan (compared with CT scan), there is much greater concern for malignancy, based on the pattern of tracer uptake. As mentioned above, diffuse uptake on PET scan is much more consistent with benign disease and has been demonstrated in multiple studies, including a large US-based study and a large Korean study that included more than 5000 patients each.[17,18] A diffuse uptake pattern only yielded a rate of malignancy of 4.4%, which is again almost identical to palpable nodules at 5%. However, focal uptake has been found to correlate with a cancer rate of 30% to 50% in most studies[17–19] and was 34.8% in the meta-analysis.[16]

Our current recommendations for the evaluation of the thyroid incidentaloma detected by PET scan are a detailed history and a physical examination (looking for risk factors for cancer, such as radiation exposure, family history of thyroid cancer), thyroid function testing (including anti-TPO antibody to look for thyroiditis manifesting as diffuse uptake on PET), and a dedicated thyroid U/S with FNABx. The American Thyroid Association guidelines, as mentioned above,[12] dictate that nodules greater than 1 cm in size be biopsied. However, they also include a suggestion that lesions less than 1 cm in size with atypical or worrisome characteristics "should be considered" for biopsy. As such, in the setting of an isolated nodule detected by positive PET scan, biopsy can be considered at a size less than 1 cm due to the high risk of malignancy.

Key points for PET scan detected incidental thyroid nodules

- The prevalence of thyroid incidentalomas found during PET scan is 1.6%.
- Risk of malignancy in a PET thyroid incidentaloma varies with PET uptake pattern but is highest with a solitary uptake pattern (30%–50%).
- Decreasing the biopsy size threshold for focal PET and thyroid incidentalomas should be considered.

NECK U/S AND CAROTID DUPLEX SCAN DETECTION OF INCIDENTAL THYROID NODULES

Neck U/Ss are often performed for non-thyroid-related indications, but yield a finding of an incidental thyroid nodule. Neck U/S may be performed for a palpable neck mass, lymphadenopathy, evaluation of parathyroid glands for targeted parathyroidectomy, and vascular access. During these examinations, the thyroid gland is typically visualized and nodules may be discovered. Prevalence based on the radiology litera-ture quotes a prevalence of thyroid nodules of 42% to 67%.[5,6] In addition, for patients undergoing a thyroid U/S for a palpable thyroid nodule, up to 48% may have an addi-tional nonpalpable (incidental) nodule seen.[20]

Neck U/S has become a routine part of minimally invasive parathyroidectomy to help localize the culprit gland preoperatively. In patients undergoing neck U/S for parathyroid disease, concomitant thyroid disease can be found in 20% to 56% (see examples in **Fig. 3**).[21] Biopsy of such nodules can lead to a diagnosis of thyroid nod-ules that requires or excludes surgical resection. If deemed necessary, the thyroidec-tomy can be performed simultaneously with parathyroidectomy, thus eliminating the need for additional surgery later or "unanticipated" intraoperative discovery of a nodule. Cancer in these lesions has been reported between 2% and 6%.[21,22]

The proximity of the common carotid artery as it lies just lateral to the thyroid gland also yields a frequent finding of thyroid nodules during carotid artery duplex. In fact, in one study,[23] thyroid nodules were found more frequently (28%) during carotid duplex than a finding of significant carotid stenosis (13%). Steele and colleagues[24] reported an incidence of thyroid cancer of 7.4% in incidental nodules found during carotid duplex. Detection of both lesions (thyroid nodule and carotid stenosis) can facilitate a combined operative approach with both thyroidectomy and carotid endarterectomy (**Fig. 4**).

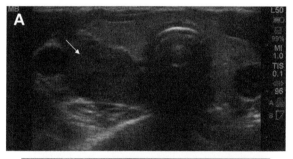

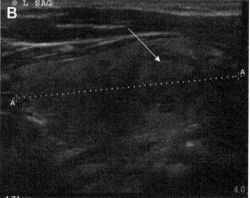

Fig. 3. (*A, B*) Patient with an incidental thyroid nodule discovered during neck U/S for hyper-parathyroidism. (*A*) Right inferior parathyroid adenoma found on neck U/S. Arrow points to hypoechoic extrathyroidal mass, consistent with a parathyroid adenoma. (*B*) Incidental (nonpalpable) left thyroid nodule in the same patient as (*A*) (*arrow* designates 2-cm left upper pole nodule, which underwent biopsy).

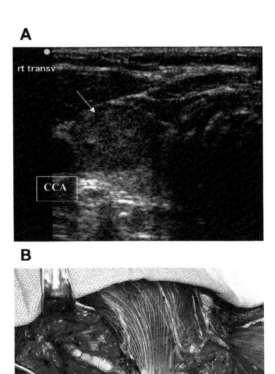

Fig. 4. (*A*) A 2-cm right thyroid nodule (*arrow*) found during carotid duplex. FNABx was consistent with a follicular neoplasm; the patient also had high-grade carotid stenosis that required carotid endarterectomy. CCA, common carotid artery. (*B*) Patient underwent combined thyroidectomy and right carotid endarterectomy.

The biggest benefit of U/S in its role in the management of the incidental thyroid nodule is not so much its detection of nodules themselves but the follow-up of nodules found on other tests. U/S is the gold standard for the accurate measurement of thyroid nodules. As mentioned above, nodules greater than 1 cm should be biopsied according to American Thyroid Association guidelines; thus, reliable measurements are critical. In addition, U/S can look for features of the nodule that may be more worrisome for malignant potential. Papini and colleagues[25] performed an excellent review of almost 500 incidental thyroid nodules. All patients referred with an incidental nodule subsequently underwent a thyroid U/S and biopsy of nodules greater than 1 cm. Two hundred ninety-five patients had a benign biopsy (no surgery needed); 92 had an inadequate biopsy, and 107 had a biopsy consistent with or suspicious for cancer and went on to surgery. Of the 107 surgical patients, 31 had cancer; 24 had a benign follicular adenoma, and 52 had other benign disease. They then went back and reviewed again the U/S findings of all surgical patients and found several markers on U/S that were more commonly found in malignant versus benign nodules (**Table 1**). Although these features cannot diagnose or rule out the chance of cancer in a thyroid nodule, they can help point out which nodules are more suspicious and at least heighten the concern to prompt an FNABx for more information. The overall

Table 1 Ultrasonographic features, malignant versus benign incidental thyroid nodules			
Ultrasonographic Feature	Malignant (%)	Benign (%)	P value
Hypoechoic	87	56	.009
Irregular borders	77	15	.0001
Vascular pattern (central hypervascularity)	74	19	.0001
Microcalcification	29	4	.0001

Data from Papini E, Guglielmi R, Bianchini A, et al. Risk of malignancy in nonpalpable thyroid nodules: predictive value of ultrasound and color-Doppler features. J Clin Endocrinol Metab 2002;87:1941–46.

rate of cancer found in incidental thyroid nodules, based on U/S in the Papini study, was 8%, but may be as high as 15% in some studies.[26]

In addition to the 4 U/S characteristics mentioned (hypoechoic lesion, irregular borders, microcalcifications, and central hypervascularity), 2 other U/S characteristics have been investigated to try to determine risk of malignancy in a thyroid nodule. These characteristics include nodule size and shape. Nodule size has been investigated in the past. There has been a great deal of controversy as to nodules broken into lesion size greater than or less than 4 cm in size. Despite multiple studies, the data remain quite controversial. For example, McHenry and colleagues[27] demonstrated that thyroid nodules greater than 4 cm actually had a higher rate of being benign as opposed to lesions closer to 3 cm in size. In contrast, Stang and Carty[28] showed nodules greater than 4 cm in size may have an increased risk of malignancy. They based this decision on FNABx rates that were more likely to miss cancer; this was thought to be due to sampling error because of the size of the lesion. In the setting of the incidental thyroid nodule where these lesions are typically smaller than 2 cm, size likely has less impact.

Nodule shape has also been shown to predict malignancy. Lesions that are taller than they are wide on U/S can indicate a growth pattern more indicative of cancer than benign disease,[29] which is also true for breast lesions imaged on U/S.[30]

Thus, it can be clearly seen that U/S is critical in the role of evaluating the incidental thyroid nodule. Based on available data, all incidental thyroid nodules, approaching 1 cm in size, regardless of study (CT scan, PET scan, carotid duplex) should undergo a formal thyroid U/S, which can determine the exact size of the lesion. U/S can also determine worrisome structural features that may impact the decision for biopsy and timing of procedures.

Key points for U/S and duplex detected incidental thyroid nodules

- The prevalence of thyroid nodules found during neck U/S is extremely high at 40% to 67%, with a risk of malignancy of 2% to 15%.
- Risk of malignancy of incidental thyroid nodules found during carotid duplex is 7.4%.
- Neck U/S plays a critical role in evaluating both size and characteristics of incidental thyroid nodules, which may impact the decision for and timing of FNABx.

THE ROLE OF THE INCIDENTAL THYROID NODULE IN THE RISING INCIDENCE OF THYROID CANCER

Thyroid cancer, along with melanoma, is 1 of the 2 most rapidly rising forms of cancer in the United States today.[31] In 2002, the American Cancer Society reported a total of 22,500 new cases of thyroid cancer in the United States. By 2012, that number had

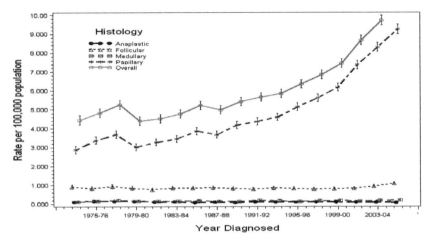

Fig. 5. Trends in thyroid cancer incidence in the United States from 1970 to 2006 based on the SEER database.[32] The rising incidence of papillary cancers mirrors and thus accounts for the general rising incidence of thyroid cancer overall.

more than doubled to 56,460 cases. The bulk of the increase in thyroid cancer is specifically due to the increasing incidence of papillary thyroid carcinoma,[32] as seen in **Fig. 5**.

Several studies have shown that the incidental thyroid nodule contributes greatly to the rising incidence of thyroid cancer. One working theory is that due to increased radiographic surveillance of all types, more and more incidental thyroid cancers are being caught. Davies and Welch[33] demonstrated that micropapillary thyroid carcinoma (that is, lesions less than 1 cm in size) accounted for 49% of the rising incidence of thyroid carcinoma in their study. Similarly, Kent and colleagues[34] showed that a large percentage of thyroid cancers discovered in the United States today are less than 2 cm in size. They did not specifically classify these as "incidental" versus traditional palpable nodules. Their studies draw to light a question as to whether small incidental thyroid lesions should be considered clinically relevant. Nevertheless, others[35] think that the increase in thyroid cancer is real and demonstrated a substantial increase in thyroid cancers larger than 2 cm in size.

This discrepancy prompted the author's group to do a data analysis of the Surveillance, Epidemiology, and End Results (SEER) database from 1973 to 2006.[32] The working theory was that if incidental thyroid nodules are the sole contributor to the rising incidence of thyroid cancer, the bulk of all thyroid cancers should be less than 2 cm in size. Data in **Table 2** show that incidental nodules classified as

Table 2				
Incidence of thyroid cancer by tumor size				
Size of Papillary Thyroid Cancer (cm)	**Rate in 1983–1984 per 100,000**	**Rate in 2005–2006 per 100,000**	**Total Change (%)**	**Percent Change (%/y)**
≤1	.79	3.48	441	19.3
1.1–2	.91	2.57	283	12.3
2.1–5	.92	2.19	237	10.3
5+	.12	.33	276	12.0

Data from Cramer JD, Fu P, Harth KC, et al. Analysis of the rising incidence of thyroid cancer using the Surveillance, Epidemiology and End Results National cancer data registry. Surgery 2010; 148(6):1147–53.

micropapillary cancers (tumors <1 cm) clearly contribute to the overall incidence of thyroid cancer. These microcancers increase the incidence of thyroid cancer by a rate of 19% per year over the 33-year study period. However, tumors of all other sizes (1 cm to >5 cm) are also increasing at a rate of 10.3% to 12.3% per year as well. This finding is evidence that there are other factors also leading to the overall rising incidence of thyroid cancer in developed countries. Factors such as obesity,[36] estrogen levels,[37,38] increased use of high-resolution CT scan,[39] and other unknown environmental factors are being considered for future research.

SUMMARY

The incidental thyroid nodule is an extremely common entity that has an overall prevalence of 1.6% to 67% depending on the radiographic test that discovered it. The rate of cancer in the traditional "palpable" thyroid nodule is generally accepted to be about 5%. The rate of malignancy in incidental nodules can again be quite variable based on how it was discovered and can range from 4% to 50% (carotid duplex 7%, neck U/S 2%–15%, CT scan 4%–11%, and PET scan 30%–50% in a solitary uptake pattern corresponding to a solitary thyroid nodule).

In 2 studies from the author's institution,[11,19] it was found that incidental thyroid nodules (regardless of mechanism of discovery) referred for evaluation harbored a risk of cancer of 15% (consistent with data from Liebeskind and colleagues).[26] Both studies accounted for personal or family history of thyroid cancer and radiation exposure and excluded micropapillary cancer in the final prevalence calculations. (Excluding micropapillary thyroid cancers from data analysis is important because these lesions may often be reported on final pathology reports that are unrelated to the actual "incidental nodule" for which that the procedure was being performed. In fact, incidental micropapillary thyroid cancers may be found in up to 13% of all thyroid pathology specimens in the United States.[40])

After exclusion of such micropapillary cancers, the data[11,19] still suggest a possible 3-fold increased risk of cancer in incidental nodules compared with the traditional palpable thyroid nodule. As such, incidental thyroid nodules do warrant proper clinical investigation. Because nodules often discovered on CT scan or PET scan can be incorrectly measured, nodules found by this mechanism should be referred for a formal thyroid U/S. Thyroid U/S is considered the gold standard for accurate measurement of thyroid nodules. U/S can also provide additional information as to characteristics of nodules, which may make them more likely to be benign versus malignant. Once solid nodules are found to be greater than 1 cm in size, they should undergo U/S-guided FNABx as currently recommended by American Thyroid Association guidelines. Consideration for biopsy of thyroid nodules less than 1 cm should be restricted to nodules with atypical U/S characteristics and potential nodules that are positive on PET scan due to their higher rate of malignancy. The term "incidental" should not be equated with the term "inconsequential" and, as such, these nodules should be referred to endocrine specialists who can carry out a thorough evaluation to determine malignant potential and proper treatment.

REFERENCES

1. Vander JB, Gaston EA, Dawber TR. The significance of nontoxic thyroid nodules: final report of a 15-year study of the incidence of thyroid malignancy. Ann Intern Med 1968;69(3):537–40.

2. Tunbridge WM, Evered DC, Hall R, et al. The Spectrum of thyroid disease in a community: the Whickham survey. Clin Endocrinol 1977;7:481–93.
3. Hegedus L. Clinical practice. The thyroid nodule. N Engl J Med 2004;351(17): 1764–71.
4. Mortensen JD, Woolner LB, Bennett WA. Gross and microscopic findings in clinically normal thyroid glands. J Clin Endocrinol Metab 1955;15:1270–80.
5. Brander A, Viikinkowski P, Nickels J, et al. Thyroid gland: US screening in a random adult population. Radiology 1991;181:683–7.
6. Ezzat S, Sarti DA, Cain DR, et al. Thyroid incidentalomas. Prevalence by palpation and ultrasonography. Ann Intern Med 1994;154:1838–40.
7. Ross DS. Editorial: nonpalpable thyroid nodules—managing an epidemic. J Clin Endocrinol Metab 2002;87(5):1938–40.
8. Yoon DY, Chang SK, Choi CS, et al. The prevalence and significance of incidental thyroid nodules identified on computerized tomography. J Comput Assist Tomogr 2008;32:810–5.
9. Youserm DM, Huang T, Loevner LA, et al. Clinical and economic impact of incidental thyroid lesions found with CT and MR. AJNR Am J Neuroradiol 1997;18(8):1423–8.
10. Frank L, Quint LE. Chest CT incidentalomas: thyroid lesions, enlarged mediastinal lymph nodes, and lung nodules. Cancer Imaging 2012;12:41–8.
11. Wilhelm SM, Robinson AV, Krishnamurthi SS, et al. Evaluation and management of incidental thyroid nodules in patients with another primary malignancy. Surgery 2007;142:581–7.
12. Cooper DS, Doherty GM, Haugen BR, et al. Revised American Thyroid Association management guidelines for patients with thyroid nodules and differentiated thyroid cancer. Thyroid 2009;19:1167–214.
13. Shetty SK, Maher MM, Hahn PF, et al. Significance of incidental thyroid lesions detected on CT: correlation among CT, sonography, and pathology. AJR Am J Roentgenol 2006;187:1349–56.
14. Jin J, McHenry CR. Thyroid incidentaloma. Best Pract Res Clin Endocrinol Metab 2012;26:83–96.
15. Lu Z, Zhu H, Luo Y, et al. Thyroid nodule macrocalcification does not mean the nodule is benign. World J Surg 2011;35:122–7.
16. Soelberg K, Bonnema SJ, Heiberg-Brix T, et al. Risk of malignancy in thyroid incidentalomas detected by 18F-flourodeoxyglucose PET: a systematic review. Thyroid 2012;22(9):918–25.
17. Cohen MS, Nuri A, Dehdashti F, et al. Risk of malignancy in thyroid incidentalomas identified by fluorodeoxyglucose-positron emission tomography. Surgery 2001;130(6):941–6.
18. Kim TY, Kim WB, Ryu JS, et al. 18F-flourodeoxyglucose uptake in thyroid from PET for evaluation of cancers patients: high prevalence of malignancy in thyroid PET incidentaloma. Laryngoscope 2005;115:1074–8.
19. Jin J, Wilhelm SM, McHenry CR. Incidental thyroid nodule: patterns of diagnosis and rate of malignancy. Am J Surg 2009;197:320–4.
20. Tan GH, Gharib H, Reading CC. Solitary thyroid nodule. Comparison between palpation and ultrasonography. Arch Intern Med 1995;155(22):2418–23.
21. Arciero CA, Shiue ZS, Gates JD, et al. Preoperative thyroid ultrasound is indicated in patients undergoing parathyroidectomy for primary hyperparathyroidism. J Cancer 2012;3:1–6.
22. Adler JT, Chen H, Schaefer S, et al. Does routine use of ultrasound result in additional thyroid procedures in patients with primary hyperparathyroidism? J Am Coll Surg 2010;211(4):536–9.

23. Rommel O, Tegenthoff M. Screening study of the thyroid gland within the scope of color-coded duplex ultrasound of brain-supplying arteries. Ultraschall Med 1996; 17(3):113–7.

24. Steele SR, Martin MJ, Mullenix PS, et al. The significance of incidental thyroid abnormalities identified during carotid duplex ultrasonography. Arch Surg 2005; 140:981–5.

25. Papini E, Guglielmi R, Bianchini A, et al. Risk of malignancy in nonpalpable thyroid nodules: predictive value of ultrasound and color-doppler features. J Clin Endocrinol Metab 2002;87:1941–6.

26. Liebeskind A, Sikore AG, Komisar A, et al. Rates of malignancy in incidentally discovered thyroid nodules evaluated with sonography and fine needle aspiration. J Ultrasound Med 2005;24:629–34.

27. McHenry CR, Huh ES, Machekano RN. Is nodule size an independent predictor of thyroid malignancy? Surgery 2008;144:1062–8.

28. Stang MT, Carty SE. Recent developments in predicting thyroid malignancy. Curr Opin Oncol 2009;21(1):11–7.

29. Kim EK, Park CS, Chung WY, et al. New sonographic criteria for recommending fine-needle aspiration biopsy of nonpalpable solid nodules of the thyroid. Am J Roentgenol 2002;178:687–91.

30. Stavros TA, Thickman D, Rapp CL, et al. Solid breast nodules: use of sonography to distinguish between benign and malignant lesions. Radiology 1995;196: 123–34.

31. Cancer trends progress report 2011-12. National Cancer Institute—United States National Institutes of Health. Available at: http://progressreport.cancer.gov/index.asp.

32. Cramer JD, Fu P, Harth KC, et al. Analysis of the rising incidence of thyroid cancer using the Surveillance, Epidemiology and End Results National cancer data registry. Surgery 2010;148(6):1147–53.

33. Davies L, Welch HG. Increasing incidence of thyroid cancer in the United States, 1973–2002. JAMA 2006;295:2164–7.

34. Kent WD, Hall SF, Isotalo PA, et al. Increased incidence of differentiated thyroid carcinoma and detection of subclinical disease. CMAJ 2007;177:1357–61.

35. Enewold L, Zhu K, Ron E, et al. Rising thyroid cancer incidence in the United States by demographic and tumor characteristics, 1980–2005. Cancer Epidemiol Biomarkers Prev 2009;18:784–91.

36. Engeland A, Tretli S, Akslen LA, et al. Body size and thyroid cancer in two million Norwegian men and women. Br J Cancer 2006;95(3):366–70.

37. Zahid M, Goldner W, Beseler CL, et al. Unbalanced estrogen metabolism in thyroid cancer. Int J Cancer 2013;133(11):2642–9.

38. Yao R, Chiu CG, Strugnell SS, et al. Gender differences in thyroid cancer. Expert Rev Endocrinol Metab 2011;6(2):215–43.

39. Smith-Bindman R, Lipson J, Marcus R, et al. Radiation dose associated with common computed tomography examinations and the associated lifetime attributable risk of cancer. Arch Intern Med 2009;169(22):2078–86.

40. Nishiyama RH, Ludwig GK, Thompson NW. The prevalence of small papillary thyroid carcinomas in 100 consecutive autopsies in an American population. Radiation-associated thyroid carcinoma. New York: Grune & Stratton; 1977. p. 123.

Follicular Lesions of the Thyroid

Aarti Mathur, MD[a], Matthew T. Olson, MD[b], Martha A. Zeiger, MD[a],*

KEYWORDS

- Follicular • Cancer • Thyroid • Neoplasms

KEY POINTS

- Follicular lesions of the thyroid gland include benign follicular adenoma, minimally invasive follicular carcinoma, widely invasive follicular carcinoma, and encapsulated and infiltrative follicular variant of papillary thyroid cancer.
- Fine-needle aspiration (FNA) biopsy is the best diagnostic test to diagnose a thyroid nodule but is indeterminate in 15% to 20% of cases, especially when follicular lesions are involved; capsular invasion, the hallmark that distinguishes benign from malignant, cannot be assessed with FNA.
- Molecular markers are a recent promising area of research to differentiate thyroid neoplasms; however, none has proved adequate in differentiating benign from malignant follicular tumors.
- At a minimum, a diagnostic thyroid lobectomy is required to assess the histologic architecture and obtain a definitive diagnosis. However, gray zones exist within the diagnostic spectrum of follicular neoplasms.
- Widely invasive and infiltrative follicular variant of papillary thyroid cancers have higher recurrence rates and metastatic potential; a total thyroidectomy is therefore indicated.
- Controversy exists for small, minimally invasive carcinomas and well-encapsulated follicular variant of papillary cancer in patients younger than 45 years; some consider a lobectomy sufficient treatment.

INTRODUCTION

Follicular lesions of the thyroid encompass a wide range of diseases, including benign follicular adenoma, malignant follicular carcinoma, and follicular variant of papillary cancer. Follicular adenoma is defined as an encapsulated, benign neoplastic proliferation of thyroid follicles.[1] Follicular carcinoma represents 10% to 15% of all thyroid

Disclosures: None.
Conflict of Interest: None.
[a] Department of Surgery, Johns Hopkins University School of Medicine, 600 North Wolfe Street, Baltimore, MD 21287, USA; [b] Department of Pathology, Johns Hopkins University School of Medicine, 600 North Wolfe Street, Baltimore, MD 21287, USA
* Corresponding author. Department of Surgery, The Johns Hopkins Hospital, 600 North Wolfe Street, Blalock 606, Baltimore, MD 21287.
E-mail address: mzeiger@jhmi.edu

http://dx.doi.org/10.1016/j.suc.2014.02.005
0039-6109/14/$ – see front matter © 2014 Elsevier Inc. All rights reserved.
surgical.theclinics.com

cancers, and has been classified by the World Health Organization as minimally invasive follicular carcinoma (MIFC) or widely invasive follicular carcinoma (WIFC).[2] Follicular variant of papillary thyroid cancer (FVPTC) is the second most common variant of papillary carcinoma after the classic variety. Because, follicular neoplasms also represent a spectrum of disease with considerable morphologic overlap rather than discreet entities, controversy exists regarding diagnoses of these histologic subtypes. These lesions have subsequently been referred to as "the bane of the pathologist."[3] Furthermore, the specific diagnosis has an impact on patient treatment and prognosis. This review addresses the clinical presentation, preoperative diagnosis in the era of molecular markers, pathologic diagnosis, treatment, and prognosis of follicular lesions, taking into account the frequent controversy about definitive histologic diagnoses.

CLINICAL PRESENTATION

Thyroid nodules are present in 60% to 70% of the US population; most are benign, and only 5% are malignant.[4] Most patients with a follicular adenoma or carcinoma present with a solitary thyroid nodule, which is either palpable or incidentally discovered on imaging in an otherwise asymptomatic patient. The nodule may also occur in association with thyroiditis or nodular hyperplasia. Patients with large tumors may complain of compressive symptoms such as dyspnea, coughing, choking sensation, dysphagia, inability to lie flat, or hoarseness. Rarely, patients may present with hyperthyroidism. Most patients with an adenoma are clinically and biochemically euthyroid. Approximately 1% of follicular adenomas are toxic adenomas, causing symptomatic hyperthyroidism, and nearly all of these lesions are benign.[5] However, hyperthyroidism usually does not occur until an adenoma is larger than 3 cm.

Follicular carcinoma typically presents as a solitary mass, usually greater than 2 cm, and is more prevalent in iodine-deficient regions.[6] It occurs most often in women. MIFC resembles a follicular adenoma with an indolent course; it tends to present in younger patients, and some have proposed that it may be a precursor to its WIFC counterpart. Conversely, WIFC is clinically recognizable as a cancer. It tends to present in older patients, with a median age of 60 years. Follicular carcinoma has a tendency for hematogeneous spread, but the patient rarely has lung or bone metastases at initial presentation.

FVPTC is a unique intermediate clinical entity, with histologic and clinical features that span the cytologic features of classic papillary thyroid cancer (PTC) and the architectural features of follicular thyroid cancer. According to a large population-based study of more than 10,000 cases,[7] the mean tumor size was larger than that of classic PTC, but smaller than follicular cancer. Extrathyroidal extension and lymph node metastases in FVPTC are seen more commonly than with follicular cancer, but less commonly than with classic PTC. Distant metastases were present in 2%, compared with 1% in patients with PTC and 4% with follicular cancer.[7]

PREOPERATIVE DIAGNOSIS
Ultrasonography

Certain sonographic features of a thyroid nodule can be used as predictors of the presence of a malignancy. Characteristics of a suspicious nodule include the following: unifocal, hypoechoic, solid, a discontinued halo, irregular margins, microcalcifications, and predominantly intranodular color flow.[8,9] Recent studies using duplex ultrasonography showed that the absence of blood flow in a follicular neoplasm is associated with a 96% negative predictive value, but its presence had only a 15% positive predictive value for carcinoma.[10] Some have proposed an ultrasonography-based malignancy score or a practical Thyroid Imaging Reporting and Data System (TIRADS) to stratify malignant risk.[8,9,11] This score incorporates ultrasonography features that are significantly associated with malignancy such as solid component, hypoechogenicity, microlobulation or irregular margins, microcalcifications, and taller-than-wide shape. As the number of suspicious features increases, the probability and risk of malignancy also increases, with a TIRADS score of 5 associated with an 88% risk of malignancy. However, prospective studies with larger patient populations are needed to verify the value of this ultrasonography-based malignancy scoring system.

The sonographic appearance of a follicular thyroid cancer differs from classic PTC. Follicular cancers tend to appear more isoechoic to hyperechoic with thick and irregular halo, and usually do not have microcalcifications.[12] PTC generally appears as a predominantly solid and hypoechoic mass with increased nodular vascularity, often with infiltrative or irregular margins and microcalcifications.

Characteristic sonographic features have also been examined to determine whether follicular carcinoma can be differentiated from follicular adenoma. In a retrospective analysis, Sillery and colleagues[13] found that although sonographic features of follicular adenoma and follicular carcinoma are similar, larger lesion size, lack of a sonographic halo, hypoechoic appearance, and absence of cystic change favored a diagnosis of follicular carcinoma. Another group found that ultrasonography features of isoechoic or hypoechoic echogenicity, predominantly solid or mixed echotexture, and microcalcifications or rim calcifications are more common in follicular cancers than in follicular adenomas.[14] Others have found that FVPTC tends to have benign sonographic features such as hypoechogenicity, well-defined margins, an oval shape, and no microcalcifications, making them difficult to diagnose on ultrasonography alone.[15]

Fine-Needle Aspiration

Although fine-needle aspiration (FNA) biopsy is the most widely used and best diagnostic test for a thyroid nodule, it falls short 15% to 20% of the time as a guide for appropriate clinical management.[4] This situation is because many FNAs are read as either indeterminate or suspicious only. However, with the exception of these biopsy results, and occasional inadequate samples, thyroid FNA is highly accurate; a benign result has a negative predictive value greater than 95%, and a malignant result has a positive predictive value that exceeds 99%.[16,17] Most FNAs of follicular neoplasms are read as either indeterminate or suspicious only because of 3 inherent limitations, which are important to know, especially in the context of this tumor type. First, morphologic evaluation is inherently subjective, so differences in risk stratification are commonplace despite the standardization of nomenclature of the Bethesda System for Reporting Thyroid Cytopathology (TBSRTC).[16,18] Second, biopsy represents only a limited sampling of a lesion that may otherwise be heterogeneous; this limitation is theoretically addressed through the use of FNA, which samples a wider range of the mass than core biopsy.[19] Finally, the sine qua non for the diagnosis of a follicular malignancy is capsular-vascular invasion, and this cannot be assessed on FNA.[20]

Because the malignant nature of follicular lesions requires histologic proof of capsular or vascular invasion, any FNA diagnosis of a follicular lesion is inherently uncertain. This uncertainty is the rationale behind the preferred use of suspicious for follicular neoplasm rather than simply follicular neoplasm in the standardized terminology of TBSRTC.[21,22] This diagnostic category carries a 15% to 30% risk for malignancy.[23] The cytologic features that lead to a specimen being classified as suspicious for a follicular neoplasm include the presence of abundant microfollicles and the absence of colloid (**Fig. 1**).

Molecular Markers

To improve on the differential diagnosis of follicular tumors, ancillary molecular tests have been investigated. Point mutations in *BRAF* and *RAS* (*H-RAS, N-RAS, K-RAS*) genes and gene rearrangements involving *RET/PTC* and *PAX8/PPARγ* have been studied extensively and identified in more than 70% of thyroid malignancies. Although these markers have a high positive predictive value and may serve as a useful adjunct to FNA in the future, current assays are still neither sensitive nor specific enough to differentiate benign from malignant follicular neoplasms.[24–29] Conversely, a gene expression classifier (GEC) was developed to identify benign lesions among patients who have morphologically atypia of undetermined significance or suspicious for a follicular neoplasms on FNA.[30] Afirma is a commercially available GEC test, developed by Veracyte (San Francisco, CA, USA) to classify indeterminate thyroid nodules as either benign or suspicious for malignancy. It uses a messenger RNA (mRNA) expression panel of 142 different genes to identify a benign signature. Duick and colleagues[31] conducted a study to evaluate the impact of Afirma results on the endocrinologist and patient decisions regarding whether to operate for an indeterminate thyroid nodule. These investigators studied 368 patients and reported a substantial reduction in the rate of thyroidectomy for these patients with the use of Afirma (from 74% to 7.6%). Alexander and colleagues[30] also studied GEC on 265 indeterminate thyroid nodules, which included many from the study by Duick and colleagues. These investigators reported that Afirma is a sensitive (92%), but nonspecific (52%) diagnostic test for detecting suspicious nodules. Therefore,

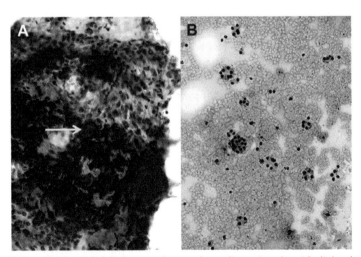

Fig. 1. (*A*) Normal thyroid follicles are large, three-dimensional epithelial spheres that contain abundant thin colloid (*arrow*) either separate from or within sheets of evenly spaced follicular cells. Benign follicular cells contain a single nucleus roughly equivalent in size to the amount of surrounding cytoplasm (papanicolau, original magnification ×40). In contrast, in (*B*), the cells of a follicular neoplasm are arranged in microfollicles that do not contain abundant colloid. The cells within the microfollicles have monotonous nuclei, with little surrounding cytoplasm (modified romanowsky [diff quick], original magnification ×40).

because of the low specificity, Afirma identifies approximately 50% of benign nodules with indeterminate cytology accurately (true negative); on the other hand, it reports the other 50% of benign nodules as suspicious (false positive). If the GEC were performed on morphologically benign nodules, it would classify a third of them as suspicious. Although the current literature shows that this test has a high negative predictive value, it is not specific enough to alter management when it is positive.[32] Although the 2009 American Thyroid Association guidelines recommend that use of molecular markers be considered for patients with indeterminate cytology, there remains a lack of consensus guidelines on how to interpret or alter surgical decision making based on these tests.[12,33]

Other proposed markers to aid in the differential diagnosis include protein-based assays such as Galectin-3, RNA-based studies such as human telomerase reverse transcriptase and microRNA analysis, detection of peripheral blood markers for thyroid-stimulating hormone receptor and thyroglobulin mRNA, and analysis of DNA copy number variation.[28,34–37] Genetic gains and losses in thyroid cancers have been extensively studied, and comparative genomic hybridization has shown that DNA copy number changes are frequent in follicular adenoma, but infrequent in FVPTC.[36]

Although a large research emphasis has been placed on this clinical problem and the literature is replete with a variety of methods to aid in the diagnosis of follicular lesions, none has proved to be adequate in differentiating a benign from malignant tumor, nor has prospectively incorporated these markers into a clinical algorithm in a blinded fashion to assess their true impact.

PATHOLOGIC DIAGNOSIS
Follicular Adenoma and Carcinoma

The histopathologic diagnosis of a follicular patterned thyroid nodule requires the recognition of key features identified with both low-power and high-power magnification. At low power, the pathologist looks for the presence or absence of capsular invasion. The benign follicular adenoma does not show invasive growth, is solitary, and is surrounded by a fibrous capsule (**Fig. 2**A). It is a solitary lesion in an otherwise normal gland. Adenomas tend to show a microfollicular or macrofollicular growth pattern and lack degenerative changes such as hemorrhage, fibrosis, and cyst formation.[3] Follicular carcinomas are defined by the presence of tumor into or through its surrounding capsule or invasion into vessels (ie, angioinvasion) (**Fig. 2**B). Consensus about what defines capsular invasion is lacking, and therefore, careful histologic examination of the tumor capsule interface is necessary.[1] Vascular invasion is defined as the presence of tumor cells within capsular vessels attached to the vessel wall.[38] Histologic examination of a minimum of 10 tissue blocks is necessary to rule out a follicular carcinoma.[39] Follicular carcinoma is further subdivided into MIFC and WIFC subtypes. Invasion limited to the tumor capsule defines MIFC, and even just an extension into the capsule is diagnostic of malignancy. MIFC, for the most part, resembles a follicular adenoma, but the diagnosis relies on identifying a nest of tumor cells that penetrate the capsule. In contrast, WIFC extends into the normal thyroid parenchyma and often lacks any defined capsule (**Fig. 2**C). These lesions usually are large and have obvious extraglandular spread, with adhesion or invasion into neighboring structures.

Follicular Variant of Papillary Cancer

Follicular variant of papillary carcinoma is defined by cytologic atypia, regardless of the presence or absence of invasive growth, and therefore, an examination of the

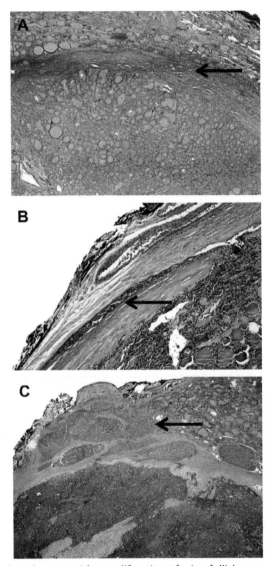

Fig. 2. (*A*) A follicular adenoma with a proliferation of microfollicles completely surrounded by a fibrous capsule (*arrow*). (*B*) This MIFC is encapsulated; however, it shows invasive growth into a capsular blood vessel (ie, angioinvasion [*arrow*]). (*C*) shows a WIFC that has a retained capsule, beyond which the tumor has invaded into the thyroid parenchyma (*arrow*) (hematoxylin-eosin, original magnification ×40). (*Courtesy of* Justin A. Bishop, MD, Baltimore, MD.)

cells lining the follicles of the nodule at high-power magnification is critical. The key cytologic features include nuclear enlargement, nuclear overlapping, chromatin clearing, and irregular nuclear contours, including longitudinal grooves and pseudoinclusions (**Fig. 3**A). FVPTC shows characteristic nuclear features of PTC with a dominant (>50%) follicular growth pattern, and is divided into 2 subtypes: encapsulated and infiltrative. Encapsulated tumors possess a fibrous capsule, whereas infiltrative

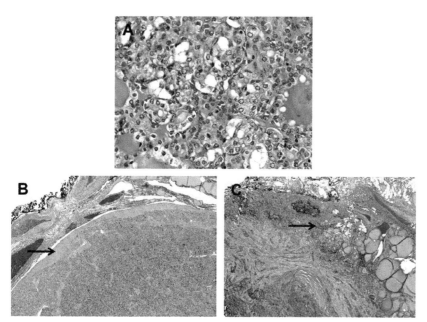

Fig. 3. (*A*) Follicular variant of papillary carcinoma is classically characterized by a purely follicular growth pattern in addition to significant nuclear atypia, including nuclear enlargement, chromatin clearing, nuclear crowding and overlapping, and irregular nuclear contours (hematoxylin-eosin, original magnification ×400). (*B*) An encapsulated follicular variant of papillary carcinoma; it does not show invasive growth and is surrounded by a fibrous capsule (*arrow*) (hematoxylin-eosin, original magnification ×40). (*C*) An infiltrative follicular variant of papillary carcinoma, in which the unencapsulated tumor invades the thyroid parenchyma (*arrow*) as follicles and cords, inducing a desmoplastic stromal reaction (hematoxylin-eosin, original magnification ×40). (*Courtesy of* Justin A. Bishop, MD, Baltimore, MD.)

tumors have absent or incomplete tumor encapsulation, with tongues of tumor infiltrating into the thyroid parenchyma (**Fig. 3**B, C). Therefore, the diagnosis of an encapsulated cancer is straightforward only when the atypical cytologic features are well developed but more difficult when the atypia is not uniformly distributed throughout the nodule.

DIFFERENTIAL DIAGNOSIS

Although pathologic definitions for each follicular lesion exist, significant observer variation in the diagnosis of these lesions has been reported in multiple studies.[2,40–43] The lack of consensus in defining capsular invasion makes diagnosing a benign adenoma versus an MIFC difficult. The absence of clear diagnostic criteria for FVPTC has led to a progressive decrease of its diagnostic threshold. Ambiguity about both in terms of the degree of nuclear atypia required for diagnosis and whether this degree of nuclear atypia is characteristic of malignancy factor into this uncertainty.[44] Fear of potential litigation may lead to overdiagnosis of cancer. If a patient with a known diagnosis of thyroid cancer develops metastases, the scenario would be described as predestined, whereas a situation in which a patient who develops metastatic thyroid cancer when they were initially believed to have benign disease would be described as litigious.[44]

TREATMENT
Surgical Management

A patient with a follicular neoplasm on FNA result should, at minimum, undergo a diagnostic thyroid lobectomy with isthmusectomy. Clinical risk factors, such as family history, multiple nodules, worrisome sonographic features, presence of hypothyroidism, and previous head/neck irradiation should be taken into consideration, and if present, total thyroidectomy offered as initial surgical management. A patient with a histopathologic final diagnosis of a follicular adenoma requires no additional therapy, whereas a total thyroidectomy is recommended for the treatment of most thyroid cancers, although this latter recommendation is controversial for MIFC and FVPTC.[39] A lobectomy with negative surgical margins can be considered adequate treatment in select patients who are young, with tumor size less than 4 cm, with a histologically confirmed MIFC.[39,45–47] Some believe that only a lobectomy is needed for an encapsulated noninvasive FVPTC, whereas others continue to recommend a total thyroidectomy for lesions larger than 1 cm.[48] Completion thyroidectomy after hemithyroidectomy may be performed within 2 weeks of initial surgery or 6 to 8 weeks later. Delay beyond 6 months after initial thyroidectomy may be associated with a higher risk of metastases and decreased survival.[49] Prophylactic central neck dissection, although controversial for PTC, has no role and is not a consideration in patients with follicular carcinoma, because less than 10% have lymph node metastases. The role of a prophylactic central neck dissection is controversial for patients with FVPTC. In a study of 115 patients who underwent prophylactic central neck dissection for FVPTPC,[50] none was found to have lymph node metastases. The ambiguity of diagnosis and the indolent nature of encapsulated FVPTC lead some to forego a prophylactic dissection. However, the aggressive nature of infiltrative tumors has led some to recommend considering a prophylactic central neck dissection, because infiltrative tumors have more of a propensity to spread to the central compartment of lymph nodes.[48]

Role of Intraoperative Frozen Section

The use of intraoperative frozen section examination during diagnostic lobectomy for a follicular neoplasm is controversial.[51–58] It offers the potential to save patients from undergoing reoperation for completion thyroidectomy by making an intraoperative diagnosis of malignancy, and thus several centers routinely perform it, quoting a sensitivity as high as 80%.[55,59] In a study from the Mayo Clinic,[55] of the 1023 patients diagnosed as having a malignancy on final pathology, the diagnosis was correctly established by frozen section in 78%, thereby permitting definitive surgical management at the first operation. However, this is a unique pathologic laboratory that uses multiple frozen sections for diagnoses. Intraoperative frozen section is suboptimal for suspected follicular lesions for several reasons. First, capsular-vascular invasion is difficult to detect and requires histologic inspection of the entirely embedded capsule, which is impractical in the setting of frozen section. Second, the histomorphologic quality of frozen tissue is substantially less than that of fixed tissue, so the potential for indeterminate or incorrect diagnoses is high. Third, tissue that has been frozen is histomorphologically compromised for the remainder of the diagnostic process. Thus, performing frozen sections on suspected follicular lesions can lead to irreversible obstacles to classification. Studies showing low reproducibility for histologic classification show increased agreement after a consensus oriented review, and this is usually not practical during frozen section.[20] For these reasons, we do not perform frozen sections on suspected follicular lesions at our institution.[5,60]

Radioactive Iodine

The absence of thyroid tissue allows administration of radioactive iodine (RAI) to ablate any remaining tumor cells. About 6 weeks postoperatively, patients with thyroid cancer are frequently treated with ^{131}I as an outpatient to ablate any residual thyroid tissue or microscopic disease and reduce the risk of recurrence. Ablation of a small amount of residual normal thyroid tissue remaining after total thyroidectomy may be considered as adjuvant therapy and facilitate the early detection of recurrence based on serum thyroglobulin measurement or RAI whole body scan (WBS).[12] [131]I ablation of an intact lobe can be considered if a patient refuses to undergo completion thyroidectomy or if complications such as recurrent laryngeal nerve injury are experienced during the initial surgery. However, remnant ablation in lieu of completion thyroidectomy is no longer recommended. Treatment with RAI is controversial in a few subtypes of indolent follicular cancers. A population-based analysis of survival among 1200 patients with MIFC[39] suggested that aggressive treatment with ^{131}I after total thyroidectomy did not improve patient outcome. In a retrospective analysis of a cohort of 102 patients with encapsulated, well-differentiated follicular patterned tumors who were treated with total thyroidectomy with or without postoperative RAI,[45] there were no deaths at an average follow-up of 12 years, showing an extremely favorable outcome. However, ^{131}I is a well-established treatment strategy for WIFC and infiltrative FVPTC.

Follow-Up

The main goal of long-term follow-up is to allow accurate surveillance for either local recurrence or presence of metastatic disease. Measurement of serum thyroglobulin (Tg) levels, ultrasonography, and WBS are all used to monitor patients for residual or recurrent disease. Serum Tg should be measured ideally in the same laboratory, using the same assay at 6 months, 12 months, and then annually if disease free. An increase or detectable level of Tg indicates recurrent disease, for which imaging modalities such as WBS and cervical ultrasonography can aid in localization. After thyroidectomy, cervical ultrasonography should be performed at 6 to 12 months and then periodically depending on the risk for recurrent disease. Ultrasonographically suspicious lymph nodes greater than 5 to 8 mm should be biopsied for cytology with Tg measurement in the needle washout fluid. A diagnostic WBS is most useful during follow-up when there is little to no remaining thyroid tissue. However, after ^{131}I, if the posttherapy scan does not show uptake outside the thyroid bed, subsequent diagnostic WBS have a low sensitivity and are usually unnecessary in low-risk patients. It may be of value in patients with intermediate-risk or high-risk disease. If Tg becomes detectable, a diagnostic scan performed after thyroxine suppression can be helpful.

PROGNOSIS

For patients with differentiated thyroid cancers, numerous systems have been developed for risk stratification and prognosis. These systems include AGES (age, tumor grade, extent, and size), AMES (age, metastasis, extent, and size), MACIS (metastasis, completeness of resection, invasion, and size), Ohio State University prognostic factors, Memorial Sloan-Kettering Cancer Center risk groups, and the TNM staging system by the American Joint Committee on Cancer. These staging systems show that the most important prognostic factors are age of the patient, tumor size and extent, and the presence of distant metastases. The TNM staging is listed in **Tables 1** and **2**. The American Cancer Society and the National Thyroid Cancer Treatment Cooperative Study Registry published 5-year relative survival rates for follicular thyroid cancer. For stages I and II, the 5-year survival rate is nearly 100%, stage III 71% to 91%, and stage IV near 50%.[61]

Table 1
Primary tumor, lymph node status, and metastases for TNM staging

Primary Tumor (T)	
T1	Tumor ≤2 cm in greatest dimension, limited to the thyroid
T2	Tumor >2 cm but ≤4 cm in greatest dimension, limited to the thyroid
T3	Tumor >4 cm in greatest dimension limited to the thyroid or any tumor with minimal extrathyroid extension (sternothyroid muscle, perithyroidal soft tissue)
T4	Tumor of any size that extends beyond thyroid capsule to invade subcutaneous soft tissues, larynx, trachea, esophagus, recurrent laryngeal nerve, prevertebral fascia, or mediastinal vessels
Nodal Status (N)	
N0	No regional lymph node metastasis
N1	Regional lymph node metastasis
Metastases (M)	
M0	No distant metastasis
M1	Distant metastasis

TUMOR HISTOLOGY
MIFC

MIFC is a less aggressive tumor with a disease-free survival that has been reported to be similar to a benign follicular adenoma. However, the presence of extensive vascular invasion has a negative impact on prognosis. A population-based analysis of survival among 1200 patients with MIFC[39] reported that distant metastases were rare and overall survival of these patients was comparable with the general US population. Lymph node metastases were present in 20% of patients, less frequent than with PTC. The disease-specific survival rate was 99.8%. However, others have reported metastases in 22% of patients, with the most common sites being lung, soft tissue, bone, and rarely, brain.[46,47] Sugino and colleagues[47] reported that distant metastatic disease-free survival was 85.6% and 70% at 10 and 20 years, respectively, and overall cause specific survival was 95% and 86.8% at 10 and 20 years, respectively. On further subgroup analysis, tumors larger than 4 cm and patient age older than 45 years were poor prognostic indicators.

Table 2
TNM staging

Stage	T	N	M
<45 y			
I	Any T	Any N	M0
II	Any T	Any N	M1
≥45 y			
I	T1	N0	M0
II	T2	N0	M0
III	T3	N0	M0
	T1–3	N1	M0
IV	T4	N0	M0
	T1–4	N1	M0
	Any T	Any N	M1

WIFC

Extrathyroidal invasion, presence of metastases at the time of diagnosis, high cancer-related mortality, and high recurrence rates have been observed in WIFC.[62,63] WIFC is aggressive and associated with a dire prognosis, with a 10-year disease-specific mortality of 15% to 25%.[64–66] The strongest poor prognostic factors for this tumor are size greater than 4 cm and presence of metastases. In a population-based study, 10-year overall survival for patients with WIFC was 86.6%, with a disease-specific survival of 94.8%.[39] In a study evaluating clinical characteristics of 243 patients with follicular carcinoma, of the 145 patients with WIFC, 3% developed lymph node metastases, 28% developed distant metastases, and the mortality was 28%.[63] Metastatic disease most commonly affects lungs and bone but can also occur in other soft tissues and lymph nodes.[46,67] Isolated lung, brain, or bone metastases that can be resected may result in improved survival.[12]

FVPTC

FVPTC has a prognosis between that of PTC and follicular cancer. A population-based study reported overall survival of 93% at 10 years and 89% at 15 years. Encapsulated, noninvasive follicular variant of papillary carcinoma has an excellent prognosis, with minimal recurrence risk or metastatic potential. In a study comparing the biological behavior of encapsulated and infiltrative FVPTCs, encapsulated tumors lacking capsular or vascular invasion were found to have virtually no metastatic potential or recurrence risk. In contrast, infiltrative tumors were found to have a significantly higher incidence of nodal metastases, positive margins, extrathyroidal extension, and risk of recurrence.[68,69] Despite this finding, bony metastases have also been reported in several patients with unifocal, well-encapsulated tumors.[70]

SUMMARY

Follicular neoplasms represent a wide clinical spectrum of disease, with tremendous overlap in clinicopathologic diagnosis, prognosis, and management. Suspicious sonographic features in conjunction with FNA biopsy of thyroid nodules provide the most accurate preoperative diagnosis to guide therapy. The use of molecular markers as an adjunct has become an extensive area of research. However, before any conclusions can be made regarding the true impact of molecular markers on the surgical management of indeterminate thyroid nodules, further prospective studies that assess the accuracy in diagnosing indeterminate or suspicious lesions, examine the cost-effectiveness of the tests, and incorporate them into a clinical management algorithm are needed. The surgical management of these lesions entails at a minimum a diagnostic lobectomy and often, total thyroidectomy followed by radioiodine treatment of the more aggressive subtypes. Even then, significant intraobserver and interobserver variability exists in the precise histopathologic diagnosis of these lesions, which in turn affects further management. It is generally accepted that patient age, gender, specific histology, size of tumor, extent of tumor, presence or absence of metastases, and surgical and postoperative treatment all affect outcome. With variations in treatment (lobectomy vs total thyroidectomy, radioiodine vs no radioiodine) as well as known uncertainties in diagnosing follicular lesions, the use of any prognostic scoring system must be considered carefully.

REFERENCES

1. Suster S. Thyroid tumors with a follicular growth pattern: problems in differential diagnosis. Arch Pathol Lab Med 2006;130(7):984–8.

2. Lloyd RV, Erickson LA, Casey MB, et al. Observer variation in the diagnosis of follicular variant of papillary thyroid carcinoma. Am J Surg Pathol 2004;28(10): 1336–40.

3. Baloch ZW, Fleisher S, LiVolsi VA, et al. Diagnosis of "follicular neoplasm": a gray zone in thyroid fine-needle aspiration cytology. Diagn Cytopathol 2002;26(1):41–4.

4. Baloch ZW, Cibas ES, Clark DP, et al. The National Cancer Institute Thyroid fine needle aspiration state of the science conference: a summation. Cytojournal 2008;5:6.

5. McHenry CR, Phitayakorn R. Follicular adenoma and carcinoma of the thyroid gland. Oncologist 2011;16(5):585–93.

6. Baloch ZW, LiVolsi VA. Our approach to follicular-patterned lesions of the thyroid. J Clin Pathol 2007;60(3):244–50.

7. Yu XM, Schneider DF, Leverson G, et al. Follicular variant of papillary thyroid carcinoma is a unique clinical entity: a population-based study of 10,740 cases. Thyroid 2013;23(10):1263–8.

8. Kwak JY, Han KH, Yoon JH, et al. Thyroid imaging reporting and data system for US features of nodules: a step in establishing better stratification of cancer risk. Radiology 2011;260(3):892–9.

9. Choi YJ, Yun JS, Kim DH. Clinical and ultrasound features of cytology diagnosed follicular neoplasm. Endocr J 2009;56(3):383–9.

10. Iared W, Shigueoka DC, Cristofoli JC, et al. Use of color Doppler ultrasonography for the prediction of malignancy in follicular thyroid neoplasms: systematic review and meta-analysis. J Ultrasound Med 2010;29(3):419–25.

11. Pompili G, Tresoldi S, Primolevo A, et al. Management of thyroid follicular proliferation: an ultrasound-based malignancy score to opt for surgical or conservative treatment. Ultrasound Med Biol 2013;39(8):1350–5.

12. American Thyroid Association (ATA) Guidelines Taskforce on Thyroid Nodules and Differentiated Thyroid Cancer, et al. Revised American Thyroid Association management guidelines for patients with thyroid nodules and differentiated thyroid cancer. Thyroid 2009;19(11):1167–214.

13. Sillery JC, Reading CC, Charboneau JW, et al. Thyroid follicular carcinoma: sonographic features of 50 cases. AJR Am J Roentgenol 2010;194(1):44–54.

14. Seo HS, Lee DH, Park SH, et al. Thyroid follicular neoplasms: can sonography distinguish between adenomas and carcinomas? J Clin Ultrasound 2009;37(9): 493–500.

15. Yoon JH, Kim EK, Hong SW, et al. Sonographic features of the follicular variant of papillary thyroid carcinoma. J Ultrasound Med 2008;27(10):1431–7.

16. Olson MT, Clark DP, Erozan YS, et al. Spectrum of risk of malignancy in subcategories of 'atypia of undetermined significance'. Acta Cytol 2011;55(6):518–25.

17. Yassa L, Cibas ES, Benson CB, et al. Long-term assessment of a multidisciplinary approach to thyroid nodule diagnostic evaluation. Cancer 2007;111(6): 508–16.

18. Olson MT, Boonyaarunnate T, Aragon Han P, et al. A tertiary center's experience with second review of 3885 thyroid cytopathology specimens. J Clin Endocrinol Metab 2013;98(4):1450–7.

19. Olson MT, Tatsas AD, Ali SZ. Cytotechnologist-attended on-site adequacy evaluation of thyroid fine-needle aspiration comparison with cytopathologists and correlation with the final interpretation. Am J Clin Pathol 2012;138(1):90–5.

20. Wang CC, Friedman L, Kennedy GC, et al. A large multicenter correlation study of thyroid nodule cytopathology and histopathology. Thyroid 2011;21(3):243–51.

21. Ali SZ. Thyroid cytopathology: Bethesda and beyond. Acta Cytol 2011;55(1):4–12.

22. Cibas ES, Ali SZ, NCI Thyroid FNA State of the Science Conference. The Bethesda system for reporting thyroid cytopathology. Am J Clin Pathol 2009; 132(5):658–65.
23. Boonyaarunnate T, Olson MT, Ali SZ. 'Suspicious for a follicular neoplasm' before and after the Bethesda system for reporting thyroid cytopathology: impact of standardized terminology. Acta Cytol 2013;57(5):455–63.
24. Nikiforov YE. Molecular diagnostics of thyroid tumors. Arch Pathol Lab Med 2011;135(5):569–77.
25. Nikiforov YE, Steward DL, Robinson-Smith TM, et al. Molecular testing for mutations in improving the fine-needle aspiration diagnosis of thyroid nodules. J Clin Endocrinol Metab 2009;94(6):2092–8.
26. Ohori NP, Nikiforova MN, Schoedel KE, et al. Contribution of molecular testing to thyroid fine-needle aspiration cytology of "follicular lesion of undetermined significance/atypia of undetermined significance". Cancer Cytopathol 2010;118(1): 17–23.
27. Yip L, Kebebew E, Milas M, et al. Summary statement: utility of molecular marker testing in thyroid cancer. Surgery 2010;148(6):1313–5.
28. Lee SR, Jung CK, Kim TE, et al. Molecular genotyping of follicular variant of papillary thyroid carcinoma correlates with diagnostic category of fine-needle aspiration cytology: values of RAS mutation testing. Thyroid 2013;23(11): 1416–22.
29. Yu XM, Patel PN, Chen H, et al. False-negative fine-needle aspiration of thyroid nodules cannot be attributed to sampling error alone. Am J Surg 2012;203(3): 331–4 [discussion: 334].
30. Alexander EK, Kennedy GC, Baloch ZW, et al. Preoperative diagnosis of benign thyroid nodules with indeterminate cytology. N Engl J Med 2012;367(8):705–15.
31. Duick DS, Klopper JP, Diggans JC, et al. The impact of benign gene expression classifier test results on the endocrinologist-patient decision to operate on patients with thyroid nodules with indeterminate fine-needle aspiration cytopathology. Thyroid 2012;22(10):996–1001.
32. Han AP, Olson MT, Fazeli R, et al. The impact of molecular testing on the surgical management of patients with thyroid nodules. Ann Surg Oncol 2014. [Epub ahead of print].
33. American Thyroid Association Surgery Working Group, et al. Consensus statement on the terminology and classification of central neck dissection for thyroid cancer. Thyroid 2009;19(11):1153–8.
34. Chiu CG, Strugnell SS, Griffith OL, et al. Diagnostic utility of galectin-3 in thyroid cancer. Am J Pathol 2010;176(5):2067–81.
35. Milas M, Shin J, Gupta M, et al. Circulating thyrotropin receptor mRNA as a novel marker of thyroid cancer: clinical applications learned from 1758 samples. Ann Surg 2010;252(4):643–51.
36. Liu Y, Cope L, Sun W, et al. DNA copy number variations characterize benign and malignant thyroid tumors. J Clin Endocrinol Metab 2013;98(3):E558–66.
37. Kitano M, Rahbari R, Patterson EE, et al. Expression profiling of difficult-to-diagnose thyroid histologic subtypes shows distinct expression profiles and identify candidate diagnostic microRNAs. Ann Surg Oncol 2011;18(12):3443–52.
38. LiVolsi VA, Baloch ZW. Follicular-patterned tumors of the thyroid: the battle of benign vs. malignant vs. so-called uncertain. Endocr Pathol 2011;22(4):184–9.
39. Goffredo P, Cheung K, Roman SA, et al. Can minimally invasive follicular thyroid cancer be approached as a benign lesion?: a population-level analysis of survival among 1,200 patients. Ann Surg Oncol 2013;20(3):767–72.

40. Elsheikh TM, Asa SL, Chan JK, et al. Interobserver and intraobserver variation among experts in the diagnosis of thyroid follicular lesions with borderline nuclear features of papillary carcinoma. Am J Clin Pathol 2008;130(5):736–44.

41. Widder S, Guggisberg K, Khalil M, et al. A pathologic re-review of follicular thyroid neoplasms: the impact of changing the threshold for the diagnosis of the follicular variant of papillary thyroid carcinoma. Surgery 2008;144(1):80–5.

42. Duggan MA, Di Francesco L, Alakija P, et al. A pathologic re-review of follicular thyroid neoplasms: the impact of changing the threshold for the diagnosis of the follicular variant of papillary thyroid carcinoma. Surgery 2009;145(6):687–8 [author reply: 688–9].

43. Cibas ES, Baloch ZW, Fellegara G, et al. A prospective assessment defining the limitations of thyroid nodule pathologic evaluation. Ann Intern Med 2013;159(5): 325–32.

44. Daniels GH. What if many follicular variant papillary thyroid carcinomas are not malignant? A review of follicular variant papillary thyroid carcinoma and a proposal for a new classification. Endocr Pract 2011;17(5):768–87.

45. Piana S, Frasoldati A, Di Felice E, et al. Encapsulated well-differentiated follicular-patterned thyroid carcinomas do not play a significant role in the fatality rates from thyroid carcinoma. Am J Surg Pathol 2010;34(6):868–72.

46. Ban EJ, Andrabi A, Grodski S, et al. Follicular thyroid cancer: minimally invasive tumours can give rise to metastases. ANZ J Surg 2012;82(3):136–9.

47. Sugino K, Ito K, Nagahama M, et al. Prognosis and prognostic factors for distant metastases and tumor mortality in follicular thyroid carcinoma. Thyroid 2011; 21(7):751–7.

48. Ghossein R. Problems and controversies in the histopathology of thyroid carcinomas of follicular cell origin. Arch Pathol Lab Med 2009;133(5):683–91.

49. Scheumann GF, Seeliger H, Musholt TJ, et al. Completion thyroidectomy in 131 patients with differentiated thyroid carcinoma. Eur J Surg 1996;162(9):677–84.

50. Salter KD, Andersen PE, Cohen JI, et al. Central nodal metastases in papillary thyroid carcinoma based on tumor histologic type and focality. Arch Otolaryngol Head Neck Surg 2010;136(7):692–6.

51. Callcut RA, Selvaggi SM, Mack E, et al. The utility of frozen section evaluation for follicular thyroid lesions. Ann Surg Oncol 2004;11(1):94–8.

52. Chen H, Nicol TL, Udelsman R. Follicular lesions of the thyroid. Does frozen section evaluation alter operative management? Ann Surg 1995;222(1):101–6.

53. LiVolsi VA, Baloch ZW. Use and abuse of frozen section in the diagnosis of follicular thyroid lesions. Endocr Pathol 2005;16(4):285–93.

54. McHenry CR, Raeburn C, Strickland T, et al. The utility of routine frozen section examination for intraoperative diagnosis of thyroid cancer. Am J Surg 1996; 172(6):658–61.

55. Paphavasit A, Thompson GB, Hay ID, et al. Follicular and Hurthle cell thyroid neoplasms. Is frozen-section evaluation worthwhile? Arch Surg 1997;132(6): 674–8 [discussion: 678–80].

56. Roach JC, Heller KS, Dubner S, et al. The value of frozen section examinations in determining the extent of thyroid surgery in patients with indeterminate fine-needle aspiration cytology. Arch Otolaryngol Head Neck Surg 2002;128(3): 263–7.

57. Wong Z, Muthu C, Craik J, et al. Role of intraoperative frozen section in the management of thyroid nodules. ANZ J Surg 2004;74(12):1052–5.

58. Kahmke R, Lee WT, Puscas L, et al. Utility of intraoperative frozen sections during thyroid surgery. Int J Otolaryngol 2013;2013:496138.

59. Liu FH, Liou MJ, Hsueh C, et al. Thyroid follicular neoplasm: analysis by fine needle aspiration cytology, frozen section, and histopathology. Diagn Cytopathol 2010; 38(11):801–5.

60. Udelsman R, Westra WH, Donovan PI, et al. Randomized prospective evaluation of frozen-section analysis for follicular neoplasms of the thyroid. Ann Surg 2001; 233(5):716–22.

61. Rios A, Rodriguez J, Ferri B, et al. Are prognostic scoring systems of value in patients with follicular thyroid carcinoma? Eur J Endocrinol 2013;169(6):821–7.

62. Kushchayeva Y, Duh QY, Kebebew E, et al. Comparison of clinical characteristics at diagnosis and during follow-up in 118 patients with Hurthle cell or follicular thyroid cancer. Am J Surg 2008;195(4):457–62.

63. Huang CC, Hsueh C, Liu FH, et al. Diagnostic and therapeutic strategies for minimally and widely invasive follicular thyroid carcinomas. Surg Oncol 2011; 20(1):1–6.

64. Ito Y, Hirokawa M, Masuoka H, et al. Distant metastasis at diagnosis and large tumor size are significant prognostic factors of widely invasive follicular thyroid carcinoma. Endocr J 2013;60(6):829–33.

65. Ito Y, Hirokawa M, Masuoka H, et al. Prognostic factors of minimally invasive follicular thyroid carcinoma: extensive vascular invasion significantly affects patient prognosis. Endocr J 2013;60(5):637–42.

66. van Heerden JA, Hay ID, Goellner JR, et al. Follicular thyroid carcinoma with capsular invasion alone: a nonthreatening malignancy. Surgery 1992;112(6): 1130–6 [discussion: 1136–8].

67. Muresan MM, Olivier P, Leclere J, et al. Bone metastases from differentiated thyroid carcinoma. Endocr Relat Cancer 2008;15(1):37–49.

68. Liu J, Singh B, Tallini G, et al. Follicular variant of papillary thyroid carcinoma: a clinicopathologic study of a problematic entity. Cancer 2006;107(6):1255–64.

69. Vivero M, Kraft S, Barletta JA. Risk stratification of follicular variant of papillary thyroid carcinoma. Thyroid 2013;23(3):273–9.

70. Baloch ZW, LiVolsi VA. Encapsulated follicular variant of papillary thyroid carcinoma with bone metastases. Mod Pathol 2000;13(8):861–5.

The Role of Genetic Markers in the Evaluation and Management of Thyroid Nodules

Sareh Parangi, MD[a],*, Hyunsuk Suh, MD[b]

KEYWORDS

- Thyroid nodules • Indeterminate cytology • Molecular markers • Genetic testing

KEY POINTS

- Genetic markers should only be used as an ancillary diagnostic tool for indeterminate thyroid nodules.
- Veracyte Afirma may improve the diagnostic accuracy for a subset of indeterminate cytologic diagnosis.
- Overall clinical, imaging, and cytopathologic evaluation in addition to patient preference should guide the management of indeterminate nodules.
- Further multicentered and independent validation studies are needed in order to prove the efficacy of commercially available genetic markers.

INTRODUCTION

Thyroid nodules are common, with increasing incidence, but only 5% to 15% of nodules are malignant. Fine-needle aspiration (FNA) with cytopathologic evaluation is the gold standard test for distinguishing benign from malignant nodules, but in about 20% of instances the test is indeterminate, often leading to diagnostic surgeries. The Bethesda System for Reporting Thyroid Cytopathology (TBSRTC) classification defines indeterminate cytology as either (1) atypical cells of undetermined significance/follicular lesion of undetermined significance (AUS/FLUS) or (2) follicular neoplasm (FN)/suspicious for a follicular neoplasm (SFN). However, the final pathology in most diagnostic surgeries proves the nodule to be benign. The risk of malignancy in the final pathology for those cytology samples deemed indeterminate can vary from

The authors have nothing to disclose.

[a] Unit of Endocrine Surgery, Massachusetts General Hospital, Harvard Medical School, Wang ACC 460, 15 Parkman Street, Boston, MA 02115, USA; [b] Department of General Surgery, Massachusetts General Hospital, Wang ACC 460, 15 Parkman Street, Boston, MA 02115, USA
* Corresponding author.
E-mail address: sparangi@partners.org

5% to 30%, depending on the category within the Bethesda classification. In contrast, FNAs that are read as suspicious for malignancy are associated with a 60% to 75% risk of malignancy, and a cytologic sample read as positive for malignancy has a 96% to 98% chance of being malignant on final pathology.[1,2] Furthermore, even within the cytologic categories, significant variability exists in the risk of malignancy between the institutions and pathologists.[3] Therefore, highly sensitive and specific diagnostic tools are essential for minimizing unnecessary diagnostic surgeries and 2-stage operations. In an effort to improve diagnostic accuracy, many existing and innovative diagnostic utilities are being actively investigated, including elastography, optical probes, serum biomarkers, and molecular tests. Among them, genetic markers have shown initial promise as a diagnostic tool that may complement standard clinical, radiologic, and FNA evaluation of thyroid nodules.

Thus far, genetic markers have been investigated at various stages of evaluation for management of thyroid nodules. Such efforts have led to a few commercially available gene-based diagnostic tools for indeterminate thyroid nodules. Because molecular testing is progressing rapidly with few publications available, readers should not use information provided here as rules or recommendations. Instead, this article is an educational launching point to further clinicians' knowledge of these state-of-the-art tests. Molecular testing in thyroid nodules is minimally invasive, and it may avoid the intervariability and intravariability often observed in cytologic or histopathologic analysis, potentially becoming the most important, cost-effective, and operator-independent diagnostic tool in the evaluation of a thyroid nodule; however, more research is needed. For the foreseeable future, the best evaluation of thyroid nodules will be achieved with a thorough physical examination, ultrasonography, and cytopathologic evaluation, coupled with the treating physician's experience and judgment. Molecular testing will supplement but not replace this comprehensive approach.

BACKGROUND

The role of commonly associated genetic mutations in thyroid cancer is being actively investigated. However, the role of genetic alterations in tumorigenesis, the clinicopathologic presentations, and their diagnostic or prognostic importance are yet to be fully defined. Thus far, no single molecular marker has shown clinically acceptable negative predictive values (NPVs) and positive predictive values (PPVs), allowing their use as a sole diagnostic tool in evaluating thyroid nodules. Nonetheless, modern high-throughput gene extraction, microarray profiling, and computational analysis have defined certain panels of genetic markers that are promising in the evaluation of thyroid nodules. Many surgical and basic science laboratories have been pioneers over the last decade by using large cohorts of patient needle aspirates, tissue, and blood samples from patients with a variety of thyroid disorders. Recent clinical studies, such as the Afirma Veracyte Trial, have validated the usefulness and efficacy of commercially available tests in diagnosis of indeterminate thyroid nodules. In addition, these studies have shown the importance of incorporation of molecular testing in the national guidelines, such as the National Comprehensive Cancer Network (NCCN). Since December of 2012, genetic testing has been poised to become a mainstream practice in the management of thyroid neoplasms.[4]

CURRENTLY AVAILABLE TECHNIQUES

The 2 most clinically promising types of molecular panels currently are (1) gene expression profiling tools that use the RNA expression profiles of thyroid FNA samples to try to rule out thyroid cancer by determining which nodules have a benign RNA expression profile, and (2) gene mutation panels that use alterations in the DNA to try to rule in patients who have a high likelihood of cancer. There are other genetic markers that use RNA, microRNA, antibodies, and blood biomarkers that have been explored with variable success; these are not be discussed here because of the small number of studies using these technologies.

GENE EXPRESSION PROFILING

Gene expression profiling uses microarray technology to detect and quantify the expression of hundreds of genes simultaneously, which enables complex analysis of gene expression patterns, including the effects of various mutations of a single target gene. The science of gene sequencing, detection methods, and amplification process has evolved greatly over the last 2 decades with the initiation of the Human Genome Project, whereas its cost has decreased substantially. Panels of genes have been identified for different types of disease processes. In breast cancer, for example, the 21-gene Recurrence Score has become a standard practice in determining the potential usefulness of chemotherapy, and distant recurrence risk in select groups of patients.[5] Similar technology was applied to the management of indeterminate thyroid nodules by several investigators, such as Arora and colleagues[6] and Chudova and colleagues,[7] in an effort to correlate the gene expression panels with the final histopathology diagnosis.

Available Gene Expression Profiling Tests

The most widely known clinically validated system is the Veracyte Afirma gene expression classifier (GEC; Veracyte, San Francisco, CA). The Afirma GEC is an RNA-based assay designed to evaluate the gene expression profile of a given thyroid nodule via 2 designated FNA samples by comparing it with the panel of 167 mRNA expression patterns (derived from 142 genes identified originally from the Affymetrix Human Exon Array) associated with benign nodules. The test uses a multidimensional proprietary algorithm with reliable accuracy in identifying benign nodules and thus is referred to as a rule-out test. Furthermore, the GEC also has incorporated a screening process for medullary thyroid cancer, as well as other secondary thyroid malignancies.[7] Veracyte currently requires 2 sets of FNA samples: one for cytologic evaluation and one for running the gene expression profiling: the Afirma GEC test. The patient's FNA sample is subjected to standardized cytologic evaluation by the company's independent cytopathologist at the Thyroid Cytopathology Partners (TCP; Austin, TX). Cytologic results are based on the Bethesda classification and are reported as nondiagnostic, benign, AUS/FLUS, FN/SFN, suspicious for malignancy, or malignant. FNA samples with Bethesda categories of benign, malignant, or suspicious for malignancy do not undergo further evaluation with Afirma GEC and only the cytologic diagnosis is forwarded to the ordering physician. Clinicians trust their local cytopathologist's evaluation and are familiar with the wording and intonations from a long-standing relationship, so they may find it difficult to familiarize themselves with the outside cytopathologic reading. Furthermore, although most community and academic cytopathologists gather quality assurance data on their department's thyroid FNA experience to present to interested clinicians, no such information is available from TCP directly to the clinician on a regular basis. Clinicians should ask for the cytology slides to be sent to their own institutional cytopathologist for review in cases in which the reading is difficult to interpret or is at odds with the previous reading. If clinicians do not find their hospital's cytopathologic evaluation useful, perhaps because of inadequate volume or experience, they may find that the Afirma's TCP group of cytopathologists provides a better service. No comments can be made about potential conflict of interest but it is hoped that ethical guidelines and professional standards set by the American College of Pathology are maintained. If the clinician's hospital has a contract with Afirma to do on-site cytologic evaluation, there will be no cytology result in the Veracyte report.

For cytologic samples with the diagnosis of AUS/FN/SFN, clinicians should expect to receive a 2-part report from Veracyte: cytologic evaluation and the GEC test result. The GEC test result is binary and reported as benign or suspicious if the samples were adequate.

The genetic material is first put through 6 different cassettes before applying the final benign versus malignant classifier. The first 6 cassettes act as filters for rare subtypes of thyroid cancer and nonfollicular cell-derived tumors (malignant melanoma, renal cell carcinoma, medullary thyroid cancer, and parathyroid tissue), which prevent the material from being scored by the main thyroid classifier.

Several clinical validation studies were performed on Afirma. Alexander and colleagues[8] performed one of the largest prospective and multicenter studies, validating the potential clinical usefulness of the Afirma GEC in a subset of indeterminate thyroid FNA categories. The overall sensitivity and specificity were 92% and 52% for indeterminate thyroid FNA samples, respectively, with a high overall NPV ranging from 85% to 95%. As a rule-out test, the assay has a high sensitivity with a low specificity for malignancy that is comparable with the diagnostic accuracy of FNA, which has high sensitivity with low specificity as well. Based on these validation studies, about 50% of the indeterminate cytologies, according to the Bethesda classification, could be accurately classified as benign nodules, potentially avoiding unnecessary diagnostic surgeries.[9] The analytical performance of this test has been validated with respect to sensitivity, specificity, and reproducibility. It is important to remember that, even as a rule-out test, the test has a false-negative rate of 5% to 15% and, therefore, a repeat assessment is important if the nodule enlarges or clinical suspicions arise. Furthermore, a PPV for a suspicious test result is only 38%.[8,10] Therefore, it is also important to remember that a suspicious test result does not mean the patient has cancer. Physicians should understand that a suspicious result needs to be reassessed and discussed with the patient for partial or total thyroidectomy, depending on the clinical scenario. In order to minimize the nondiagnostic test results, caused by poor sample quality, Afirma requests 2 FNA samples.

Which Patients Should Be Considered for Afirma Testing?

Thus far, limited data and clinical validation studies suggest that Veracyte can be used in all indeterminate FNA samples including AUS/FLUS and FN/SFN with high NPV. The sensitivity of the Afirma test was good for both the AUS/FLUS and FN/SNF groups at 90%, whereas the specificities of the tests were low, as expected, at 53% for AUS/FLUS and 49% for FN/SNF (**Table 1**).

Among the 265 samples ultimately selected for the study, the rate of malignancy was nearly equivalent in AUS/FLUS and FN/SFN groups (24% vs 25%). This rate is not representative of the general risk of malignancy observed, based on the TBSRTC for AUS/FLUS (5%–15%).[1] Thus, the AUS/FLUS group in the study may not be representative of the general population. As mentioned earlier, the observed false-negative rate of 5% to 15% in the study is similar to the overall risk of malignancy observed in the AUS/FLUS category in TBSRTC. This risk is equivalent to classifying the AUS/FLUS group as benign with a 5% to 15% false-negative rate. At this point, the potential statistical significance of having 2 independent negative test results (FNA and Afirma) has not been studied.

Table 1
Patients who should be considered for Afirma testing

Cytologic Diagnosis	% of FNAs	Risk of Malignancy (%)	Afirma Sensitivity (%)	Afirma Specificity (%)	False-negative Rate (%)	NPV	PPV
Nondiagnostic	10	1–4	—	—	—	—	—
Benign	60	0–3	—	—	—	—	—
AUS/FLUS	10–15	5–15	90	53	9.7	95	38
FNS/SFN	10–15	15–30	90	49	10	94	37
Suspicious for malignancy	3–5	60–75	94	52	5.9	85	76
Malignant	5–7	97–99	—	—	—	—	—

Given the findings discussed earlier and the false-positive rate of 50% to 60%, we think that the test does not add any benefit to the AUS/FLUS category with a low prevalence of malignancy. The high false-positive rate may confound the evaluation and management of benign nodules. Furthermore, the existing Bethesda guideline recommends repeat FNA for the AUS/FLUS category, which can reclassify about 50% of AUS/FLUS cytology to the benign category. However, in cases of a minimal clinical suspicion for malignancy in the AUS/FLUS category, there may be a potential benefit of performing the Afirma and avoiding diagnostic surgery, while providing reasonable assurance if the results are benign (see **Fig. 3**).

Which Patients Should Not Undergo Afirma Testing?

There are no established guidelines for Afirma. As a rule-out test for indeterminate nodules, the test is only beneficial for people with benign test results. Afirma GEC is not indicated or necessary in certain instances, including nodules that should be managed with hemithyroidectomy or total thyroidectomy based on validated data from clinical or ultrasonography criteria (**Box 1**).

Timing and Details of Sample Collection for Afirma Testing

Similar to mutational testing, routine collection of an additional specimen for GEC Afirma at the time of initial FNA biopsy would require at least 2 additional needle sticks per nodule, which would be unnecessary in most patients. As an alternative, a repeat FNA for molecular analysis can be performed at a later date after an FN/SFN cytology

Box 1
Patients who should not undergo Afirma testing

Do not consider Afirma:

Nodules larger than 4 to 5 cm, a size at which sampling error increases and nodules can effectively hide malignancies

Nodules with local or compressive symptoms, for which surgery would be required regardless

Nodules with strong clinical or ultrasonographic findings concerning for malignancy

Patients younger than 21 years of age because the Afirma test has not been validated in this patient population

Patients who prefer to have surgery and would not be comfortable with expectant management of a nodule regardless of the Afirma results diagnosis is received or in patients with AUS/FLUS category with any clinical suspicion or leaning toward diagnostic lobectomy. Afirma test may serve as a reassurance and avoid diagnostic surgeries. If a repeat FNA is performed, cytologic evaluation should again be carefully considered.

At present, only a select group of academic centers may send a sample for Afirma testing, bypassing the Veracyte TCP evaluation based on the in-house cytopathology results. This requirement may provide standardized evaluation and quality control for all samples. It is also a duplicate effort, which may undermine the collaboration between the institutional and regional cytopathologists, as well as the endocrinologists and surgeons, where the treatment and follow-up will occur. Alexander and colleagues[8] found there was 14% discordance between the institutions and the Veracyte TCP. In such cases, we recommend repeating the institutional cytologic review, which may result in a benign classification.

MUTATIONAL PANELS

Mutation testing involves using the thyroid tissue or cytologic samples to detect common genetic mutations known to be present in certain nonmedullary forms of thyroid cancer. Mutational panel testing is generally considered a rule-in test, which means that it has a higher specificity for the presence of malignancy, thus yielding a high PPV, whereas its sensitivity and NPV are low. This phenomenon is caused by the known DNA mutations being seen only in approximately 50% of thyroid cancers. Some mutations are present only in malignancies with near 100% specificity, whereas some mutations are seen in benign thyroid tumors. It is important that clinicians understand these important differences so as not to mislead themselves and their patients. The presence of mutations does not always equate to malignancy. The mutations listed later are being studied for their effects on tumorigenesis, proliferation, and dedifferentiation (**Fig. 1**). New driver mutations in development of benign and malignant thyroid lesions are being revealed as whole-exome sequencing, RNA, and protein profiling of thyroid tumors and matched normal tissue is underway in large cohorts such as The Cancer Genome Atlas Project (www.genome.gov; National Human Genome Research Institute). Reliability, reproducibility, and overall accuracy of mutational testing on FNA, tissue, and blood samples are being actively investigated.

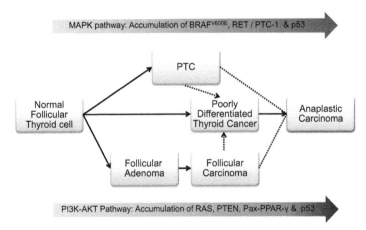

Fig. 1. The mutations being studied for their effects on tumorigenesis, proliferation, and dedifferentiation. MAPK, mitogen-activated protein kinase.

BRAF Mutations

BRAF is a member of the mitogen-activated protein kinase (MAPK) pathway and there are more than 40 mutational variations. The most common mutational variant (BRAF V600E) is the 1799-loci single-nucleotide T to A conversion with subsequent amino acid change from glutamate to valine, which causes constitutive activation of serine/threonine kinase (**Fig. 2**). BRAF mutations are commonly found in papillary thyroid cancer (PTC, 50%), less commonly in follicular variant of papillary thyroid cancer (FVPTC, 24%), and rarely (1.4%) in follicular thyroid cancer. BRAF mutation is highly specific for malignancy (false-positive rate of 0.2%) but, because of its low sensitivity, absence of mutation does not rule out the presence of thyroid cancer. Given its high specificity, if an FNA sample is positive for BRAF mutation, the nodule should be considered malignant and patients should undergo a total thyroidectomy even when the FNA cytology is indeterminate.[4,11–15]

Although some studies have shown that BRAF-mutated thyroid cancers may show more aggressive tumor behavior and confer worse clinical outcome, their role as independent prognostic indicators has not been well established and is controversial at this point.[16,17] Although there is limited evidence that BRAF-mutated thyroid cancers have a higher incidence of lymph node metastasis, routine prophylactic central neck dissection has not shown any benefit in disease-free recurrence or overall survival benefit and no decisions about addition of central neck dissection to the surgical intervention should be made based on BRAF status of the FNA at this point in time.[18] A role for targeted systemic therapy such as BRAF inhibitors is being investigated for

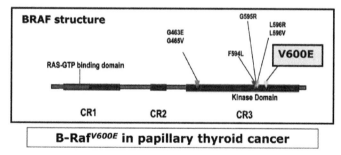

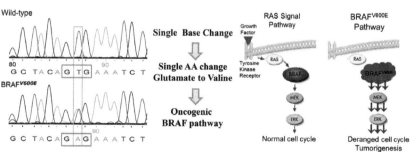

Fig. 2. A single-nucleotide change in the DNA of thyroid cells leads to overactivation of the B-Raf kinase. This DNA analysis pherogram shows the T1796A (V600E) activating point mutation of the B-Raf gene in thyroid cancer tissue from a patient with human papillary thyroid carcinoma.

patients who have advanced thyroid cancer with BRAF mutation. BRAF testing can be performed from formalin-fixed pathologic tissue, which may guide the therapeutic options.

RAS Oncogenes

The RAS oncoprotein is also involved in MAPK pathway as well as phosphatidylinositol-3-kinase (PI3K)–AKT pathway found in thyroid cancer tumorigenesis, especially in follicular adenomas. There are 3 known RAS mutations (HRAS, KRAS, and NRAS), which all lead to a constitutively activated RAS signaling mechanism caused by the loss of an intrinsic GTPase function that normally converts the RAS to an inactive state.[19,20] RAS mutations can be found in up to 40% of differentiated thyroid malignancies, particularly in follicular subtypes (FTC and FVPTC). However, RAS mutations are not too specific, because they are also found in benign follicular adenomas in 20% to 40% of cases. Hence, the low PPV of RAS mutations precludes reliable clinical use for the diagnosis of thyroid malignancy.[21,22]

Rearrangment during transfection/PTC proto-oncogene rearrangements

The rearrangment during transfection (RET) proto-oncogene is located on chromosome 10q11.2, which encodes for a receptor tyrosine kinase (RTK). RET was initially recognized and isolated in the 1980s during a transfection process in which a DNA rearrangement led to the proto-oncogene activation.[23] RET is involved in multiple endocrine neoplasia type 2 syndromes, thereby predisposing it to medullary thyroid carcinoma, whereas the RET/PTC rearrangement leads to constitutive activation of both PI3K and MAPK pathways leading to classic and FVPTCs as well as follicular adenomas. Although several variations of RET/PTC mutations have been described, RET/PTC1 and RET/PTC3 seem to have the most clinical relevance in thyroid cancer. RET/PTC rearrangements are found more commonly in children, or after radiation exposure, and they are present in only 20% to 40% of adults with PTC.[24,25]

PAX8/PPARG rearrangements

Rearrangements of the PAX8/PPARG genes produce a fusion product that is a transcription factor and a nuclear hormone receptor controlling cell differentiation. The PAX/PPARG rearrangement has been reported to occur in about 20% to 40% of follicular carcinomas, whereas only 8% of Hürthle cell cancers harbor this rearrangement. The exact frequency is not known but PAX8/PPARG rearrangements are also detected in follicular adenomas, thereby affecting its specificity.[26,27]

Telomerase reverse transcriptase promoter mutations

Telomerase reverse transcriptase (TERT) mutation involves an alteration of telomerase expression and cell immortalization; recent studies have shown increased prevalence of TERT mutations in advanced thyroid cancers (ATC) and in poorly differentiated thyroid cancers (PDTC) compared with the differentiated papillary thyroid cancers. Furthermore, comparative increase in prevalence of TERT mutations in the presence of known mutations such as BRAF, RAS, and RET/PTC in these ATC and PDTC suggest that TERT mutation may represent a progressive end-stage mutation in thyroid cancer tumorigenesis.[28,29]

AVAILABLE MUTATIONAL PANEL TESTS

There are 2 main commercially available platforms for mutational analysis:

1. Quest Diagnostics (Madison, NJ) Thyroid Cancer Mutation Panel.
2. Asuragen miR*Inform* (Austin, TX) mutation analysis assay.

Using an FNA sample, both of these panels assess for known genetic alterations such as BRAF and RAS mutations, as well as rearrangements of RET/PTC and PAX8/PPAR. More specifically, miR*Inform* assesses for 17 genetic alterations plus a panel of microRNA in identifying malignant tumors. Positive results in these mutational or rearrangement panels confer a high likelihood of malignancy, although not all cases are malignant. Negative results do not rule out cancer.[11,30] At present, there are no robust clinical studies validating the usefulness of these platforms because the validities of these mutation panels are strictly based on published results from seminal and ongoing studies by Nikiforov and colleagues[31] and Ohori and colleagues.[32]

Which Patients Should Be Considered for Mutational Testing?

Several studies have shown the efficacy of mutational testing in indeterminate thyroid nodules. A single-institutional prospective study on more than 1000 FNA samples with indeterminate cytology by Nikiforov and colleagues[31] showed that, compared with cytology alone, identification of mutations including RAS, BRAF, PAX8/PARG, and RET/PTC increased the risk of malignancy being present in the nodules from 14% to 88% in the AUS/FLUS cytology group and from 27% to 87% in the FN/SFN group. If no mutations were identified, the risk of cancer decreased to 5.9% in the AUS/FLUS group and 14% for the FN/SFN group.[31]

Thus, as a rule-in test, a positive mutational test significantly improves specificity and allows total thyroidectomy to be recommended as initial surgery instead of staged diagnostic lobectomy followed by a completion thyroidectomy. However, routine mutational testing on a group with low prevalence for malignancy may not be cost-effective. Furthermore, NPV remains low, although the false-negative rate is slightly improved compared with cytology alone, because of the low sensitivity.

Therefore, for patients with AUS/FLUS diagnosis, clinicians may consider performing the mutational panel only if there is a suspicious result from a GEC test, such as Afirma. In such cases, a higher proportion of benign patients are already ruled out because of a high NPV and resultant increase in the prevalence of cancer (**Fig. 3**). For patients with cytology findings suspicious for PTC, immediate mutational testing would be reasonable given the high cancer prevalence only if the surgeon or the patient is not already committed to a total thyroidectomy based on the clinical findings.

Which Patients Should Not Get Mutational Testing?

Mutational testing should not be done on patients with known thyroid malignancy, cervical lymph node positivity, distant metastases, malignant or benign FNA results, or functional nodules. Furthermore, patients with clinical indications or strong preference for a total thyroidectomy do not benefit from mutational testing.

Timing and Details of Sample Collection for Mutational Testing

Asuragen samples are collected in a separate fixative tube provided by the company. The timing for obtaining the FNA sample for DNA testing is controversial. Although some companies advocate routine collection for an additional specimen for molecular analysis on every thyroid nodule sample, this requires an additional FNA specimen that is unnecessary 70% to 80% of the time (ie, in those FNAs that return benign or malignant results).[1] If there are multiple nodules in a patient, this exposes the patient to increased discomfort and risk involved with the procedure. In contrast, the collection of 2 separate samples on different days raises the possibility that the specimens subjected to molecular analysis may not originate from the same lesion or represent the same cellular makeup as the specimens examined by the cytopathologist.

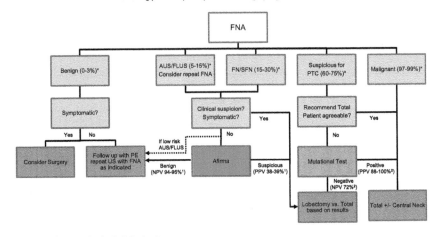

Possible pathway for patients with thyroid nodule if
•Age > 21**
•Nodules < 4-5cm***
•Normal TSH
•No strong clinical and radiologic suspicion for malignancy
•No strong personal predisposition to surgery regardless of the test results

* Risk of malignancy based on the Bethesda system
** Afirma not clinical validated in pediatric population;
   please refer to pediatric guidelines
*** Increased risk of sampling error. Consider lobectomy
    or mutational testing for possible total thyroidectomy

Fig. 3. Possible pathway for patients with thyroid nodule. (*Data from* Alexander EK, Kennedy GC, Baloch ZW, et al. Preoperative diagnosis of benign thyroid nodules with indeterminate cytology. N Engl J Med 2012;367(8):705–15; and Nikiforov YE, Ohori NP, Hodak SP, et al. Impact of mutational testing on the diagnosis and management of patients with cytologically indeterminate thyroid nodules: a prospective analysis of 1056 FNA samples. J Clin Endocrinol Metab 2011;96(11):3390–7.)

Mutational testing is therefore most useful in patients with suspicious malignancy results from a rule-out test, such as Afirma, or patients with cytologic diagnosis suspicious for PTC who prefer to have a diagnostic lobectomy (see **Fig. 3**).

For an optimal sample, repeat FNA for molecular analysis should be delayed for about 3 months based on the TBSRTC guidelines; this also allows time for review of the initial cytologic sample at an academic center with high-volume thyroid cytopathology, which in some cases might alter the cytopathologic diagnosis.[33]

Clinicians using the Quest mutational panel testing have the option of ordering the mutational panel on the same fixed cytologic material that was analyzed by the cytopathologist. Quest's technique, although not published or detailed anywhere, supposedly obtains DNA from scraping cells off the cytologic slides. The benefits of this are that the same cells analyzed by the cytopathologist are being analyzed for mutations, but the sample is destroyed, hindering further analysis later. To the best of our knowledge, there are no publications on this technique directly from Quest and thus no reliable data to be vetted.

DISCUSSION

Molecular markers, including genetic testing and expression profiling, are an important part of cancer diagnosis and management. In particular, mutational panel and gene expression profiling hold great promise in diagnostic, prognostic, and perhaps even therapeutic management of patients with thyroid nodules. With the recent development and clinical validation of genetic expression profiling systems, such as Afirma, genetic testing has been integrated into thyroid nodule evaluation as a viable option. However, molecular profiling is just one of many steps that might be undertaken in the evaluation of a thyroid nodule at this point. The best evidence suggests that Afirma may be beneficial in a subset of thyroid nodules with an indeterminate cytology category. This test may improve the accuracy of the current diagnostic standard FNA in minimizing unnecessary surgeries. Clinicians must continue to use the entire spectrum of tests available to them when evaluating a thyroid nodule instead of relying on any single test. Patient characteristics such as age and gender, physical examination, thyroid ultrasonography, and FNA biopsy, as well as sound clinical judgment, should be applied in a balanced manner. As such, clinicians should consider using Afirma as an ancillary diagnostic tool in patients with thyroid nodules of between 1 cm and 4 to 5 cm in whom an adequate FNA biopsy has been performed yielding a cytologic diagnosis of FN or Hürthle cell neoplasm/SFN. At present, no molecular testing could replace cytopathologic diagnosis in the management of thyroid cancer. Mutational testing of a nodule with an indeterminate or suspicious for PTC FNA that undergoes mutational panel testing and is positive for BRAF or RET/PTC is best treated with total thyroidectomy instead of a diagnostic hemithyroidectomy.

Cost-effectiveness

As discussed earlier, the need for molecular diagnosis only occurs when the cytologic diagnosis is indeterminate, which represents the minority of cases. Therefore, both the routine sampling at the time of initial FNA biopsy and selective repeat FNA biopsy for molecular testing are associated with extra time and effort by the physician and patient plus the additional cost. However, within this selective group of indeterminate cytology, a negative result might obviate diagnostic surgery in reportedly more than 50% of indeterminate cases.[9] Preliminary cost analysis has suggested that such an approach might be cost-effective based on the study parameters.[34] A cost analysis has suggested that use of the mutation panel alone might be cost-effective by reducing the need for completion thyroidectomy.[35] However, no cost analysis has been undertaken to determine whether the use of both tests in conjunction with initial total thyroidectomy is more cost-effective than the 2-stage thyroidectomy approach. The combined cost of Afirma (US$4200.00) followed by Asuragen (US$1500.00) could be prohibitive at the present rate.

Based on the meta-analysis of TBSRTC by Bongiovanni and colleagues,[1] 39.2% of AUS/FLUS cases and approximately 70% of FN/SFN cases underwent a diagnostic surgery purely based on the cytologic diagnosis with 15.9% and 26.1% risk of malignancy, respectively. When evaluating the efficacy and cost-effectiveness of molecular tests, it is important to remember that not all indeterminate cases lead to diagnostic surgeries, and that the management for the AUS/FLUS category may be different from the management for the FN/SFN category in a clinical practice. Although performing Afirma testing in all indeterminate nodules may reduce overall cost by decreasing unnecessary surgery, most of this benefit may be derived only from nodules in the FN/SFN group, and inclusion of a large group of patients with AUS/FLUS with a higher false-positive rate may lead to higher costs. Thus, routine or reflexive molecular testing for all indeterminate patients may partially negate the beneficial aspect of the Afirma test.

FUTURE DIRECTION

Ideal genetic markers should encompass both high diagnostic efficacy and independent prognostic value, which eliminates the indeterminate category from the thyroid

H&E staining   BRAF staining

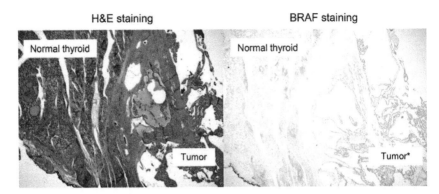

* A positive BRAF staining of a thyroid nodule
demonstrates distinctive pattern compared to the
surrounding normal thyroid tissue

Fig. 4. An example of the recent development of antibodies that can stain mutated BRAF with a high level of accuracy on pathologic thyroid tissue (hematoxylin-eosin [H&E], original magnification ×40). (*Courtesy of* Dr Peter Sadow).

nodule diagnosis and leads to a cost-effective overall management of thyroid malignancy. New tests are continually being developed, although some are simpler and more cost-effective than others. One such example is the recent development of antibodies that can stain mutated BRAF with a high level of accuracy on pathologic thyroid tissue (**Fig. 4**). If this BRAF staining can be adjusted to stain cytologic samples, then this significantly cheaper test (less than US$100) may replace the much more expensive sequencing methods traditionally used to find the BRAF mutation. Several academic institutions (eg, Nikiforov's laboratory in the University of Pittsburgh Medical Center), as well as established molecular genetics biotech companies, such as Illumina and Life Technology, are trying to develop more economical, streamlined, targeted, and more accurate molecular maker tests (eg, Targeted Next-generation Sequencing panel/ThyroSeq and Ion AmpliSeq panel).[36] We expect to see continuous progress in the future fueled by ongoing scientific endeavors elucidating driver mutations and molecular markers in thyroid cancer, as well as ongoing robust clinical validation studies.

REFERENCES

1. Bongiovanni M, Spitale A, Faquin WC, et al. The Bethesda System for Reporting Thyroid Cytopathology: a meta-analysis. Acta Cytol 2012;56(4):333–9.
2. Cibas ES, Ali SZ, NCI Thyroid FNA State of the Science Conference. The Bethesda System for reporting thyroid cytopathology. Am J Clin Pathol 2009; 132(5):658–65.
3. Wang CC, Friedman L, Kennedy GC, et al. A large multicenter correlation study of thyroid nodule cytopathology and histopathology. Thyroid 2011;21(3):243–51.
4. Cohen Y, Rosenbaum E, Clark DP, et al. Mutational analysis of BRAF in fine needle aspiration biopsies of the thyroid: a potential application for the preoperative assessment of thyroid nodules. Clin Cancer Res 2004;10(8):2761–5.
5. Harris L, Fritsche H, Mennel R, et al. American Society of Clinical Oncology 2007 update of recommendations for the use of tumor markers in breast cancer. J Clin Oncol 2007;25(33):5287–312.

6. Arora N, Scognamiglio T, Lubitz CC, et al. Identification of borderline thyroid tumors by gene expression array analysis. Cancer 2009;115(23):5421–31.
7. Chudova D, Wilde JI, Wang ET, et al. Molecular classification of thyroid nodules using high-dimensionality genomic data. J Clin Endocrinol Metab 2010;95(12): 5296–304.
8. Alexander EK, Kennedy GC, Baloch ZW, et al. Preoperative diagnosis of benign thyroid nodules with indeterminate cytology. N Engl J Med 2012; 367(8):705–15.
9. Duick DS, Klopper JP, Diggans JC, et al. The impact of benign gene expression classifier test results on the endocrinologist-patient decision to operate on patients with thyroid nodules with indeterminate fine-needle aspiration cytopathology. Thyroid 2012;22(10):996–1001.
10. Faquin WC. Can a gene-expression classifier with high negative predictive value solve the indeterminate thyroid fine-needle aspiration dilemma? Cancer Cytopathol 2013;121(3):116–9.
11. Nikiforova MN, Nikiforov YE. Molecular diagnostics and predictors in thyroid cancer. Thyroid 2009;19(12):1351–61.
12. Xing M. Molecular pathogenesis and mechanisms of thyroid cancer. Nat Rev Cancer 2013;13(3):184–99.
13. Kebebew E, Weng J, Bauer J, et al. The prevalence and prognostic value of BRAF mutation in thyroid cancer. Ann Surg 2007;246(3):466–70 [discussion: 470–1].
14. Ito Y, Yoshida H, Maruo R, et al. BRAF mutation in papillary thyroid carcinoma in a Japanese population: its lack of correlation with high-risk clinicopathological features and disease-free survival of patients. Endocr J 2009;56(1):89–97.
15. Kouniavsky G, Zeiger MA. The quest for diagnostic molecular markers for thyroid nodules with indeterminate or suspicious cytology. J Surg Oncol 2012;105(5): 438–43.
16. Prescott JD, Sadow PM, Hodin RA, et al. BRAF V600E status adds incremental value to current risk classification systems in predicting papillary thyroid carcinoma recurrence. Surgery 2012;152(6):984–90.
17. Xing M, Alzahrani AS, Carson KA, et al. Association between BRAF V600E mutation and mortality in patients with papillary thyroid cancer. JAMA 2013;309(14): 1493–501.
18. Gouveia C, Can NT, Bostrom A, et al. Lack of association of BRAF mutation with negative prognostic indicators in papillary thyroid carcinoma: the University of California, San Francisco, experience. JAMA Otolaryngol Head Neck Surg 2013;139(11):1164–70.
19. Abubaker J, Jehan Z, Bavi P, et al. Clinicopathological analysis of papillary thyroid cancer with PIK3CA alterations in a Middle Eastern population. J Clin Endocrinol Metab 2008;93(2):611–8.
20. Liu Z, Hou P, Ji M, et al. Highly prevalent genetic alterations in receptor tyrosine kinases and phosphatidylinositol 3-kinase/akt and mitogen-activated protein kinase pathways in anaplastic and follicular thyroid cancers. J Clin Endocrinol Metab 2008;93(8):3106–16.
21. Suarez HG, du Villard JA, Severino M, et al. Presence of mutations in all three ras genes in human thyroid tumors. Oncogene 1990;5(4):565–70.
22. Esapa CT, Johnson SJ, Kendall-Taylor P, et al. Prevalence of Ras mutations in thyroid neoplasia. Clin Endocrinol (Oxf) 1999;50(4):529–35.
23. Takahashi M, Ritz J, Cooper GM. Activation of a novel human transforming gene, ret, by DNA rearrangement. Cell 1985;42(2):581–8.

24. Marx SJ. Molecular genetics of multiple endocrine neoplasia types 1 and 2. Nat Rev Cancer 2005;5(5):367–75.

25. Marotta V, Guerra A, Sapio MR, et al. RET/PTC rearrangement in benign and malignant thyroid diseases: a clinical standpoint. Eur J Endocrinol 2011;165(4): 499–507.

26. Castro P, Rebocho AP, Soares RJ, et al. PAX8-PPARgamma rearrangement is frequently detected in the follicular variant of papillary thyroid carcinoma. J Clin Endocrinol Metab 2006;91(1):213–20.

27. Kroll TG, Sarraf P, Pecciarini L, et al. PAX8-PPARgamma1 fusion oncogene in human thyroid carcinoma [corrected]. Science 2000;289(5483):1357–60.

28. Landa I, Ganly I, Chan TA, et al. Frequent somatic TERT promoter mutations in thyroid cancer: higher prevalence in advanced forms of the disease. J Clin Endocrinol Metab 2013;98(9):E1562–6.

29. Liu X, Bishop J, Shan Y, et al. Highly prevalent TERT promoter mutations in aggressive thyroid cancers. Endocr Relat Cancer 2013;20(4):603–10.

30. Cantara S, Capezzone M, Marchisotta S, et al. Impact of proto-oncogene mutation detection in cytological specimens from thyroid nodules improves the diagnostic accuracy of cytology. J Clin Endocrinol Metab 2010;95(3):1365–9.

31. Nikiforov YE, Ohori NP, Hodak SP, et al. Impact of mutational testing on the diagnosis and management of patients with cytologically indeterminate thyroid nodules: a prospective analysis of 1056 FNA samples. J Clin Endocrinol Metab 2011;96(11):3390–7.

32. Ohori NP, Nikiforova MN, Schoedel KE, et al. Contribution of molecular testing to thyroid fine-needle aspiration cytology of "follicular lesion of undetermined significance/atypia of undetermined significance". Cancer Cytopathol 2010;118(1): 17–23.

33. American Thyroid Association (ATA) Guidelines Taskforce on Thyroid Nodules and Differentiated Thyroid Cancer, Cooper DS, et al. Revised American Thyroid Association management guidelines for patients with thyroid nodules and differentiated thyroid cancer. Thyroid 2009;19(11):1167–214.

34. Li H, Robinson KA, Anton B, et al. Cost-effectiveness of a novel molecular test for cytologically indeterminate thyroid nodules. J Clin Endocrinol Metab 2011;96(11): E1719–26.

35. Yip L, Farris C, Kabaker AS, et al. Cost impact of molecular testing for indeterminate thyroid nodule fine-needle aspiration biopsies. J Clin Endocrinol Metab 2012;97(6):1905–12.

36. Nikiforova MN, Wald AI, Roy S, et al. Targeted next-generation sequencing panel (ThyroSeq) for detection of mutations in thyroid cancer. J Clin Endocrinol Metab 2013;98(11):E1852–60.

Prophylactic Central Compartment Neck Dissection for Papillary Thyroid Cancer

Christopher R. McHenry, MD[a],*, Jonah J. Stulberg, MD, PhD, MPH[b]

KEYWORDS

- Prophylactic central compartment neck dissection • Papillary thyroid cancer
- Differentiated thyroid cancer

KEY POINTS

- Controversy exists regarding the benefit of prophylactic central compartment neck dissection (pCCND) in papillary thyroid cancer (PTC), as there are no prospective randomized trials or other high-level evidence to guide decision making.
- Performing a large enough randomized controlled trial would be cost prohibitive and will therefore likely not be accomplished.
- This article presents a summary of the available data examining the controversy for and against pCCND, and concludes that the balance between the risks and potential benefits favors total thyroidectomy alone for patients with clinically node-negative PTC. There is no proven benefit for pCCND.

INTRODUCTION

A central compartment neck dissection (CCND) consists of removal of all lymph nodes and fibrofatty tissue between the common carotid arteries laterally from the hyoid bone superiorly to the innominate artery inferiorly (**Fig. 1**). The lymph nodes that are removed include the prelaryngeal, pretracheal, and paratracheal lymph nodes, otherwise known as level VI lymph nodes, and the anterior superior mediastinal lymph nodes along the innominate artery, referred to as level VII lymph nodes (see **Fig. 1**). Some investigators describe an ipsilateral CCND, which is defined as removal of the pretracheal, prelaryngeal, and the paratracheal lymph nodes from the side of the cancer only; the contralateral paratracheal lymph nodes are not removed. The

[a] Department of Surgery, MetroHealth Medical Center, Case Western Reserve University School of Medicine, 2500 MetroHealth Drive, Cleveland, OH 44109, USA; [b] Department of Surgery, University Hospitals, Case Medical Center, 11100 Euclid Avenue, Cleveland, OH 44106, USA
* Corresponding author.
E-mail address: cmchenry@metrohealth.org

Surg Clin N Am 94 (2014) 529–540
http://dx.doi.org/10.1016/j.suc.2014.02.003
0039-6109/14/$ – see front matter © 2014 Elsevier Inc. All rights reserved.

surgical.theclinics.com

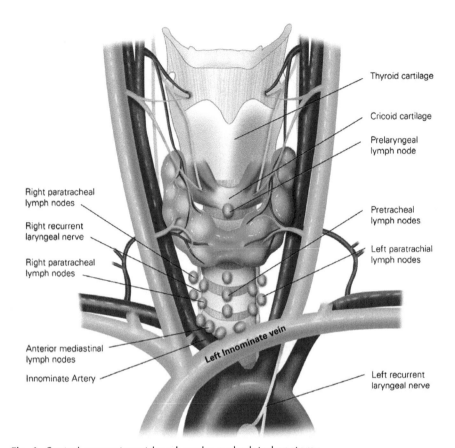

Fig. 1. Central compartment lymph nodes and related anatomy.

mean size and number of metastatic lymph nodes removed during a pCCND is 0.35 cm and 2.6 ± 3 out of a mean 13 ± 5 lymph nodes removed, respectively.[1,2]

All major endocrine societies agree that a therapeutic CCND is recommended in all patients with clinically node-positive papillary thyroid cancer (PTC).[3–7] However, there are differences in the guidelines regarding a prophylactic central compartment node dissection (pCCND). A pCCND is defined as a CCND in a patient with thyroid cancer who has no clinical, sonographic, or intraoperative evidence of abnormal lymph nodes. Whether pCCND should be performed in all patients with clinically node-negative PTC is controversial, and the arguments for and against pCCND are detailed in this article.

The controversy regarding pCCND originated from the management guidelines for patients with thyroid nodules and differentiated thyroid cancer, published in 2006 by the American Thyroid Association (ATA).[7] It was recommended that "routine" CCND be considered for all patients with PTC. The strength of the recommendation was given a rating of B, indicating it was based on fair evidence that CCND may improve health outcomes. At the same time in 2006, a European consensus statement on pCCND was endorsed by the European Thyroid Association and read, "there is no evidence that pCCND improves recurrence or mortality rates, but it does allow an accurate staging of the disease that may guide subsequent treatment and follow-up.[8]" In 2009, the revised ATA guidelines were published with a modification in the recommendation for CCND.[6] Recommendation 27B was modified to read "prophylactic CCND (ipsilateral or bilateral) may be performed in patients with PTC with clinically uninvolved central neck lymph nodes, especially for advanced primary tumors (T3 or T4)." The strength of the recommendation was lowered to C, meaning that this was based on expert opinion.

How is it that 2 reputable organizations can come up with almost polarly opposite recommendations regarding pCCND? In part, the explanation is related to the fact that no randomized controlled trial exists to evaluate pCCND for treatment of PTC. A feasibility study completed by the ATA estimated that a randomized trial would require 5840 patients and would cost approximately US$15 million.[9] In addition, the controversy over whether to perform pCCND also relates to the differing interpretations of existing data.

Those who advocate pCCND do so for its potential benefits, including reduced rates of recurrence, lower postoperative serum thyroglobulin (Tg) levels, accurate staging to help modify indications for radioiodine ablation and radioactive iodine dosing, and reduced reoperation in the central neck with its potential for higher morbidity. Those who oppose pCCND do so because there is no proven oncologic benefit, and there is concern for an increased risk for recurrent laryngeal nerve injury and hypoparathyroidism. In this article, the data regarding the effect of pCCND on recurrence in the central compartment of the neck, postoperative serum Tg levels, postoperative radioiodine uptake, recommendations for radioiodine ablation and dosing of radioactive iodine, and postoperative morbidity are examined.

LYMPH NODE METASTASES IN PATIENTS WITH PAPILLARY THYROID CANCER

Lymph node metastases are common in patients with PTC. At the time of initial surgery, approximately 35% of patients with PTC have macroscopic lymph node metastases and up to 80% have microscopic lymph node metastases.[10–13] Clinically apparent lymph nodes are more common at the extremes of age. The yield of metastatic lymph nodes in the central and lateral neck is significantly related to the number of lymph nodes in the neck dissection,[14,15] and also is likely related to the extent of pathologic examination.

It is important to recognize that all lymph node metastases are not the same in terms of their implications for recurrence and mortality. Macroscopic lymph node metastases in patients with PTC are associated with higher recurrence rates, and an increased mortality rate has been observed in patients with lymph node metastases who are 45 years or older.[16,17] Lundgren and colleagues,[16] in a large population-based, case-control study, reported a 3-fold higher disease-related mortality in patients with differentiated thyroid cancer and lymph node metastases. Sugitani and colleagues[18] demonstrated an increased disease-specific mortality in older patients with PTC and lymph node metastases greater than 3 cm. By contrast, microscopic lymph node metastases do not affect patient survival and are associated with much lower rates of recurrence. The effect on locoregional recurrence is the main end point that is being evaluated in patients with PTC being treated with total thyroidectomy with or without pCCND.

It is standard practice to obtain an ultrasonographic examination to evaluate the central and lateral compartments of the neck for abnormal lymph nodes before thyroidectomy in patients with PTC.[6] Sonographic features raising suspicion for metastatic lymph nodes include: a diameter greater than 1 cm; loss of the normal fatty hilum; an irregular rounded contour with a long-access to short-access ratio of less than 1.5; heterogeneous echogenicity; microcalcifications; hypervascularity; and cystic change. Ultrasonography is much more sensitive for detection of metastatic lymph nodes in the lateral neck than in the central neck, with sensitivities varying from 82% to 94% and 30% to 60%, respectively.[19–21]

Kouvaraki and colleagues[22] demonstrated that physical examination will miss macroscopic lymph node metastases in 40% of patients with PTC, emphasizing the role of ultrasonography in the surgical management of patients with PTC. Stulak and colleagues[23] from the Mayo clinic performed ultrasonographic examination before thyroidectomy in 486 patients with PTC, and found nonpalpable lymph node metastases in 14% of patients. Sensitivity, specificity, and positive predictive value of 84%, 98%, and 89%, respectively, were reported for lymph node metastases.

There is evidence that lymphadenectomy reduces recurrence and may improve survival in patients with macroscopic nodal disease.[24] The ATA and National Comprehensive Cancer Network guidelines recommend a compartment-oriented neck dissection for patients with macroscopic lymph node metastases in the central and lateral neck.[4,6] By contrast, removal of microscopic lymph node metastases has not been shown to reduce recurrence in the central compartment of the neck or improve survival. Despite occult lymph node micrometastases being found in the central compartment of the neck in 38% to 80% of patients with PTC, the median rate of recurrence for patients with clinically node-negative disease is 2%, whether or not a CCND is performed.[25,26] This finding suggests that most micrometastases remain dormant and rarely become clinically significant, or alternatively that radioiodine ablation is adequate for the treatment of micrometastatic disease.

CENTRAL COMPARTMENT RECURRENCE FOR CLINICALLY NODE-NEGATIVE PTC WITH OR WITHOUT PCCND

There have been multiple studies comparing recurrence in the central neck in patients who underwent thyroidectomy with pCCND in comparison with patients who underwent thyroidectomy without pCCND for clinically node-negative PTC (**Table 1**).[24,27–46] Although there is variability in the rates of recurrence in the central neck among the individual series, there is no significant difference in the rate of recurrence whether a CCND is performed or not. This finding has been substantiated by Zetoune and colleagues[47] in a large meta-analysis of patients with PTC, in which no difference was

Table 1
Central compartment recurrence of papillary thyroid cancer (PTC) following total thyroidectomy (TT) versus TT with prophylactic central compartment node dissection (pCCND)

Authors,[Ref.] Year	N	TT Only	TT + pCCND	Recurrence with TT	Recurrence with TT + pCCND
Barczyński et al,[27] 2013	640	282	358	22 (7.8%)	2 (0.6%)
Besic et al,[43] 2009	89	83	6	0 (0.0%)	0 (0.0%)
Costa et al,[31] 2009	244	118	126	4 (3.4%)	4 (3.2%)
Gemsenjäger et al,[39] 2003	159	88	71	2 (2.3%)	4 (5.6%)
Hughes et al,[49] 2010	143	65	78	2 (3.1%)	2 (2.6%)
Lang et al,[28] 2012	185	103	82	0 (0.0%)	0 (0.0%)
Moo et al,[30] 2010	81	36	45	2 (5.6%)	1 (2.2%)
Moreno et al,[58] 2012	252	133	119	3 (2.3%)	2 (1.7%)
Roh et al,[41] 2009	197	49	148	0 (0.0%)	0 (0.0%)
Roh et al,[40] 2007	113	73	40	3 (4.1%)	1 (2.5%)
Sywak et al,[33] 2006	447	391	56	7 (1.8%)	0 (0.0%)

found in locoregional recurrence whether or not a pCCND was performed. A 1.9% locoregional recurrence rate was reported in the group who underwent pCCND versus 1.7% in the group that underwent thyroidectomy alone. A significantly higher incidence of temporary postoperative hypoparathyroidism occurred in patients who underwent pCCND.

Furthermore, 2 other systematic reviews and meta-analyses focusing on locoregional recurrence after thyroidectomy with CCND versus thyroidectomy alone found no difference in recurrence and confirmed a higher incidence of transient postoperative hypocalcemia.[25,26] These meta-analyses represent the results from high-volume surgeons at high-volume centers, and substantiate that CCND in patients with clinically node-negative PTC does not reduce locoregional recurrence. A major reason for performing routine pCCND, suggested by its proponents, has been to reduce the need for reoperation in the central compartment of the neck for recurrence, which is technically more challenging and is associated with increased morbidity. Given that recurrence rates are not different whether a pCCND is performed or not, this does not seem to be a legitimate reason for advocating routine pCCND.

EFFECT OF PCCND ON POSTOPERATIVE SERUM THYROGLOBULIN LEVELS AND RADIOIODINE UPTAKE

Sywak and colleagues[33] have reported lower serum Tg levels and a higher rate of athyroglobulinemia with pCCND. However, they performed their study with the goal of reducing serum Tg levels, and compared their results with those of patients operated on before institution of the study. It is conceivable that their results were due to a more complete total thyroidectomy rather than a pCCND.

Yoo and colleagues[48] from Rhode Island Hospital and Hughes and colleagues[49] from the University of Michigan showed no difference in serum Tg levels in patients with clinically node-negative PTC who underwent total thyroidectomy with pCCND versus total thyroidectomy alone. Yoo and colleagues[48] also showed that there was no difference in preablation radioiodine uptake or the number of foci of radioiodine activity in the neck whether or not a CCND was performed, this despite the fact that 60% of patients who underwent total thyroidectomy and CCND had nodal metastases. Radioiodine uptake was 1.2% in 190 patients with clinically node-negative PTC who underwent total thyroidectomy alone versus 0.93% in the 87 who underwent total thyroidectomy and pCCND. Although normalization of serum Tg levels is an admirable goal, it is less important than the change in Tg over time.

EFFECT OF PCCND ON INDICATIONS FOR RADIOIODINE ABLATION AND DOSING OF [131]I

The 2009 ATA guidelines recommend selective use of radioiodine ablation for patients with distant metastases, extrathyroidal tumor spread, and tumors larger than 4 cm.[6] The strength of the recommendations are category A for distant metastases and category B for extrathyroidal tumor spread and tumors larger than 4 cm, meaning that there is good and fair evidence, respectively, that the intervention will improve health outcomes. Radioiodine ablation is also recommended for patients with tumors 1 to 4 cm in size with lymph node metastases or intermediate-risk or high-risk tumors. The strength of the recommendation is category C, or based on expert opinion alone. Radioiodine ablation is not recommended for patients with PTC smaller than 1 cm that is confined to the thyroid gland without evidence of metastases.[6]

Three retrospective studies have suggested that accurate staging of PTC using pCCND may be used to determine the need for ^{131}I therapy and dosing in patients with PTC.[14,49,50] Hughes and colleagues[49] performed a retrospective cohort study of patients with clinically node-negative PTC, comparing 65 patients who underwent total thyroidectomy with 78 patients who underwent total thyroidectomy and pCCND. Central lymph node metastases were found in 62% of patients. The median dose of radioiodine given was 30 mCi in the total thyroidectomy group versus 150 mCi in the total thyroidectomy plus pCCND group. However, even with pCCND and higher doses of radioiodine, locoregional recurrence was 4.6% in the group that underwent total thyroidectomy alone versus 5.1% in the group that underwent total thyroidectomy and bilateral CCND. Central compartment recurrence was 3.0% and 2.6%, respectively, for the 2 groups, and there was no difference in postablative Tg levels 1 year after treatment. Hughes and colleagues[49] concluded that pCCND is of value for determining doses of radioiodine. An alternative conclusion is that pCCND leads to the administration of higher doses of radioiodine without apparent benefit. This point is important to consider because radioiodine is associated with its own morbidity, including salivary and lacrimal gland dysfunction, dysphagia, and second malignancies.

Bonnet and colleagues[50] reported that lymph node staging by pCCND and ipsilateral lateral neck dissection in 115 patients with clinically node-negative T1 PTC modified the indication for radioiodine ablation in 25 (21.7%) patients, 12 (10%) patients with tumors smaller than 1 cm with microscopic lymph node metastases who were given radioiodine, and 13 (11%) patients with tumors 1 to 2 cm in size without lymph node metastases who did not receive radioiodine. Hartl and colleagues[14] performed pCCND and level III and IV lateral neck dissection in 317 patients with clinically node-negative PTC;184 (58%) patients with pathologic node-negative disease received a median 30-mCi dose of radioiodine, compared with 100 mCi for 133 (42%) patients with pathologic node-positive disease.

It is difficult to determine the value of these studies because the efficacy of radioiodine for the treatment of lymph node micrometastases remains unclear, and high-level evidence supporting more aggressive use of radioiodine based on information obtained from a pCCND is lacking. Sawka and colleagues,[51] in a systematic review of the literature, were unable to show a significant and consistent benefit of ^{131}I ablation in decreasing cause-specific mortality or recurrence. The lack of efficacy of radioiodine for the treatment of lymph node metastases is, in part, related to the facts that only 70% to 75% of PTCs concentrate radioiodine, and that this decreases with age.[52]

MORBIDITY OF CCND

A significantly higher incidence of transient hypocalcemia following total thyroidectomy and CCND versus total thyroidectomy alone has been confirmed in 3 large meta-analyses.[25,26,47] This result is not unexpected, because more extensive dissection in the central neck may interfere with the blood supply to the parathyroid glands, particularly the inferior parathyroid glands. However, the addition of CCND did not result in a significant increase in the incidence of permanent complications.

Giordano and colleagues[53] compared the rates of recurrent laryngeal nerve injury and hypoparathyroidism in 3 groups of patients with clinically node-negative PTC: those treated with total thyroidectomy alone, total thyroidectomy with ipsilateral CCND, and total thyroidectomy with bilateral CCND. There was a higher rate of permanent recurrent laryngeal nerve injury in patients who underwent bilateral CCND, which was not statically significant. The investigators also reported a significantly higher rate of permanent hypoparathyroidism, 16% in patients who underwent bilateral CCND compared with 6% and 7% in patients who underwent no CCND or an ipsilateral CCND, respectively. There are multiple other smaller series that have examined the morbidity in patients undergoing thyroidectomy with or without pCCND (**Table 2**).

Table 2
Defining the morbidity of central neck dissection

Authors,[Ref.] Year	TT + CCND	TT Only	Recurrent Laryngeal Nerve Paralysis		Permanent Hypoparathyroidism	
			TT + CCND	TT Only	TT + CCND	TT Only
Henry et al,[59] 1998	50	50	0	0	2 (4%)	0
Gemsenjäger et al,[39] 2003	88	71	4 (5.6%)	0	1 (1.4%)	0
Rosenbaum & McHenry,[42] 2009	22	88	0	1 (1.1%)	1 (4.5%)	0
Hughes et al,[49] 2010	78	65	0	2 (3.1%)	2 (2.6%)	0
Giordano et al,[53] 2012	308	394	7 (2.3%)	4 (1%)	50 (16.2%)	25 (6.3%)
Pereira et al,[60] 2005	43	0	0	—	2 (4.6%)	—

Although some series document a higher incidence of recurrent laryngeal nerve injury with pCCND, essentially all series report a higher incidence of permanent hypoparathyroidism. However, the studies have been underpowered to establish significance.

It is important to recognize the influence of publication bias on the outcome of pCCND for clinically node-negative PTC. The reported morbidity for pCCND comes from expert endocrine surgeons at specialized centers. However, in the United States low-volume surgeons, defined as surgeons who perform fewer than 3 thyroidectomies per year, perform the majority of thyroid surgery and treat most patients with thyroid cancer.[54,55] Recognizing the technical challenges of performing a CCND, it is reasonable to assume that the complications are actually higher than are reported in the literature.

Specialized endocrine surgery units have reported that secondary CCND can be performed in patients for metastatic disease after initial thyroidectomy, with no additional morbidity.[45,56] It has been suggested that patients with tiny nonpalpable nodal recurrences smaller than 1 cm in the central neck can be followed without surgical therapy to assess the tumor biology. Rondeau and colleagues[57] have reported that nodal recurrences less than 1 cm in the previously operated central neck rarely show clinically significant progression. For this reason, recurrence in the central neck is best managed by referral to specialized centers with expertise in endocrine surgery.

SUMMARY

The only potential benefit of pCCND may be precise lymph node staging to help determine the need for radioiodine ablation and the dose of ^{131}I, although the efficacy remains suspect because high-level evidence is lacking for such an approach. The high price of hypoparathyroidism is not offset by any measurable oncologic benefit. It is better for experienced surgeons to perform therapeutic operations for rare recurrences in the central neck than for inexperienced surgeons to perform pCCND in all patients. In conclusion, the balance between the risks and benefits favors total thyroidectomy alone for patients with clinically node-negative PTC. There is no proven benefit for pCCND.

REFERENCES

1. So YK, Son YI, Hong SD, et al. Subclinical lymph node metastasis in papillary thyroid microcarcinoma: a study of 551 resections. Surgery 2010;148(3): 526–31. Available at: http://www.ncbi.nlm.nih.gov/pubmed/20189620. Accessed November 13, 2013.

2. Roh JL, Kim JM, Park CI. Central cervical nodal metastasis from papillary thyroid microcarcinoma: pattern and factors predictive of nodal metastasis. Ann Surg Oncol 2008;15(9):2482–6. Available at: http://www.ncbi.nlm.nih.gov/pubmed/18612697. Accessed November 13, 2013.

3. Robbins KT, Shaha AR, Medina JE, et al. Consensus statement on the classification and terminology of neck dissection. Arch Otolaryngol Head Neck Surg 2008; 134(5):536–8. Available at: http://www.ncbi.nlm.nih.gov/pubmed/20096215.

4. National Comprehensive Cancer Network. Thyroid carcinoma. 2012. Available at: http://www.nccn.org/professionals/physician_gls/. Accessed October 22, 2013.

5. Carty SE, Cooper DS, Doherty GM, et al. Consensus statement on the terminology and classification of central neck dissection for thyroid cancer. Thyroid 2009; 19(11):1153–8. Available at: http://www.ncbi.nlm.nih.gov/pubmed/20096215.

6. Cooper DS, Doherty GM, Haugen BR, et al. Revised American Thyroid Association management guidelines for patients with thyroid nodules and differentiated thyroid cancer. Thyroid 2009;19(11):1167–214. Available at: http://www.ncbi.nlm.nih.gov/pubmed/19860577. Accessed September 30, 2013.

7. Cooper DS, Doherty GM, Haugen BR, et al. Management guidelines for patients with thyroid nodules and differentiated thyroid cancer. Thyroid 2006;16(2): 109–42. Available at: http://www.ncbi.nlm.nih.gov/pubmed/16420177. Accessed September 25, 2013.

8. Pacini F, Schlumberger M, Dralle H, et al. European consensus for the management of patients with differentiated thyroid carcinoma of the follicular epithelium. Eur J Endocrinol 2006;154(6):787–803. Available at: http://www.ncbi.nlm.nih.gov/pubmed/16728537. Accessed October 22, 2013.

9. Carling T, Carty SE, Ciarleglio MM, et al. American Thyroid Association design and feasibility of a prospective randomized controlled trial of prophylactic central lymph node dissection for papillary thyroid carcinoma. Thyroid 2012;22(3): 237–44. Available at: http://www.ncbi.nlm.nih.gov/pubmed/22313454. Accessed October 22, 2013.

10. Schlumberger M. Papillary and follicular thyroid carcinoma. N Engl J Med 1998; 338:297–306. Available at: http://www.nejm.org/doi/full/10.1056/NEJM199801293380506. Accessed October 23, 2013.

11. Noguchi S, Murakami N. The value of lymph-node dissection in patients with differentiated thyroid cancer. Surg Clin North Am 1987;67:251–61.

12. Cranshaw IM, Carnaille B. Micrometastases in thyroid cancer. An important finding? Surg Oncol 2008;17(3):253–8. Available at: http://www.ncbi.nlm.nih.gov/pubmed/18504121. Accessed October 23, 2013.

13. Randolph GW, Duh QY, Heller KS, et al. The prognostic significance of nodal metastases from papillary thyroid carcinoma can be stratified based on the size and number of metastatic lymph nodes, as well as the presence of extranodal extension. Thyroid 2012;22(11):1144–52. Available at: http://www.ncbi.nlm.nih.gov/pubmed/23083442. Accessed October 23, 2013.

14. Hartl DM, Leboulleux S, Al Ghuzlan A, et al. Optimization of staging of the neck with prophylactic central and lateral neck dissection for papillary thyroid carcinoma. Ann Surg 2012;255(4):777–83. Available at: http://www.ncbi.nlm.nih.gov/pubmed/22418010. Accessed October 28, 2013.

15. Köhler HF, Kowalski LP. How many nodes are needed to stage a neck? A critical appraisal. Eur Arch Otorhinolaryngol 2010;267(5):785–91. Available at: http://www.ncbi.nlm.nih.gov/pubmed/19904547. Accessed November 12, 2013.

16. Lundgren CI, Hall P, Dickman PW, et al. Clinically significant prognostic factors for differentiated thyroid carcinoma: a population-based, nested case-control

study. Cancer 2006;106(3):524–31. Available at: http://www.ncbi.nlm.nih.gov/pubmed/16369995. Accessed September 30, 2013.

17. Zaydfudim V, Feurer ID, Griffin MR, et al. The impact of lymph node involvement on survival in patients with papillary and follicular thyroid carcinoma. Surgery 2008;144(6):1070–7 [discussion: 1077–8]. Available at: http://www.ncbi.nlm.nih.gov/pubmed/19041020. Accessed October 23, 2013.

18. Sugitani I, Kasai N, Fujimoto Y, et al. A novel classification system for patients with PTC: addition of the new variables of large (3 cm or greater) nodal metastases and reclassification during the follow-up period. Surgery 2004;135(2):139–48. Available at: http://linkinghub.elsevier.com/retrieve/pii/S0039606003003842. Accessed November 12, 2013.

19. Hwang HS, Orloff LA. Efficacy of preoperative neck ultrasound in the detection of cervical lymph node metastasis from thyroid cancer. Laryngoscope 2011;121(3):487–91. Available at: http://www.ncbi.nlm.nih.gov/pubmed/21344423. Accessed November 13, 2013.

20. Morita S, Mizoguchi K, Suzuki M, et al. The accuracy of (18)[F]-fluoro-2-deoxy-D-glucose-positron emission tomography/computed tomography, ultrasonography, and enhanced computed tomography alone in the preoperative diagnosis of cervical lymph node metastasis in patients with papillary thyroid carcinoma. World J Surg 2010;34(11):2564–9. Available at: http://www.ncbi.nlm.nih.gov/pubmed/20645089. Accessed November 13, 2013.

21. Choi JS, Kim J, Kwak JY, et al. Preoperative staging of papillary thyroid carcinoma: comparison of ultrasound imaging and CT. AJR Am J Roentgenol 2009;193(3):871–8. Available at: http://www.ncbi.nlm.nih.gov/pubmed/19696304. Accessed November 13, 2013.

22. Kouvaraki MA, Shapiro SE, Fornage BD, et al. Role of preoperative ultrasonography in the surgical management of patients with thyroid cancer. Surgery 2003;134(6):946–54. Available at: http://linkinghub.elsevier.com/retrieve/pii/S0039606003004240. Accessed October 23, 2013.

23. Stulak JM, Grant CS, Farley DR, et al. Value of preoperative ultrasonography in the surgical management of initial and reoperative papillary thyroid cancer. Arch Surg 2006;141(5):489–94 [discussion: 494–6]. Available at: http://www.ncbi.nlm.nih.gov/pubmed/16702521.

24. Hughes DT, Laird AM, Miller BS, et al. Reoperative lymph node dissection for recurrent papillary thyroid cancer and effect on serum thyroglobulin. Ann Surg Oncol 2012;19(9):2951–7. Available at: http://www.ncbi.nlm.nih.gov/pubmed/22526913. Accessed October 22, 2013.

25. Shan CX, Zhang W, Jiang DZ, et al. Routine central neck dissection in differentiated thyroid carcinoma: a systematic review and meta-analysis. Laryngoscope 2012;122(4):797–804. Available at: http://www.ncbi.nlm.nih.gov/pubmed/22294492. Accessed October 17, 2013.

26. Wang TS, Cheung K, Farrokhyar F, et al. A meta-analysis of the effect of prophylactic central compartment neck dissection on locoregional recurrence rates in patients with papillary thyroid cancer. Ann Surg Oncol 2013;20(11):3477–83. Available at: http://www.ncbi.nlm.nih.gov/pubmed/23846784. Accessed October 20, 2013.

27. Barczyński M, Konturek A, Stopa M, et al. Prophylactic central neck dissection for papillary thyroid cancer. Br J Surg 2013;100(3):410–8. Available at: http://www.ncbi.nlm.nih.gov/pubmed/23188784. Accessed October 22, 2013.

28. Lang BH, Yih PC, Shek TW, et al. Factors affecting the adequacy of lymph node yield in prophylactic unilateral central neck dissection for papillary thyroid

carcinoma. J Surg Oncol 2012;106(8):966–71. Available at: http://www.ncbi.nlm.
nih.gov/pubmed/22718439. Accessed October 23, 2013.

29. Lang BH, Wong KP, Wan KY, et al. Impact of routine unilateral central neck
dissection on preablative and postablative stimulated thyroglobulin levels after
total thyroidectomy in papillary thyroid carcinoma. Ann Surg Oncol 2012;
19(1):60–7. Available at: http://www.pubmedcentral.nih.gov/articlerender.fcgi?
artid=3251780&tool=pmcentrez&rendertype=abstract. Accessed October
23, 2013.

30. Moo TA, McGill J, Allendorf J, et al. Impact of prophylactic central neck lymph
node dissection on early recurrence in papillary thyroid carcinoma. World J
Surg 2010;34(6):1187–91. Available at: http://www.ncbi.nlm.nih.gov/pubmed/
20130868. Accessed October 22, 2013.

31. Costa S, Giugliano G, Santoro L, et al. Role of prophylactic central neck dissection in cN0 papillary thyroid cancer Il ruolo dello svuotamento profi lattico del
compartimento centrale del collo. Acta Otorhinolaryngol Ital 2009;29:61–9.

32. Son Y, Jeong H, Baek C, et al. Extent of prophylactic lymph node dissection in
the central neck area of the patients with papillary thyroid carcinoma: comparison of limited versus comprehensive lymph node dissection in a 2-year safety
study. Ann Surg Oncol 2008;15(7):2020–6.

33. Sywak M, Cornford L, Roach P, et al. Routine ipsilateral level VI lymphadenectomy reduces postoperative thyroglobulin levels in papillary thyroid cancer. Surgery 2006;140(6):1000–5 [discussion: 1005–7]. Available at: http://www.ncbi.
nlm.nih.gov/pubmed/17188149. Accessed October 23, 2013.

34. Koo BS, Choi EC, Yoon YH, et al. Predictive factors for ipsilateral or contralateral
central lymph node metastasis in unilateral papillary thyroid carcinoma. Ann
Surg 2009;249(5):840–4. Available at: http://www.ncbi.nlm.nih.gov/pubmed/
19387316. Accessed October 23, 2013.

35. Roh JL, Kim JM, Park CI. Central lymph node metastasis of unilateral papillary
thyroid carcinoma: patterns and factors predictive of nodal metastasis,
morbidity, and recurrence. Ann Surg Oncol 2011;18(8):2245–50. Available at:
http://www.ncbi.nlm.nih.gov/pubmed/21327454. Accessed October 23, 2013.

36. Laird AM, Gauger PG, Miller BS, et al. Evaluation of postoperative radioactive
iodine scans in patients who underwent prophylactic central lymph node
dissection. World J Surg 2012;36(6):1268–73. Available at: http://www.ncbi.
nlm.nih.gov/pubmed/22270997. Accessed October 23, 2013.

37. Davidson HC, Park BJ, Johnson JT. Papillary thyroid cancer: controversies in the
management of neck metastasis. Laryngoscope 2008;118(12):2161–5. Available at: http://www.ncbi.nlm.nih.gov/pubmed/19029855. Accessed October
23, 2013.

38. Wada N, Duh Q, Sugino K, et al. Lymph node metastasis from 259 papillary thyroid microcarcinomas frequency, pattern of occurrence and recurrence, and
optimal. Ann Surg 2003;237(3):399–407.

39. Gemsenjäger E, Perren A, Seifert B, et al. Lymph node surgery in papillary thyroid carcinoma. J Am Coll Surg 2003;197(2):182–90. Available at: http://www.
ncbi.nlm.nih.gov/pubmed/12892795. Accessed October 23, 2013.

40. Roh JL, Park JY, Park CI. Total thyroidectomy plus neck dissection in differentiated papillary thyroid carcinoma patients: pattern of nodal metastasis,
morbidity, recurrence, and postoperative levels of serum parathyroid hormone.
Ann Surg 2007;245(4):604–10. Available at: http://www.pubmedcentral.nih.gov/
articlerender.fcgi?artid=1877043&tool=pmcentrez&rendertype=abstract. Accessed October 22, 2013.

41. Roh JL, Park JY, Park CI. Prevention of postoperative hypocalcemia with routine oral calcium and vitamin D supplements in patients with differentiated papillary thyroid carcinoma undergoing total thyroidectomy plus central neck dissection. Cancer 2009;115(2):251–8. Available at: http://www.ncbi.nlm.nih.gov/pubmed/19117033. Accessed October 23, 2013.

42. Rosenbaum MA, McHenry CR. Central neck dissection for papillary thyroid cancer. Arch Otolaryngol Head Neck Surg 2009;135(11):1092–7. Available at: http://www.ncbi.nlm.nih.gov/pubmed/19917920.

43. Besic N, Zgajnar J, Hocevar M, et al. Extent of thyroidectomy and lymphadenectomy in 254 patients with papillary thyroid microcarcinoma: a single-institution experience. Ann Surg Oncol 2009;16(4):920–8. Available at: http://www.ncbi.nlm.nih.gov/pubmed/19189188. Accessed October 23, 2013.

44. Zuniga S, Sanabria A. Prophylactic central neck dissection in stage N0 papillary thyroid carcinoma. Arch Otolaryngol Head Neck Surg 2009;135(11):1087–91. Available at: http://www.ncbi.nlm.nih.gov/pubmed/19917919.

45. Shen W, Ogawa L, Ruan D, et al. Central neck lymph node dissection for papillary thyroid cancer. Arch Surg 2010;145(3):272–5.

46. Perrino M, Vannucchi G, Vicentini L, et al. Outcome predictors and impact of central node dissection and radiometabolic treatments in papillary thyroid cancers < or =2 cm. Endocr Relat Cancer 2009;16(1):201–10. Available at: http://www.ncbi.nlm.nih.gov/pubmed/19106146. Accessed October 23, 2013.

47. Zetoune T, Keutgen X, Buitrago D, et al. Prophylactic central neck dissection and local recurrence in papillary thyroid cancer: a meta-analysis. Ann Surg Oncol 2010;17(12):3287–93. Available at: http://www.ncbi.nlm.nih.gov/pubmed/20596784. Accessed October 23, 2013.

48. Yoo D, Ajmal S, Gowda S, et al. Level VI lymph node dissection does not decrease radioiodine uptake in patients undergoing radioiodine ablation for differentiated thyroid cancer. World J Surg 2012;36(6):1255–61. Available at: http://www.ncbi.nlm.nih.gov/pubmed/22430670. Accessed November 13, 2013.

49. Hughes DT, White ML, Miller BS, et al. Influence of prophylactic central lymph node dissection on postoperative thyroglobulin levels and radioiodine treatment in papillary thyroid cancer. Surgery 2010;148(6):1100–6 [discussion: 1006–7]. Available at: http://www.ncbi.nlm.nih.gov/pubmed/21134539. Accessed November 4, 2013.

50. Bonnet S, Hartl D, Leboulleux S, et al. Prophylactic lymph node dissection for papillary thyroid cancer less than 2 cm: implications for radioiodine treatment. J Clin Endocrinol Metab 2009;94(4):1162–7. Available at: http://www.ncbi.nlm.nih.gov/pubmed/19116234. Accessed October 28, 2013.

51. Sawka AM, Rilkoff H, Tsang RW, et al. The rationale of patients with early-stage papillary thyroid cancer for accepting or rejecting radioactive iodine remnant ablation. Thyroid 2013;23(2):246–7. Available at: http://www.ncbi.nlm.nih.gov/pubmed/23009127. Accessed November 13, 2013.

52. Durante C, Haddy N, Baudin E, et al. Long-term outcome of 444 patients with distant metastases from papillary and follicular thyroid carcinoma: benefits and limits of radioiodine therapy. J Clin Endocrinol Metab 2006;91(8):2892–9. Available at: http://www.ncbi.nlm.nih.gov/pubmed/16684830. Accessed November 13, 2013.

53. Giordano D, Valcavi R, Thompson GB, et al. Complications of central neck dissection in patients with papillary thyroid carcinoma: results of a study on 1087 patients and review of the literature. Thyroid 2012;22(9):911–7. Available at: http://www.ncbi.nlm.nih.gov/pubmed/22827494. Accessed October 22, 2013.

54. Stavrakis AI, Ituarte PH, Ko CY, et al. Surgeon volume as a predictor of outcomes in inpatient and outpatient endocrine surgery. Surgery 2007;142(6): 887–99 [discussion: 887–99]. Available at: http://www.ncbi.nlm.nih.gov/pubmed/18063073. Accessed November 14, 2013.

55. Saunders BD, Wainess RM, Dimick JB, et al. Who performs endocrine operations in the United States? Surgery 2003;134(6):924–31. Available at: http://linkinghub.elsevier.com/retrieve/pii/S0039606003004203. Accessed November 14, 2013.

56. Alvarado R, Sywak MS, Delbridge L, et al. Central lymph node dissection as a secondary procedure for papillary thyroid cancer: is there added morbidity? Surgery 2009;145(5):514–8. Available at: http://www.ncbi.nlm.nih.gov/pubmed/19375610. Accessed November 13, 2013.

57. Rondeau G, Fish S, Hann LE, et al. Ultrasonographically detected small thyroid bed nodules identified after total thyroidectomy for differentiated thyroid cancer seldom show clinically significant structural progression. Thyroid 2011;21(8): 845–53. Available at: http://www.ncbi.nlm.nih.gov/pubmed/21809914. Accessed November 13, 2013.

58. Moreno MA, Edeiken-Monroe BS, Siegel ER, et al. In papillary thyroid cancer, preoperative central neck ultrasound detects only macroscopic surgical disease, but negative findings predict excellent long-term regional control and survival. Thyroid 2012;22(4):347–55.

59. Henry JF, Gramatica L, Denizot A, et al. Morbidity of prophylactic lymph node dissection in the central neck area in patients with papillary thyroid carcinoma. Langenbecks Arch Surg 1998;383(2):167–9.

60. Pereira JA, Jimeno J, Miquel J, et al. Nodal yield, morbidity, and recurrence after central neck dissection for papillary thyroid carcinoma. Surgery 2005;138(6): 1095–100 [discussion: 1100–1].

Medical Therapy for Advanced Forms of Thyroid Cancer

Uma Rajhbeharrysingh, MD[a], Matthew Taylor, MD[b],
Mira Milas, MD[c],*

KEYWORDS

- Advanced thyroid cancer • Targeted therapy • Clinical trials • Chemotherapy
- Anaplastic • Medullary and differentiated thyroid cancer • Medical therapy

KEY POINTS

- Patients with unresectable or metastatic thyroid cancer are candidates for systemic treatment with targeted therapeutics.
- Classes of targeted therapeutic agents tested in clinical trials for thyroid cancer include selective tyrosine kinase inhibitors, multikinase inhibitors, proteasome inhibitors, inhibitors of angiogenesis, histone deacetylase inhibitors, and inhibitors of DNA methylation.
- Drugs inducing differentiation of thyroid tumors to increase susceptibility to radioiodine ablation have shown a good initial response.
- Newer trials involve combinations of drugs.
- Three drugs have received Federal Drug Administration approval: vandetanib and cabozantinib (XL184) for medullary thyroid cancer and sorafenib for papillary thyroid cancer.

INTRODUCTION

In 2013, it is estimated that 60,220 new individuals (75% women) will be diagnosed with thyroid cancer and 1850 patients will die of thyroid cancer (Surveillance, Epidemiology, and End Results Program[1]). Thyroid cancer represents 4% of all new cancer cases and is the fifth most common cancer in women. There has been an increase in the incidence of thyroid cancer since the mid 1990s, especially in the female population. This increase is partly attributed to incidentalomas found on radiology studies

Disclaimer: Drug dosages are presented to the best of current knowledge and for general illustration. Readers are advised to confirm the dosage if considering therapy.

[a] Department of Surgery, Oregon Health and Science University, 3181 Southwest Sam Jackson Park Road, Portland, OR 97239, USA; [b] Division of Hematology & Medical Oncology, Knight Cancer Institute, Oregon Health and Science University, 3181 Southwest Sam Jackson Park Road, Portland, OR 97239, USA; [c] Department of Surgery, Knight Cancer Institute, Oregon Health and Science University, 3181 Southwest Sam Jackson Park Road, L619, Portland, OR 97239, USA
* Corresponding author.
E-mail address: milas@ohsu.edu

used in general medical care. Primary thyroid cancer can be classified into 3 major histopathologic types: differentiated thyroid cancers (DTC), including papillary (PTC, 85% of cases) and follicular (FTC, 5%–10%); medullary thyroid cancer (MTC, 5%); and anaplastic thyroid cancer (ATC, 1%).[2] Even though the general prognosis of thyroid cancer is excellent, 10% to 20% of patients with DTC have advanced cancer either at the initial presentation or as a recurrence. Advanced presentations can be broadly defined as those with metastatic disease or extensive regional invasion of major anatomic structures, such as the aerodigestive tract (larynx, trachea, esophagus, recurrent laryngeal nerve), spine, or large cervical blood vessels. Conventional medical therapy for thyroid cancer is used in these cases, including radioactive iodine (RAI) and high-dose levothyroxine replacement therapy for thyroid-stimulating hormone (TSH) suppression. It is estimated, however, that about half of these patients with advanced disease will not respond adequately to the conventional therapy. One reason may be the dedifferentiation of the tumor, resulting in the inability to transport RAI into the tumor cell. Long-term survival for patients presenting with stage IV DTC is about 51% compared with nearly 100% for patients with stage I (American Cancer Society, www.cancer.org). The long-term overall survival decreases to 10% to 15% in patients with RAI-resistant disease.[3,4] RAI insensitivity/resistance also exists in ATC whereby cells are either dedifferentiated or undifferentiated and in MTC whereby parafollicular cells do not participate in iodine uptake. Treatment options, therefore, for thyroid tumors that cannot be managed either by surgical intervention or RAI have been very limited.

Over the last decade, there has been an exponential growth in biomolecular information focused on cell signaling pathways resulting in cell growth, proliferation, differentiation, migration, and survival. This has identified various genetic mutations in multiple pathways, which can lead to thyroid cancer. Mutations in the RAS, RET, and RAF genes were among the most common mutations noted in DTC and MTC; additionally, several somatic mutations have been described in ATC, including the genes of the MAP kinase (MAPK, more commonly referred to as MEK in published literature) and PI3K/AKT pathways and TP53. The major cell signaling pathways affected by these mutations include but are not limited to the RAS/RAF/MEK/ERK pathway, PI3K/AKT/mTOR pathway, JAK/STAT3, and NFkb pathways (**Fig. 1**), which in turn affect cell growth, proliferation, and survival. EGFR is a receptor tyrosine kinase (RTK) that acts downstream through the activation of several cascades, including MAPK, AKT, and JAK. The inhibition of one or more of the kinases in these pathways, in epigenetic mechanisms, angiogenesis, or cellular mechanics involved in cell division are likely targets that can result in tumor regression.[5] In 2004, new targeted therapies for these advanced thyroid cancers came to light, creating an upsurge in clinical trials and off-label use of these drugs soon after. Thus far, the Food and Drug Administration (FDA) has approved 2 drugs for use in advanced MTC: vandetanib (in 2011) and cabozantinib (in 2012). The purpose of this article is to provide a contemporary summary of available targeted therapies for advanced thyroid cancer, corresponding clinical trials, and innovative drugs on the horizon.

HISTORICAL OVERVIEW

There has been quite an evolution regarding innovative medical therapies for advanced thyroid cancer. The authors would like to take this opportunity to provide a timeline highlighting major events to date (**Fig. 2**). **Tables 1–7** reference specific publications with the year of publication in an effort to add to the timeline associated with a therapy. Medical therapy in the form of RAI was first reported for use in thyroid cancer

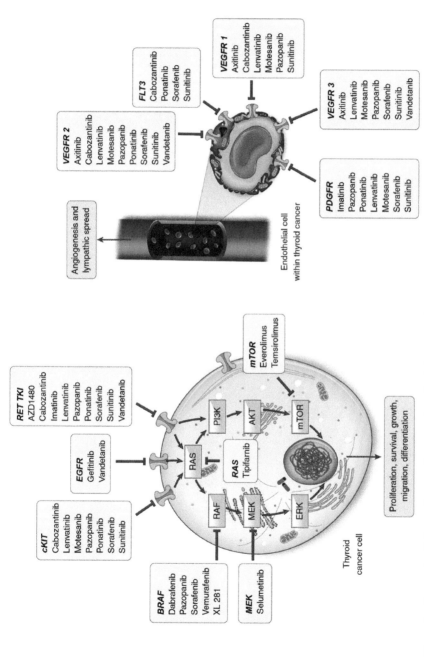

Fig. 1. Sites of action and cellular pathways of targeted medical therapies for thyroid cancer. TKI, tyrosine kinase inhibitor.

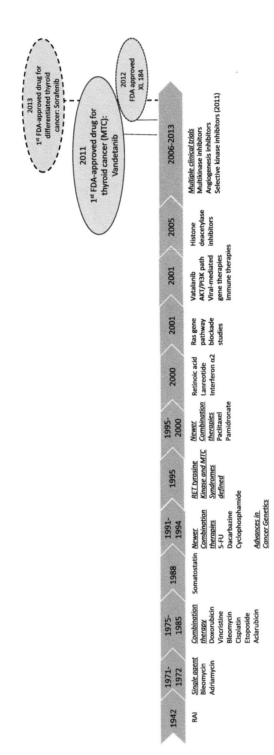

Fig. 2. Timeline of targeted therapy development for thyroid cancer. 5-FU, fluorouracil.

Table 1
Targets of selective tyrosine kinase inhibitors

Drug	RET	BRAF	RAS	MEK	mTOR	EGFR
AZD 1480	x	–	–	–	–	–
Dabrafenib	–	x	–	–	–	–
Vemurafenib	–	x	–	–	–	–
XL 281	–	x	–	–	–	–
Tipifarnib	–	–	x	–	–	–
Selumetinib	–	–	–	x	–	–
Temsirolimus	–	–	–	–	x	–
Gefitinib	–	–	–	–	–	x

between 1942 and 1946. About 30 years later, in the 1970s, conventional chemotherapy was applied for advanced thyroid cancers, usually as single-agent therapy with bleomycin or doxorubicin. During the 1980s and 1990s, combinations of chemotherapeutic agents including paclitaxel and fluorouracil (5-FU) were used; somatostatin was introduced for symptomatic control of metastatic MTC.[6] It was only in 2004 that therapies were targeted to known genetic mutations and specific pathways involved in thyroid cancer, and the first clinical trials started in 2005. The first targeted therapy drug tested in animals was vatalinib, a vascular endothelial growth factor (VEGF) inhibitor. The first clinical trials occurred between 2006 and 2008.[7] The first multikinase inhibitor to be systematically evaluated in DTC was motesanib, and tumor shrinkage in several patients with DTC was noted in this phase I trial.[8] Vandetanib became the first FDA-approved therapeutic agent for thyroid cancer, in this case for MTC, in 2011. Sorafenib became the first FDA-approved agent for DTC (PTC, FTC) in November 2013. It is remarkable that 50 years of thyroid cancer care would pass for these achievements to be realized.

MEDICAL THERAPY FOR ADVANCED DTC

Despite being derived from the same cell (thyroid follicular cell), PTC and FTC accumulate distinct and mutually exclusive genetic abnormalities during malignant transformation. For instance, most PTCs are associated with RET/PTC rearrangements and BRAF mutations. There is a high prevalence of RAS mutations and PAX8/PPARγ rearrangements in follicular patterned carcinomas (FTCs and follicular variant of PTCs).[9]

Targets and Mechanisms

Abnormal activation of the RET/RAS/RAF/MAPK pathway is one of the most studied mechanisms in thyroid tumorigenesis (see **Fig. 1**). Although MAPK is technically a correct denotation for this pathway, it is more routinely referred to as MEK in clinical practice; the drugs targeting this are called MEK inhibitors. The following is a summary of the rationale for target selection in this thyroid cancer subtype.

- The RET proto-oncogene is located on chromosome 10q11-2. It encodes for a tyrosine kinase transmembrane receptor. The proto-oncogene is normally expressed in a variety of neural cell lineages, including thyroid C cells and adrenal medulla; but it is not expressed, or it is expressed at very low levels, in normal thyroid follicular cells. The RET oncogene activation may be generated either by a fusion rearrangement or by activating point mutations. RET/PTC fusion

Table 2
Targets of multikinase inhibitors

Drugs	RET and RET/PTC	VEGFR 1	VEGFR 2	VEGFR 3	EGFR	FGFR	PDGFR	Bcr-Abl	BRAF	MET	FLT3	cKIT
Axitinib	–	x	x	x	–	–	–	–	–	–	–	–
Cabozantinib	x	x	x	–	–	–	–	–	–	x	x	x
Imatinib	x	–	–	–	–	–	x	x	–	–	–	x
Lenvatinib	x	x	x	x	–	–	x	–	–	–	–	x
Motesanib	–	x	x	x	–	–	x	–	–	–	–	x
Pazopanib	x	x	x	x	–	–	x	–	x	–	–	x
Ponatinib	x	–	x	–	–	x	x	x	–	–	x	x
Sorafenib	x	–	x	x	–	–	x	–	x	–	x	x
Sunitinib	x	x	x	x	–	–	x	–	–	–	x	x
Vandetanib	x	–	x	x	x	–	–	–	–	–	–	–

Table 3
Targeted medical therapy for thyroid cancer by pathways

MAPK/ERK	PI3K/AKT/ mTOR	Angiogenesis	Other
AZD 1480	AZD 1480	Axitinib	Azacytidine (DNA methylation inhibitor)
Cabozantinib	Cabozantinib	Bortezomib	Bortezomib (proteosome inhibitor)
Dabrafenib	Gefitinib	Cabozantinib	Decitabine (DNA methylation inhibitor)
Gefitinib	Imatinib	Combretastatin 4A	Romidepsin (histone deacetylase inhibitor)
Imatinib	Lenvatinib	Fosbretabulin	Valproic acid (histone deacetylase inhibitor)
Lenvatinib	Ponatinib	Lenvatinib	
Ponatinib	Temsirolimus	Motesanib	
Selumetinib	Vandetanib	Pazopanib	
Sorafenib		Ponatinib	
Sunitinib		Sunitinib	
Tipifarnib		Thalidomide	
Vandetanib		Vandetanib	
Vemurafenib			
XL 281			

Table 4
Targeted medical therapy for thyroid cancers by histologic types

Drug	DTC	PTC	FTC	MTC	ATC
Axitinib	x	x	x	x	–
AZD 1480	x	x	–	x	–
Bortezomib	x	x	–	x	x
Cabozantinib	–	–	–	x	–
Dabrafenib	x	x	–	–	–
Fosbretabulin	–	–	–	–	x
Gefitinib	x	x	x	x	–
Imatinib	–	–	–	x	x
Lenvatinib	x	–	–	–	–
Motesanib	x	–	–	x	–
Pazopanib	x	x	x	–	–
Ponatinib	–	–	–	x	–
Romidepsin	x	–	–	–	–
Selumetinib	x	x	–	–	–
Sorafenib	x	x	x	x	x
Sunitinib	x	x	x	x	–
Temsirolimus	x	x	–	–	–
Thalidomide	x	x	x	x	–
Tipifarnib	x	x	x	x	–
Valproic acid	x	x	–	–	x
Vandetanib	x	x	–	x	–
Vemurafenib	x	–	–	–	–
XL 281	–	x	–	–	x

Table 5
Clinical trials of targeted therapies in DTC

Drugs	Phase of Study	Author/Publication Year	Number of Patients	Dosage	Subtype	Response to Therapy
Selective tyrosine kinase inhibitors						
Dabrafenib	Phase 2	NCT01723302[46]	Ongoing	150 mg bid	DTC	—
Everolimus	Phase 2	NCT01118065[47]	Ongoing	—	DTC, MTC, ATC	—
	Phase 2	NCT01164176[48]	Ongoing	—	DTC, MTC, ATC	—
Everolimus and pasireotide	Phase 2	NCT01270321[49]	Ongoing	—	DTC, MTC	—
Everolimus and sorafenib	Phase 2	NCT01263951[50]	Ongoing	Everolimus 5 mg daily; sorafenib 200 mg bid	DTC	—
Gefitinib	Phase 2	Pennell et al,[51] 2008	27	250 mg daily	DTC, MTC, ATC	SD 12%
Selumetinib	Open label	Ho et al,[52] 2013	20	75 mg bid	DTC	PR 25%, SD 15%
Temsirolimus and sorafenib	Phase 2	NCT01025453[53]	Ongoing (n ≈ 37)	Temsirolimus 25 IV weekly; sorafenib 200 mg bid	DTC, MTC, ATC	PR 22%, SD 57%
Tipifarnib and sorafenib	Phase 1	Hong et al,[54] 2011	22	Tipifarnib 100 mg bid, sorafenib 400 mg in AM, 200 mg in PM	DTC, MTC	PR 4.5%, SD 36%
Vemurafenib	Phase 1	Kim et al,[55] 2013	3	720 mg bid	DTC	PR 33%, SD 66%
	Phase 2	NCT01286753[56]	Ongoing	960 mg bid	DTC, PTC	—
XL 281	Phase 1	NCT00451880[57]	5	150 mg daily	DTC, PTC	SD 100%
Multi-target tyrosine kinase inhibitors						
Axitinib	Phase 2	Cohen et al,[13] 2008	60	5 mg bid	DTC, MTC, ATC	PR 30%, SD 38%
Lenvatinib	Phase 3	NCT01321554[17]	Ongoing	24 mg daily	DTC	—
Motesanib	Phase 1	Rosen et al,[58] 2007	7	125 mg daily	DTC, MTC, ATC	PR 50%
	Phase 2	Sherman et al,[59] 2008	93	125 mg daily	DTC	PR 14%, SD 35%
Pazopanib	Phase 2	Bible et al,[60] 2010	37	800 mg od	DTC	PR 49%, PFS 71%
	Phase 2	NCT00625846[61]	Ongoing	800 mg od	DTC, MTC	—

Drug	Phase	Study	N	Dose	Type	Results
Sorafenib	Phase 2	Gupta-Abramson et al,[62] 2008	30	400 mg bid	DTC	PR 23%, SD 53%
	Phase 2	Kloos et al,[63] 2009	41	400 mg bid	DTC	PR 15%, SD 56%
	Phase 2	Hoftijzer et al,[64] 2009	31	400 mg bid	DTC	PR 25%, SD 34%, PD 22%
	Phase 3 (RDBCT)	NCT00984282[15,65]	Ongoing	400 mg bid	DTC	CT
	Off label	Cabanillas et al,[3] 2010	15	400 mg bid	DTC	PR 20%, SD 60%, PD 20%
	Phase 2	Ahmed et al,[66] 2011	34	400 mg bid	DTC, MTC	PR 21%, SD 65%, PD 14%
	Open label, retrospective	Capdevila et al,[67] 2012	34	400 mg bid	DTC, MTC, ATC	PR 32%, SD 41%
	Phase 3 RCDBT	DECISION trial[15]	Ongoing (n≈417)	400 mg bid	DTC	—
	Phase 2	Schneider et al,[68] 2012	31	400 mg bid	DTC	PR 31%, SD 42%
Sunitinib	Phase 2	Cohen et al,[69] 2008	37	50 mg daily	DTC	PR 13%, SD 68%, PD 10%
	Phase 2	Goulart et al,[70] 2008	18	—	DTC, MTC	RR 44%
	Phase 2	Ravaud et al,[71] 2010 (THYSU trial)	Ongoing (n≈15)	—	DTC, MTC, ATC	PR 33%, SD 26%
	Phase 2	Carr et al,[72] 2010	35	37.5 mg daily	DTC, MTC	CR 3%, PR 28%, SD 46%, PD 17%
Vandetanib	Phase 2 (RCT)	Leboulleux et al,[73] 2012	72	300 mg daily	DTC	HR 0.63
Proteosome inhibitor						
Bortezomib	Phase 2	Putzer et al,[21] 2012	7	—	DTC	SD 57%, PD 17%
	Phase 2	NCT00104871[74]	Ongoing	—	DTC	
Angiogenesis inhibitors						
Cediranib, lenalidomide	Phase 1/2	NCT01208051[75]	Ongoing	—	DTC	—
Thalidomide	Phase 2	Ain et al,[76] 2007	28	800 mg daily	DTC, MTC	PR 18%, SD 32%
	Phase 2	NCT00026533[77]	Ongoing	800 mg daily	DTC, MTC	—
COX 2 inhibitor						
Celecoxib	Phase 2	Mrozek et al,[78] 2006	32	400 mg bid	DTC	PR 3%, SD, 3%, PD 71%

(continued on next page)

Table 5
(continued)

Drugs	Phase of Study	Author/Publication Year	Number of Patients	Dosage	Subtype	Response to Therapy
Histone deacetylase inhibitors						
Romidepsin	Phase 1	Piekarz et al,[79] 2008	9	—	DTC	SD 66%
	Phase 1	Amiri-Kordestani et al,[80] 2013	11	—	DTC	SD 54%
	Phase 2	Sherman et al,[81] 2013	20	—	DTC	SD 65%, PD 35%
	Phase 2	NCT00098813[82]	Ongoing	—	DTC	—
Valproic acid	Phase 2	NCT01182285[83]	Ongoing	—	DTC	—
Vorinostat	Phase 2	Woyach et al,[84] 2009	19	200 mg bid	DTC, MTC	SD 54%, PD 36%
Inhibitors of DNA methylation						
Azacytidine	Phase 1	NCT00004062[85]	Ongoing	—	DTC, MTC, ATC	—
Decitabine	Phase 2	NCT00085293[86]	Ongoing	—	DTC	—

Abbreviations: CR, complete response; COX 2, cyclooxygenase 2; HR, hazard ratio; IV, intravenous; PD, progressive disease; PFS, progression-free survival; PR, partial response; RCT, randomized controlled trial; RR, response rate; SD, stable disease.

rearrangements have been reported only in PTC and in some cases of benign follicular adenomas; these are related to ionizing radiation exposure, which is a well-recognized risk factor for PTC.[10] Activating RET point mutations have been exclusively found in MTC. The point mutation determines a constitutive activation of the tyrosine kinase receptor and consequently continuous stimulus to cell proliferation.[10]

- The RAS oncogene point mutations account for nearly 40% of benign and malignant follicular thyroid tumors and about 20% to 23% in poorly differentiated thyroid tumors. RAS plays an important role in the intracellular signal transduction from the cell surface to the nucleus where it is able to activate gene expression that induces cell proliferation, differentiation, and survival. There are 3 members of the RAS family (K-, N-, and H-RAS) that share 85% amino acid sequence identity. K-RAS is the most frequent mutation (at about 85% of the total), followed by N-RAS (at about 15%) and HRAS (at <1%).[10] Point mutations in codons 12 and 13 cause an increase in the RAS and GTP affinity, and a point mutation in codon 61 inactivates the RAS autocatalytic GTPase function.[11] RAS mutations are more frequent in thyroid tumors of patients living in countries where iodine intake is inadequate.[10]

- The activating mutation of the B isoform of the RAF kinase gene, located on exon 15, results from a valine to glutamic acid substitution at amino acid 600 (BRAF V600E mutation). This mutation is the most common mutation in PTC; varying between 29% and 69% of patients with PTC.[9,10] BRAF, together with ARAF and CRAF, constitute the RAF family of serine/threonine kinases. RAF proteins are intermediate members of the MAPK/ERK pathway, which links extracellular signals to the cell, ultimately controlling cellular processes, such as proliferation, differentiation, survival, and apoptosis. BRAF mutations are associated with older age of patients, extrathyroidal extension, higher cancer staging, and recurrence.[8] The BRAF V600E mutation correlated with the presence of multifocality; more aggressive histologic variants; or the infiltration of the tumor capsule, an unfavorable prognostic factor.[12] BRAF mutation is a negative prognostic marker, which may reflect, at least in part, the diminished radioiodine avidity of cells carrying such a mutation.[9]

- Downstream activation of MAPK kinase (MEK) is a common mediator of mutant RET/PTC, RAS, or BRAF kinases, leading to the numerous stimulated effects of MEK signaling, including cell proliferation, survival, differentiation, motility, and angiogenesis. Thus, selective therapeutic targeting of either the specific mutated upstream oncogenic kinase or MEK itself is being extensively explored.[8] Targeted inhibition of the PI3K/AKT/mTOR pathway has also been an attractive therapeutic concept, given that many advanced DTC tumors demonstrate activation of signaling because of diminished expression of PTEN or mutation, amplification, or overexpression of either PI3K or AKT, resulting in enhanced tumor proliferation, migration, and survival. Inhibition of mTOR complex in mutant thyroid cell lines resulted in growth inhibition and cell cycle arrest. However, feedback activation of both ERK and AKT was observed, suggesting that compensatory mechanisms might rapidly bypass the drug's effect. Xenograft models demonstrated findings consistent with a cytostatic rather than cytotoxic effect of mTOR inhibition.[8]

- A common element to thyroid cancers is their associated vascularity, with elevated levels of VEGF compared with normal thyroid tissue. Microvessel density is also higher in PTC than in normal thyroid. VEGF levels are correlated with stage, large tumor size, nodal involvement (especially with stimulation of VEGF3), extrathyroidal invasion, and distant metastasis. In PTC, VEGF is also associated

Table 6
Clinical trials of targeted therapies in MTC

Drugs	Phase of Study	Author/Publication Year	Number of Patients	Dosage	Subtype	Response to Therapy
Selective tyrosine kinase inhibitors						
Everolimus	Phase 2	NCT01118065[47]	Ongoing	—	DTC, MTC, ATC	—
	Phase 2	NCT01164176[48]	Ongoing	—	DTC, MTC, ATC	—
Everolimus and pasireotide	Phase 2	NCT01270321[49]	Ongoing	—	MTC, DTC	—
Gefitinib	Phase 2	Pennell et al,[51] 2008	27	250 mg daily	DTC, MTC, ATC	SD 12%
Pasireotide	Phase 2	NCT01625520[87]	Ongoing	60 mg/m	MTC	—
Temsirolimus and sorafenib	Phase 2	NCT01025453[53]	Ongoing (n ≈ 37)	Temsirolimus 25 IV weekly; sorafenib 200 mg bid	DTC, MTC, ATC	PR 22%, SD 57%
Tipifarnib and sorafenib	Phase 1	Hong et al,[54] 2011	22	Tipifarnib 100 mg bid; sorafenib 400 mg in AM, 200 mg in PM	MTC, DTC	PR 38%, SD 31%
Multi-kinase inhibitors						
Axitinib	Phase 2	Cohen et al,[13] 2008	60	5 mg bid	DTC, MTC, ATC	PR 30%, SD 38%
Cabozantinib	Phase 1	Kurzrock et al,[88] 2011	37	140 mg daily	MTC	PR 68%, SD 41%
	Phase 3	Schoffski et al,[89] 2012 (EXAM trial)	330	140 mg daily	MTC	HR 0.28
Imatinib	Open label	Frank-Raue et al,[90] 2007	8	600 mg daily	MTC	SD 12%
Imatinib and dacarbazine, capecitabine	Phase 1/2	NCT00354523[91]	Ongoing	—	MTC	—
Lenvatinib	Phase 2	Schlumberger et al,[92] 2012	59	24 mg daily	MTC	PR 36%,

Drug	Phase	Study	n	Dose	Disease	Response
Motesanib	Phase 1	Rosen et al,[58] 2007	6	125 mg daily	DTC, MTC, ATC	PR 50%
	Phase 2	Sclumberger et al,[93] 2009	91	125 mg daily	MTC	PR 2%, SD 47%
Pazopanib	Phase 2	NCT00625846[61]	Ongoing	—	MTC, DTC	—
Ponatinib	Phase 2	NCT01838642[94]	Ongoing	45 mg daily	MTC	—
Sorafenib	Phase 2	Ahmed et al,[66] 2011	34	400 mg bid	MTC, DTC	PR 21%, SD 65%, PD 14%
	Open label, retrospective	Capdevila et al,[67] 2012	34	400 mg bid	DTC, MTC, ATC	PR 32%, SD 41%
	Phase 2	Lam et al,[95] 2010	16	400 mg bid	MTC	PR 6%, SD 87%
	Phase 2	NCT00390325[96]	Ongoing	400 mg bid	MTC	—
Sunitinib	—	Cohen et al,[69] 2008	6	50 mg daily	MTC	SD 83%, PD 17%
	Phase 2	Goulart et al,[70] 2008	18	—	MTC, DTC	RR 44%
	Phase 2	Ravaud et al,[71] 2010 (THYSU trial)	Ongoing (n≈15)	—	DTC, MTC, ATC	PR 33%, SD 26%
	Phase 2	Carr et al,[72] 2010	35	37.5 mg daily	MTC, DTC	CR 3%, PR 28%, SD 46%, PD 17%
Vandetanib	Phase 2	Robinson et al,[97] 2010	19	100 mg daily	MTC	PR 16%, SD 53%
	Phase 3 (RDBCT)	Wells et al,[98] 2012 (ZETA trial)	331	300 mg daily	MTC	HR 0.46
	Phase 4 (RDBCT)	NCT01496313[99]	Ongoing	300 mg and 150 mg daily	MTC	—
Angiogenesis inhibitors						
Thalidomide	Phase 2	Ain et al,[76] 2007	28	800 mg daily	MTC, DTC	PR 18%, SD 32%
	Phase 2	NCT00026533[77]	Ongoing	800 mg daily	MTC, DTC	—
Histone deacetylase inhibitor						
Vorinostat	Phase 2	Woyach et al,[84] 2009	19	200 mg bid	MTC, DTC	SD 54%, PD 36%
DNA methylation inhibitor						
Azacytidine	Phase 1	NCT00004062[85]	Ongoing	—	DTC, MTC, ATC	—

Abbreviations: CR, complete response; HR, hazard ratio; IV, intravenous; PD, progressive disease; PR, partial response; RR, response rate; SD, stable disease.

Table 7
Clinical trials of targeted therapies in ATC

Drugs	Phase of Study	Author/Year of Publication	Number of Patients	Dosage and Length of Trial	Subtype	RECIST/HR
Selective kinase inhibitors						
Everolimus	Phase 2	NCT01118065[47]	Ongoing	—	DTC, MTC, ATC	—
Everolimus	Phase 2	NCT01164176[48]	Ongoing	—	DTC, MTC, ATC	—
Gefitinib	Phase 2	Pennell et al,[51] 2008	27	250 mg daily	DTC, MTC ATC	SD 12%
Temsirolimus and sorafenib	Phase 2	NCT01025453[53]	Ongoing (n≈37)	Temsirolimus 25 IV weekly; sorafenib 200 mg bid	DTC, MTC, ATC	PR 22%, SD 57%
Multi-kinase inhibitor						
Imatinib	Phase 2	Ha et al,[100] 2010	11	400 mg bid	ATC	PR 18%, SD 36%
Pazopanib	Phase 2	Bible et al,[31] 2012	15	800 mg once daily	ATC	PD 80%
Pazopanib	Phase 2	NCT00625846[61]	Ongoing	800 mg once daily	DTC, MTC, ATC	—
Sorafenib	Open label, retrospective	Capdevila et al,[67] 2012	34	400 mg bid	DTC, MTC, ATC	PR 32%, SD 41%
Sorafenib	Phase 2	Savvides et al,[101] 2013	20	400 mg bid	ATC	PR 10%, SD 25%
Sorafenib	Phase 2	Nagaiah et al,[102] 2009	16	400 mg bid	ATC	PR 13%, SD 27%
Angiogenesis inhibitors						
Combretastatin A4	Phase 2	NCT00060242[103]	Ongoing	—	ATC	—
Combretastatin A4	Phase 2	Cooney et al,[104] 2006	18	—	ATC	SD 18%, PD 66%
Crolibulin and cisplatin	Phase 1, 2	NCT01240590[105]	Ongoing	—	ATC	—
Fosbretabulin	Phase 2	Mooney et al,[106] 2009	26	—	ATC	SD 27%, median survival 12.3 mo
Fosbretabulin, carboplatin, paclitaxel	Phase 2, 3	Sosa et al,[108] 2013 (FACT trial)	80	—	ATC	HR 0.66 (phase 2) HR 0.73 (phase 3)
Fosbretabulin, carboplatin, paclitaxel	Phase 3	NCT01701349[107]	Ongoing	—	ATC	—
DNA methylation inhibitor						
Azacytidine	Phase 1	NCT00004062[85]	Ongoing	—	DTC, MTC, ATC	—

Abbreviations: HR, hazard ratio; IV, intravenous; PD, progressive disease; PR, partial response; RECIST, Response Evaluation Criteria in Solid Tumors; SD, stable disease.

with risk of recurrence and worse recurrence-free survival.[13] Targeted agents against the VEGF receptor and the MAPK pathway (tyrosine kinase inhibitors [TKIs]) are among the most promising thus far.[10]

Therapeutic Agents

Medical therapy for advanced DTC is summarized in **Tables 1–7** according to classes of drugs, mechanism of action/target, available clinical trials, and commonly reported side effects. Briefly, these are also noted as follows.

1. Selective TKIs

   The mechanism of action of small-molecule TKIs is based on the principle that sterically blocking the ATP-binding pocket results in impaired phosphorylation activity, inhibits signal transduction, and prevents activation of intracellular signaling pathways relevant to tumor growth and angiogenesis.[9] Selective TKIs inhibit one step in the signaling pathway, whereas the multiple TKIs inhibit multiple tyrosine kinases in the signaling pathway.

   - RAS inhibition via farnesyltransferase inhibitors (FTI)
     - Tipifarnib
   - BRAF inhibitors
     - Vemurafenib (PLX-4032)
     - Dabrafenib (GSK2118436)
     - XL 281
   - MEK inhibitors
     - Trametinib
     - Selumetinib (AZD6244, ARRY 142886)
   - mTOR inhibitors
     - Everolimus (Afintor)
     - Temsirolimus
   - EGFR inhibitor
     - Gefitinib (Iressa)

Early preclinical studies focused on combining inhibition of the MAPK and PI3K pathways, both to synergize blockade of proliferation pathways as well as to bypass mechanisms of resistance. There are also clinical trials combining selective TKI with multiple TKIs, for example, the phase II studies of temsirolimus and sorafenib.[8] Trametinib is the first FDA-approved MEK inhibitor for use in other solid cancers and is currently in trials for thyroid cancer. Refer to **Table 5** for individual responses to therapy as well as clinical trial information.

2. Multi-TKIs

   Several multi-TKIs have entered clinical trials for patients with advanced or progressing metastatic thyroid cancers.[14–18] Because of the similarity between RET and VEGF receptor kinases, most TKIs affect both. Many of the commercially available multi-TKIs have similar targets and mechanisms of action as well as similar therapeutic and toxicity profiles.[2]

   Multi-targeted kinase inhibitors used in clinical trials for patients with advanced DTC

   - Motesanib
   - Sorafenib (Nexavar)
   - Sunitinib (Sutent)
   - Vandetanib (Caprelsa)
   - Axitinib (AG013736, Inlyta)
   - Pazopanib (Votrient)

Table 8
Common side effects of targeted medical therapies for thyroid cancer

Drugs	Dermatologic Change	Gastrointestinal Effects	Fatigue	HTN	Cardiac Effects	Mucositis	Hematologic Effects	Other
Cabozantinib	Palmar erythema, skin infection	Nausea, vomiting, diarrhea, anorexia	x	x	–	x	–	Elevated LFTs, headache, electrolyte imbalance
Fosbretabulin	–	–	–	–	QTC prolonged	–	Leukopenia, lymphopenia	Headache
Pazopanib	–	–	–	x	–	x	–	Headache, elevated LFTs
Dabrafenib	Hand-foot syndrome, papilloma, alopecia, rash	Constipation	–	–	–	–	–	Headache, pyrexia, arthralgia, myalgia, flulike symptoms
Imatinib	Rash	Diarrhea, nausea	–	–	–	–	–	Laryngeal edema
Valproic acid	–	–	–	–	–	–	Thrombocytopenia	Liver impairment, pancreatic dysfunction, renal dysfunction
Selumetinib	Rash	Diarrhea	x	–	–	–	–	Peripheral edema
Bortezomib	–	Melena	–	–	–	–	Neutropenia, leukopenia, thrombocytopenia	Peripheral neuropathy
Lenvatinib	–	Diarrhea	x	x	–	–	–	Proteinuria, weight loss
Tipifarnib	Rash	Diarrhea	–	x	–	–	–	Increase in amylase/lipase
Temsirolimus	Rash	Nausea, loss of appetite	x	–	–	x	Anemia, lymphopenia	Increase in blood sugar levels, cholesterol and liver enzymes

Thalidomide	–	Constipation	–	–	–	–	–	Somnolence, peripheral neuropathy, dizziness	Weight loss, electrolyte imbalance
Sorafenib	Squamous cell cancer, keratoacanthomas, Hand-foot syndrome, rash, alopecia	Diarrhea	x	MI, CHF	x	Leukopenia, thrombocytopenia	–	–	–
Vemurafenib	Rash, pruritus, photosensitivity	Nausea	x	–	–	–	–	–	–
XL 281	Squamous cell cancer, keratoacanthomas	Nausea, vomiting, Diarrhea	–	–	–	–	–	–	–
Motesanib	–	Nausea, diarrhea	x	–	–	–	–	–	–
Sunitinib	Hand-foot syndrome	Diarrhea, GI bleed	x	Atrial fibrillation	x	Leukopenia, neutropenia, thrombocytopenia	–	–	–
Vandetanib	Rash, photosensitivity	Diarrhea, nausea	x	QT prolonged	–	–	–	–	–
Axitinib	–	Diarrhea, nausea	x	–	x	–	–	–	–
Gefitinib	Exanthema, acne, pruritus	Nausea, vomiting, diarrhea, anorexia	–	–	–	–	–	–	–
Romidepsin	–	–	–	Cardiac toxicity, sudden death, pulmonary embolism	–	–	–	–	–

Abbreviations: CHF, congestive heart failure; GI, gastrointestinal; HTN, hypertension; LFT, liver function tests; MI, myocardial infarction.

- Imatinib (Gleevac)
- Cabozantinib (XL 184, Exelixis, Cometriq)
- Lenvantinib (E7080)

One of the largest international trials done thus far in patients with DTC, and still ongoing, is the DECISION trial with 417 patients using sorafenib. Findings from this trial were presented at the 2013 annual meeting of the American Society of Clinical Oncology (ASCO 2013). The findings included a hazard ratio (HR) of 0.58 (confidence interval [CI] 95% and $P<.0001$) with a progression-free survival (PFS) of 10.8 months (sorafenib) versus 5.8 months (placebo).[15,16] In November 2013, the FDA issued approval for the use of sorafenib to treat progressive, advanced thyroid cancer.

Another multi-TKI showing a lot of promise in RAI refractory DTC is lenvatinib or E7080. Here too, preliminary results were highlighted at the annual meeting of the ASCO in 2011. A phase II trial of the effects of lenvatinib on RAI refractory DTC at that time revealed a response rate (RR) of 50% and median PFS of 12.6 months. This trial then progressed to a phase III trial, where the study is ongoing. Currently, the phase II study is completed, and phase III is closed to enrollment.[17,18] Please refer to **Table 5**.

The general toxicity profile for these agents includes multiorgan effects: cardiovascular (hypertension, QT prolongation, instances of torsades with vandetanib, congestive heart failure); renal (proteinuria), hepatic (elevated liver enzymes); hematologic (bone marrow suppression, thrombosis, tumor-related hemorrhage); and dermatologic (hand, foot, skin reactions; keratoacanthoma-type squamous cell carcinomas).[2] Please refer to **Table 8**.

Of interest, a recent study compared the effect of 4 TKIs (axitinib, sunitinib, vandetanib, and XL184) on cell proliferation, RET expression and autophosphorylation, and ERK activation in cell lines with MEN2A, MEN 2B, and RET/PTC mutations. Cabozantinib and vandetanib most effectively inhibited cell proliferation and RET autophosphorylation. XL184 was the most potent inhibitor in MEN2A and PTC, and vandetanib was the most effective in MEN2B in vitro.[19]

3. Proteasome inhibitors
    - Bortezomib is a first-in-class reversible inhibitor of the 26S proteasome, which leads to apoptosis through multiple mechanisms. It is approved by the FDA for the treatment of multiple myeloma and relapsed mantle cell lymphoma.[20] It is currently in trials for use either alone or in combination with multi-TKIs to treat thyroid cancer. Successful combinations have been noted in vitro with sunitinib or sorafenib.[21]
4. Angiogenesis inhibitors
    Beyond direct inhibitors of angiogenic kinases, such as VEGFR (as seen earlier), other drugs are capable of either inhibiting angiogenesis or disrupt existing tumor vasculature.
    Drugs used in clinical trials for DTC
    - Thalidomide
    - Lenalidomide (less toxic than thalidomide)
5. Inhibition of hypoxia-induced angiogenesis via cyclooxygenase 2 (COX 2) inhibition. This lacks efficacy and presents concerns about cardiovascular toxicity.[5]
    - Celecoxib
6. Target against epigenetic mechanisms
    DNA hypermethylation and histone deacetylation are 2 common epigenetic mechanisms that have been implicated in the progression of thyroid carcinoma, particularly the loss of radioiodine avidity.

- Inhibitors of histone deacetylases used in clinical trials for DTC
  - Romidepsin
  - Vorinostat
  - Valproic acid
- Inhibitors of DNA methylation
  - Azacytidine
  - Decitabine

7. Improving radioiodine uptake

As DTC becomes dedifferentiated or poorly differentiated, follicular cells lose the ability to transport iodine within the cell, which becomes RAI insensitive. Novel therapies have been developed to restore radioiodine uptake in cells:

- Retinoic acid increased uptake in about 26% to 40% of patients.[16]
- Rosiglitazone, a PPARγ agonist (also activates PTEN, which inhibits the PI3K pathway), increased radioiodine uptake in 26% to 40% of patients with DTC in a small study.[22]
- Selumetinib: The first report of efficacy of this agent for DTC was in 2013, as shown in **Table 5**.

8. Chemotherapy agents

Several cytotoxic chemotherapy drugs have been tested in clinical trials but have shown relatively poor response rates. For instance, doxorubicin as a single agent had a response rate of about 17% and, in combination with cisplatin, had variable response rates of 9% to 26%.[23] The more common conventional cytotoxic chemotherapeutic drugs historically used in advanced DTC are as follows:

- Doxorubicin
- Cisplatin
- 5-FU
- Capecitabine

MEDICAL THERAPY FOR ADVANCED MTC

MTC accounts for approximately 4% to 5% of all thyroid malignancies. The sporadic form of MTC occurs in about 75% of patients with MTC, whereas 25% of patients have the hereditary form. It is derived from the parafollicular or C cells of the thyroid gland that compose 1% to 3% of cells in the thyroid and are primarily concentrated in the upper posterior one-third of each lobe of the thyroid gland. C cells do not express the sodium-iodide symporter and, thus, do not concentrate radioiodine.[24] The neural crest origin is responsible for the amine precursor uptake and decarboxylating activity of MTC and its ability to secrete neurohumoral peptides, including calcitonin, carcinoembryonic antigen (CEA), serotonin, adrenocorticotrophic stimulating hormone, chromogranin A, somatostatin, neurotensin, pro-opiomelanocortin, prostaglandins, kinins, histaminase, and vasoactive intestinal peptide.[24]

In contrast to DTC, MTC is more aggressive than DTC and manifests higher rate of recurrence and mortality. It commonly metastasizes to cervical lymph nodes and cure of the disease depends on resection of lymph node metastases.[24] The management of MTC, therefore, has depended highly on surgery for both primary and regional disease, as RAI and thyroxine suppression cannot be used in this tumor of neuroendocrine origin.[5]

The prognosis of MTC is directly associated with the age at the diagnosis. Although early diagnosis and treatment is associated with a favorable outcome (5-year and 15-year survival rates of 95% and 86%, respectively), a late diagnosis is associated with a reduced 5-year survival rate to 40% or less in patients with locally advanced or metastatic disease. The aggressiveness of MTC can be predicted by the presence of certain RET mutations and the levels of calcitonin and CEA. The loss of calcitonin expression with high CEA levels or a rapid CEA and/or calcitonin doubling time are markers of poorly differentiated and progressive disease.[25,26]

Targets and Mechanisms

Activating point mutations in the RET gene has been noted primarily in MTC.[24] The intracellular domain of the RET receptor contains 2 tyrosine kinase regions that activate intracellular signal transduction pathways. RET activation triggers autophosphorylation of tyrosine residues, that serve as docking sites for adaptor proteins, which coordinate cellular signal transduction pathways (eg, MAPK pathway, PI3K pathway, Jun N-terminal kinase, extracellular signal-regulated protein kinase), which are important in the regulation of cell growth.[27]

Activating mutations of the tyrosine kinase receptor RET have been reported in nearly all hereditary cases of MTC and in 30% to 50 % of sporadic tumor cases.[19] In sporadic MTC, 10% of patients have a de novo RET germline mutation, and 25% to 40% of patients develop somatic mutations,[28] thus, occurring later in life. The somatic mutation (especially the M918T mutation) is associated with more aggressive disease characterized by lymph node metastases, persistent disease, and lower overall survival.

Because of the activation of RET mutations, the PI3K/AKT/mTOR intracellular signaling pathway is functionally active resulting in cellular growth and proliferation. In RET-negative patients with sporadic MTC, there is a predominance of activating point mutations in H-RAS and K-RAS.[26] VEGF-A, VEGFR1, and VEGFR2 receptors are overexpressed in 90% of patients with MTC. VEGFR2 has been implicated with tumor growth and metastases and plays a role in cell proliferation, migration, survival, and induction of neovascularization. Thirteen percent of primary MTC tumors overexpress EGFR. MTC also exhibits somatostatin receptors.[27]

Therapeutic Agents

Targeted therapies, such as TKIs, offer a treatment option to patients with metastatic, unresectable MTC. Vandetanib and cabozantinib are currently the only FDA-approved TKIs for MTC. However, similar to DTC, several commercially available drugs are being used in clinical practice in patients who are intolerant to the FDA-approved drugs or who have progressed on these agents (sorafenib, sunitinib, and pazopanib); additional medications are being studied in clinical trials.[2]

Classes of drugs tested in MTC

1. Selective TKIs
   - RAS inhibition via FTI
     ○ Tipifarnib
   - RET-activated thyroid cancer inhibition via JAK inhibitor[29]
     ○ AZD 1480
   - mTOR inhibitor
     ○ Everolimus
   - EGFR inhibitor
     ○ Gefitinib
2. Multi-targeted TKIs
   - Axitinib
   - Cabozantinib (FDA approved for MTC, 2012)
   - Imatinib
   - Motesanib

- Ponatinib
- Sorafenib
- Sunitinib
- Vandetanib (FDA approved for MTC 2011)[30]
3. Somatostatin analogue
   - Pasireotide
   - Pentetreotide
4. Proteasome inhibitor
   - Bortezomib
5. Angiogenesis inhibitors
   - Thalidomide
6. Conventional chemotherapeutic agents
   - Doxorubicin
   - 5-FU, capecitabine
   - Streptozocin
   - Dacarbazine

MEDICAL THERAPY FOR ATC

ATC is among the most deadly of all human malignancies, with an overall incidence worldwide of 1 to 2 cases per million.[24] ATC is a follicular cell-derived tumor that arises from dedifferentiation of DTC or de novo from normal thyroid tissue, which rapidly loses its normal differentiation. ATC does not retain any of the functional characteristics of the follicular cell, including synthesis of thyroglobulin (Tg) and radioiodine uptake.[24] The historical median overall survival, regardless of stage, is only about 5 to 6 months from diagnosis and less than 20% 1-year survival.[31] Approximately 10% of patients with ATC present with only an intrathyroidal tumor, whereas 40% have extrathyroidal invasion and/or lymph node metastasis, with the remainder of patients presenting with widely metastatic disease.[32] All patients with ATC are classified as stage IV, with the primary lesion restricted to the thyroid gland in stage IVA; locoregional lymph nodes may exist in IVA/IVB, and stage IVC disease is defined by distant metastases. Good prognostic factors of ATC include age less than 60 years, size of tumor less than 7 cm, and less extensive disease on presentation.[31]

Targets and Mechanisms

Our understanding of the molecular pathogenesis of ATC has included mutations in ATC include AXIN1, TP53 (tumor protein 53) (59%–55%), CTNNB1 (38%), and BRAF (26%).[33] Other mutations were noted in RAS, PIK3CA, PTEN, and APC. PI3K catalytic subunit (PIK3CA) mutations were found to be more common in ATC compared with DTC, and this pathway was activated (pAkt) in the aggressive tumors.[33] Furthermore, 35% of the tumors with PIK3CA mutations also had BRAF mutations, and 30% of these tumors had both PIK3CA and Ras mutations.[6]

Activation of the MAPK pathway is commonly found in ATC. The BRAF V600E mutation is also present in 20% to 30% of patients with ATC. Some researchers suggest that this mutation may be restricted to ATC where the well-differentiated PTC counterpart is present.[8,9]

Therapeutic Agents

Even though there is no standard therapy for ATC, multimodality treatment (ie, surgery, chemotherapy, and radiotherapy) is generally recommended for ATC. Some studies have suggested an improvement in survival for patients treated in such an aggressive manner.[34] This finding is especially so for patients with stage IVA disease. The role of targeted agents in this patient population has yet to be established, although some reports suggest benefit.[35]

Several cytotoxic chemotherapy agents have shown modest antitumor activity in ATC including taxanes, combretastatin family members, and anthracyclines, namely, doxorubicin. In vitro studies of differing therapies revealed imatinib and docetaxel induced apoptosis in ATC cell lines.[34] However, clinical response rates to cytotoxic chemotherapy are low and typically short-lived.[31] Approximately 30% of patients achieve a partial remission with doxorubicin. Combination therapies in small clinical trials have demonstrated improved tumor responses but with added toxicity, as summarized by Wein and colleagues[34]: Doxorubicin plus cisplatin versus doxorubicin alone produced more complete responses and a decreased tumor volume up to 50.7%.

Targeted agents that have been suggested in ATC

- Selective TKIs
  - BRAF inhibitor
    - XL 281
  - RAS inhibitors
    - AAL881, LBT – 613
- Multi-kinase TKIs
  - Axitinib
  - Imatinib
  - Sorafenib
- Angiogenesis inhibitors, tubulin inhibitors
  - Fosbretabulin
  - Combretastatin 4A phosphate
  - Crolibulin
- Proteasome inhibitors
  - Bortezomib (in ATC cell lines)
- Histone deacetylase inhibitors
  - Valproic acid
- Chemotherapeutic agents
  - Doxorubicin
  - Cisplatin
  - Carboplatin
  - Docetaxel
  - Paclitaxel

The largest prospective, randomized, multicenter, open-label trial conducted in metastatic ATC evaluated the therapeutic role of combretastatin-A4 (Fosbretabulin), which is a novel vascular disrupting agent able to block neoangiogenesis. Eighty patients were randomized to receive up to 6 cycles of carboplatin and paclitaxel with CA4P (CP/fosbretabulin) or without CA4P (control arm or the CP arm). Median OS was 5.2 months (95% CI) for the CP/fosbretabulin arm and 4.0 months (95% CI) for the CP arm, $P = .22$. HR was 0.73 (95% CI). One-year survival for CP/fosbretabulin versus CP was 26% versus 9%, respectively.[35,36]

INNOVATIVE STUDIES IN PROSPECTIVE DRUGS
Advanced DTC and MTC

- Dasatinib is a new Src family kinase (SFK) inhibitor and is a multifunctional non-RTK family inhibitor that regulates a variety of cellular processes, including growth, survival, migration, and invasion, via activation of downstream signaling pathways, including MAPK/ERK, PI3K, Stat3, p130Cas, paxillin, and focal adhesion kinase (FAK). Elevated levels of phospho-SFK and FAK are present in thyroid cancer cell lines leading to the rationale for investigating this drug.[36]

- AZD 1480 is a RET inhibitor and JAK 1,2 inhibitor. AZD1480 can block the growth and induce cell death of thyroid cancer cell lines harboring distinct forms of oncogenic RET in vitro and in vivo. In these cells, AZD1480 likely inhibits RET directly, leading to the blockade of the PI3K/AKT/mTOR pathway, which seems to be the preferential oncogenic force driving RET-activated cells.[29] AZD 1480 is being studied with both PTC and MTC cell lines.
- Ponatinib is an oral multi-TKI that potently inhibits BCR-ABL and additional protein tyrosine kinases, including SRC-related kinases, and members of the III/IV/V tyrosine kinase receptor classes, such as FLT3 (fms-related tyrosine kinase 3), KIT, fibroblast growth factor receptor 1, PDGFR, and VEGFR-2/KDR. Ponatinib has been tested on MTC cell lines.[37]

ATC

- Aurora kinase inhibitors are proteins implicated in the regulation of multiple aspects of chromosome segregation during the mitotic phase of the cell cycle. They are overexpressed in many human thyroid tissues, and their degradation at the end of mitosis is determined by the ubiquitin-proteasome pathway. Examples of these inhibitors are MLN8054, VX680, and AZD1152.
- In vitro testing has shown that the administration of MLN8054 resulted in an increase of apoptotic cells, decreased histone H3 phosphorylation, and induced cell cycle arrest. In vivo, treatment of ATC by MLN8054 resulted in an up to 86% reduced tumor volume and 89% reduced tumor vascularity.[38]
- Chrysin demonstrated inhibition of cell growth by activation of the Notch1 signaling pathway in ATC cells both in vitro and in vivo.[32]
- 17AAG/tanespimycin is a heat shock protein (HSP90) inhibitor. HSP90 is a molecular chaperone that stabilizes growth factor receptors and signaling molecules. Disruption of this action inhibits the MAPK and PI3K cascades and can induce cancer cell death. Anaplastic and follicular cell lines were sensitive to 17AAG.[38]

ALGORITHM FOR MANAGEMENT: TARGETED THERAPY FOR THYROID CANCER
Advanced DTC

Clinical trials are suggested as a best first step in advising further therapy for patients with metastatic or advanced disease. Specifically, systemic medical therapy in the context of a clinical trial is indicated for patients with rapidly progressive or symptomatic metastatic/unresectable RAI-refractory disease. For patients who are not eligible for participation in a clinical trial but are candidates for systemic therapy, off-label treatment with drugs, such as sunitinib, sorafenib, and pazopanib, may be considered.[39,40] Sorafenib recently became FDA approved for advanced, progressive states of DTC.

MTC

Patients with metastatic, unresectable MTC must be accurately characterized concerning all clinical prognostic indicators, including age, performance status, histology, disease extent, location, and progression rate. In patients with metastatic MTC that is asymptomatic and stable for long periods (usually 6–12 months), the benefits of novel therapies may be largely outweighed by drug toxicities and the rigors of clinical trial participation.[41]

Also, because there is no evidence that the efficacy of these novel therapies is higher at an early stage, treatment can be postponed in most patients until symptomatic or radiographic disease progression.[41] All other options of interventions for local control (excision, ablation, and embolization) should be considered before initiation of any systemic treatment.

Diagnostic procedures in patients with advanced MTC should include spiral computed tomographic scanning or magnetic resonance imaging of the brain, ultrasonography of the neck, contrast-enhanced spiral computed tomographic scanning of the neck and chest, triple-phase computed tomographic scanning or preferably magnetic resonance imaging of the liver (because liver metastases may be difficult to visualize with computed tomography during antiangiogenic treatment), bone scintigraphy, and magnetic resonance imaging of the spine and pelvis. Fluorodeoxyglucose uptake on positron emission tomography scanning is usually associated with low sensitivity in MTC.[40,42,43]

Candidates for systemic medical therapy are patients with symptomatic, advanced, measurable, and unresectable disease that cannot be alleviated with surgery or external beam radiation. Again, the starting preference is to advise participation in a clinical trial. If patients are unable to participate in the trial, the next treatment options are cabozantinib or vandetanib (FDA approved) or, alternatively, off-label treatment with sunitinib or sorafenib based on available clinical trial data. To determine patient eligibility, the progression rate can also be evaluated by doubling times of serum markers, calcitonin, and CEA levels; but progression should always be confirmed by imaging.[41]

ATC

When possible, surgical en bloc excision should be performed initially with postoperative chemoradiation therapy given subsequently depending on overall outcome. In fact, following essentially all surgery (for R0, R1, selected R2, and unresectable disease), radiation therapy with or without chemotherapy is advised for those patients with good performance status and desiring an aggressive strategy.[43] It is safe to commence radiation therapy (with or without chemotherapy) as early as 2 to 3 weeks after surgery. Following definitive radiation therapy (with or without chemotherapy) in patients with previously unresectable disease, the recommendation is to reconsider the patients for surgical extirpation if feasible. Commonly used chemotherapy regimens for concurrent chemoradiation include anthracyclines, taxanes, and platinum agents. Patients with stage IVC disease should be offered participation in a clinical trial if available. Otherwise, these patients may be offered palliative systemic therapy with cytotoxic chemotherapy as single agents or in combination. Frequently used chemotherapy treatments include taxanes, platinums, and anthracyclines. At all times, palliative care and hospice should be considered as an alternative.[44,45]

EFFICACY OF MEDICAL THERAPY FOR ADVANCED THYROID CANCER

In clinical trials that have been performed on patients with advanced thyroid cancer thus far, very few complete responses (CRs) to therapy have been achieved. Most clinical trials have used the RECIST (Response Evaluation Criteria in Solid Tumors) criteria to evaluate the response to these targeted therapies. At baseline, up to 5 target lesions are selected, and the sum of the longest diameters (SLD) is calculated (the short axis is used for lymph node metastases in RECIST). A CR indicates the disappearance of all sites of disease. A partial response (PR) indicates at least a 30% decrease in the SLD. Progressive disease is determined by at least 20% growth of the SLD. Stable disease (SD) includes changes between 20% growth and 30% decrease in the SLD. Durable response is evaluated as SD or PR for at least 6 months; and the clinical benefit is SD plus PR.[3] Additional outcome metrics include PFS with HR. HR is the effect of the variable (treatment/medication) on the hazard or risk of mortality in thyroid cancer: An HR of 1 implies the same as having no treatment. An HR greater than 1 implies that the treatment caused harm. An HR less than 1 implies a treatment benefit.

The overall PR in trials with DTC has ranged between 4.5% and 49.0%, as seen in **Table 5**. Commercially available drugs include sorafenib, sunitinib, and pazopanib. **Table 6** shows that most drugs used thus far in patients with MTC resulted in a good response, with PR ranging between 2% and 68% and SD between 12% and 83%. Kurzrock and colleagues[88] reported in 2011 that cabozantinib, in a phase I trial with 37 patients, achieved 68% PR (see **Table 6**).[89] FDA-approved drugs are vandetanib and cabozantinib. In ATC, PR has ranged between 10% and 32% (see **Table 7**), with better responses seen in patients on sorafenib and temsirolimus or sorafenib alone. The SD rates have varied between 12% and 57%, with good responses noted in sorafenib, temsirolimus, and imatinib. Many current trials are actively recruiting patients with ATC, including a trial using fosbretabulin. Sosa and colleagues reported HRs of 0.66 and 0.73, respectively, from a phase II and III trial of fosbretabulin in combination with chemotherapeutic agents (see **Table 7**).[108]

SUMMARY

More options than ever before are currently available for medical therapy in patients who present with advanced thyroid cancer or develop surgically unresectable recurrences or symptomatic or progressive disease. The newer medical therapies have addressed the need to find effective therapies beyond the conventional treatment with RAI, TSH suppression, and palliative cytotoxic chemotherapy for patients with advanced thyroid cancer. Modern targeted therapies evolved from an understanding of cellular signaling pathways, angiogenesis, cellular mechanisms of division, and epigenetic events in thyroid cancer. The main pathways involved as targets for these drugs include the MAPK pathway, the PI3K pathway, and angiogenesis via VEGFR, PDGFR, and FLT3 receptors. Current medical therapies are classified by their mechanism of action or inhibition related to these and other cellular pathways. Although tumor responses to these medical therapies vary by type of thyroid cancer and type of therapy selected, they remain encouraging and provide therapeutic options for selected patients while new drugs are in development.

REFERENCES

1. Howlader N, Noone AM, Krapcho M, et al. SEER cancer statistics review, 1975-2010. Bethesda (MD): National Cancer Institute; 2013. Available at: http://seer.cancer.gov/csr/1975_2010/. based on November 2012 SEER data submission. Posted to the SEER Web site, 2013.
2. Carhill AA, Cabanillas ME, Jimenez C, et al. The noninvestigational use of tyrosine kinase inhibitors in thyroid cancer: establishing a standard for patient safety and monitoring. J Clin Endocrinol Metab 2013;98(1):31–42.
3. Cabanillas ME, Waguespack SG, Bronstein Y, et al. Treatment with tyrosine kinase inhibitors for patients with differentiated thyroid cancer: the M. D. Anderson experience. J Clin Endocrinol Metab 2010;95(6):2588–95.

4. Durante C, Haddy N, Baudin E, et al. Long-term outcome of 444 patients with distant metastases from papillary and follicular thyroid carcinoma: benefits and limits of radioiodine therapy. J Clin Endocrinol Metab 2006;91(8): 2892–9.

5. Sherman SI. Targeted therapy of thyroid cancer. Biochem Pharmacol 2010; 80(5):592–601.

6. Leeper RD, Shimaoka K. Treatment of metastatic thyroid cancer. Clin Endocrinol Metab 1980;9(2):383–404.

7. Gild ML, Bullock M, Robinson BG, et al. Multikinase inhibitors: a new option for the treatment of thyroid cancer. Nat Rev Endocrinol 2011;7:617–24.

8. Haugen BR, Sherman SI. Evolving approaches to patients with advanced differentiated thyroid cancer. Endocr Rev 2013;34(3):439–55.

9. Couto PJ, Prazeres H, Castro P, et al. How molecular pathology is changing and will change the therapeutics of patients with follicular cell-derived thyroid cancer. J Clin Pathol 2009;62(5):414–21.

10. Giuffrida D, Prestifilippo A, Scarfia A, et al. New treatment in advanced thyroid cancer. J Oncol 2012;2012:391629.

11. Chang YS, Lin IL, Yeh KT, et al. Rapid detection of K-, N-, H-RAS, and BRAF hotspot mutations in thyroid cancer using the multiplex primer extension. Clin Biochem 2013;46(15):1572–7.

12. Elisei R, Viola D, Torregrossa L, et al. The BRAF (V600E) mutation is an independent, poor prognostic factor for the outcome of patients with low-risk intrathyroid papillary thyroid carcinoma: single-institution results from a large cohort study. J Clin Endocrinol Metab 2012;97(12):4390–8.

13. Cohen EE, Rosen LS, Vokes EE, et al. Axitinib is an active treatment for all histologic subtypes of advanced thyroid cancer: results from a phase II study. J Clin Oncol 2008;26(29):4708–13.

14. Cabanillas ME, Hu MI, Durand JB, et al. Challenges associated with tyrosine kinase inhibitor therapy for metastatic thyroid cancer. J Thyroid Res 2011;2011: 985780.

15. DECISION trial Nexavar® versus placebo in locally advanced/metastatic RAI-refractory differentiated thyroid cancer. Available at: ClinicalTrials.gov.

16. Brose MS, Nutting C, Jarzab B. Sorafenib in locally advanced or metastatic patients with radioactive iodine-refractory differentiated thyroid cancer: the phase III DECISION trial. J Clin Oncol 2013;31S(4).

17. A multicenter, randomized, double-blind, placebo-controlled, phase 3 trial of lenvatinib (E7080) in 131I-refractory differentiated thyroid cancer. Available at: ClinicalTrials.gov.

18. Sherman SI, Jarzab B, Cabanillas ME, et al. A phase II trial of the multitargeted kinase inhibitor E7080 in advanced radioiodine (RAI)-refractory differentiated thyroid cancer (DTC). J Clin Oncol 2011;29(15S):5503.

19. Fallahi P, Ferrari SM, Santini F, et al. Sorafenib and thyroid cancer. BioDrugs 2013;27(6):615–28.

20. Harvey RD, Owonikoko TK, Lewis CM, et al. A phase 1 Bayesian dose selection study of bortezomib and sunitinib in patients with refractory solid tumor malignancies. Br J Cancer 2013;108(4):762–5.

21. Putzer D, Gabriel M, Kroiss A, et al. First experience with proteasome inhibitor treatment of radioiodine nonavid thyroid cancer using bortezomib. Clin Nucl Med 2012;37(6):539–44.

22. Kapiteijn E, Schneider TC, Morreau H, et al. New treatment modalities in advanced thyroid cancer. Ann Oncol 2012;23(1):10–8.

23. Argiris A, Agarwala SS, Karamouzis MV, et al. A phase II trial of doxorubicin and interferon alpha 2b in advanced, non-medullary thyroid cancer. Invest New Drugs 2008;26(2):183–8.

24. Jin J, Phitayakorn R, Wilhelm SM, et al. Advances in management of thyroid cancer. Curr Probl Surg 2013;50(6):241–89.

25. Grabowski P, Briest F, Baum RP, et al. Vandetanib therapy in medullary thyroid cancer. Drugs Today (Barc) 2012;48(11):723–33.

26. Almeida MQ, Hoff AO. Recent advances in the molecular pathogenesis and targeted therapies of medullary thyroid carcinoma. Curr Opin Oncol 2012;24(3): 229–34.

27. Antonelli A, Bocci G, La Motta C, et al. Novel pyrazolopyrimidine derivatives as tyrosine kinase inhibitors with antitumoral activity in vitro and in vivo in papillary dedifferentiated thyroid cancer. J Clin Endocrinol Metab 2011;96(2):E288–96.

28. Ciampi R, Romei C, Cosci B, et al. Chromosome 10 and RET gene copy number alterations in hereditary and sporadic medullary thyroid carcinoma. Mol Cell Endocrinol 2012;348(1):176–82.

29. Couto JP, Almeida A, Daly L, et al. AZD1480 blocks growth and tumorigenesis of RET- activated thyroid cancer cell lines. PLoS One 2012;7(10):e46869.

30. Campbell MJ, Seib CD, Gosnell J. Vandetanib and the management of advanced medullary thyroid cancer. Curr Opin Oncol 2013;25(1):39–43.

31. Bible KC, Suman VJ, Menefee ME, et al. A multi-institutional phase 2 trial of pazopanib monotherapy in advanced anaplastic thyroid cancer. J Clin Endocrinol Metab 2012;97(9):3179–84.

32. Granata R, Locati L, Licitra L. Therapeutic strategies in the management of patients with metastatic anaplastic thyroid cancer: review of the current literature. Curr Opin Oncol 2013;25(3):224–8.

33. Kebebew E. Anaplastic thyroid cancer: rare, fatal, and neglected. Surgery 2012; 152(6):1088–9.

34. Wein RO, Weber RS. Anaplastic thyroid carcinoma: palliation or treatment? Curr Opin Otolaryngol Head Neck Surg 2011;19(2):113–8.

35. Deshpande HA, Roman S, Sosa JA. New targeted therapies and other advances in the management of anaplastic thyroid cancer. Curr Opin Oncol 2013;25(1):44–9.

36. Chan CM, Jing X, Pike LA, et al. Targeted inhibition of Src kinase with dasatinib blocks thyroid cancer growth and metastasis. Clin Cancer Res 2012;18(13): 3580–91.

37. De Falco V, Buonocore P, Muthu M, et al. Ponatinib (AP24534) is a novel potent inhibitor of oncogenic RET mutants associated with thyroid cancer. J Clin Endocrinol Metab 2013;98(5):E811–9.

38. Wunderlich A, Roth S, Ramaswamy A, et al. Combined inhibition of cellular pathways as a future therapeutic option in fatal anaplastic thyroid cancer. Endocrine 2012;42(3):637–46.

39. American Thyroid Association (ATA) Guidelines Taskforce on Thyroid Nodules and Differentiated Thyroid Cancer, Cooper DS, Doherty GM, et al. Revised American Thyroid Association management guidelines for patients with thyroid nodules and differentiated thyroid cancer. Thyroid 2009;19(11):1167–214.

40. National Cancer Institute - Clinical trials for treatment of thyroid cancer. Available at: http://www.cancer.gov/clinicaltrials/search/results?protocolsearchid=12047419.

41. Schlumberger M, Massicotte MH, Nascimento CL, et al. Kinase inhibitors for advanced medullary thyroid carcinoma. Clinics (Sao Paulo) 2012;67(Suppl 1): 125–9.

42. American Thyroid Association Guidelines Task Force, Kloos RT, Eng C, et al. Medullary thyroid cancer: management guidelines of the American Thyroid Association. Thyroid 2009;19(6):565–612.

43. Smallridge RC, Ain KB, Asa SL, et al. American Thyroid Association guidelines for management of patients with anaplastic thyroid cancer. Thyroid 2012;22(11): 1104–39.

44. O'Neill JP, Shaha AR. Anaplastic thyroid cancer. Oral Oncol 2013;49(7):702–6.

45. National Cancer Institute - palliative chemotherapy. Available at: http://www.cancer.gov/cancertopics/pdq/treatment/thyroid/HealthProfessional/page7.

46. Dabrafenib with or without trametinib in treating patients with recurrent thyroid cancer. Available at: ClinicalTrials.gov.

47. Everolimus in treating patients with progressive or recurrent, unresectable, or metastatic thyroid cancer. Available at: ClinicalTrials.gov.

48. Everolimus in treating patients with locally advanced or metastatic thyroid cancer. Available at: ClinicalTrials.gov.

49. A trial of pasireotide and everolimus in adult patients with radioiodine-refractory differentiated and medullary thyroid cancer. Available at: ClinicalTrials.gov.

50. Study of everolimus and sorafenib in patients with advanced thyroid cancer who progressed on sorafenib alone. Available at: ClinicalTrials.gov.

51. Pennell NA, Daniels GH, Haddad RI, et al. A phase II study of gefitinib in patients with advanced thyroid cancer. Thyroid 2008;18(3):317–23.

52. Ho AL, Grewal RK, Leboeuf R, et al. Selumetinib-enhanced radioiodine uptake in advanced thyroid cancer. N Engl J Med 2013;368(7):623–32.

53. Combination of temsirolimus and sorafenib in the treatment of radioactive iodine refractory thyroid cancer. Available at: ClinicalTrials.gov.

54. Hong DS, Cabanillas ME, Wheler J, et al. Inhibition of the Ras/Raf/MEK/ERK and RET kinase pathways with the combination of the multikinase inhibitor sorafenib and the farnesyltransferase inhibitor tipifarnib in medullary and differentiated thyroid malignancies. J Clin Endocrinol Metab 2011;96(4): 997–1005.

55. Kim KB, Cabanillas ME, Lazar AJ, et al. Clinical responses to vemurafenib in patients with metastatic papillary thyroid cancer harboring BRAF (V600E) mutation. Thyroid 2013;23(10):1277–83.

56. A study of RO5185426 (vemurafenib) in patients with metastatic or unresectable papillary thyroid cancer positive for the BRAF V600 mutation. Available at: ClinicalTrials.gov.

57. Study of XL281 in adults with solid tumors. Available at: ClinicalTrials.gov.

58. Rosen LS, Kurzrock R, Mulay M, et al. Safety, pharmacokinetics, and efficacy of AMG 706, an oral multikinase inhibitor, in patients with advanced solid tumors. J Clin Oncol 2007;25(17):2369–76.

59. Sherman SI, Wirth LJ, Droz JM, et al. Motesanib diphosphate in progressive differentiated thyroid cancer. N Engl J Med 2008;359(1):31–42.

60. Bible KC, Suman VJ, Molina JR, et al. Efficacy of pazopanib in progressive, radioiodine-refractory, metastatic differentiated thyroid cancers: results of a phase 2 consortium study. Lancet Oncol 2010;11(10):962–72.

61. Pazopanib hydrochloride in treating patients with advanced thyroid cancer. Available at: ClinicalTrials.gov.

62. Gupta-Abramson V, Troxel AB, Nellore A, et al. Phase II trial of sorafenib in advanced thyroid cancer. J Clin Oncol 2008;26(29):4714–9.

63. Kloos RT, Ringel MD, Knopp MV, et al. Phase II trial of sorafenib in metastatic thyroid cancer. J Clin Oncol 2009;27(10):1675–84.

64. Hoftijzer H, Heemstra KA, Morreau H, et al. Beneficial effects of sorafenib on tumor progression, but not on radioiodine uptake, in patients with differentiated thyroid carcinoma. Eur J Endocrinol 2009;161(6):923–31.
65. Nexavar® versus placebo in locally advanced/metastatic RAI-refractory differentiated thyroid cancer. Available at: ClinicalTrials.gov.
66. Ahmed M, Barbachano Y, Riddell A, et al. Analysis of the efficacy and toxicity of sorafenib in thyroid cancer: a phase II study in a UK based population. Eur J Endocrinol 2011;165(2):315–22.
67. Capdevila J, Iglesias L, Halperin I, et al. Sorafenib in metastatic thyroid cancer. Endocr Relat Cancer 2012;19(2):209–16.
68. Schneider TC, Abdulrahman RM, Corssmit EP, et al. Long-term analysis of the efficacy and tolerability of sorafenib in advanced radio-iodine refractory differentiated thyroid carcinoma: final results of a phase II trial. Eur J Endocrinol 2012;167(5):643–50.
69. Cohen BM, Needles KJ, Cullen SJ, et al. Phase 2 study of sunitinib in refractory thyroid cancer. J Clin Oncol 2008;28(15):6025.
70. Goulart B, Carr L, Martins RG, et al. Phase II study of sunitinib in iodine refractory, well-differentiated thyroid cancer (WDTC) and metastatic medullary thyroid carcinoma (MTC). J Clin Oncol 2008;26(15):6062.
71. Ravaud A, de la Fouchardiere C, Asselineau J, et al. Efficacy of sunitinib in advanced medullary thyroid carcinoma: intermediate results of phase II THYSU. Oncologist 2010;15(2):212–3 [author reply: 214].
72. Carr LL, Mankoff DA, Goulart BH, et al. Phase II study of daily sunitinib in FDG-PET-positive, iodine-refractory differentiated thyroid cancer and metastatic medullary carcinoma of the thyroid with functional imaging correlation. Clin Cancer Res 2010;16(21):5260–8.
73. Leboulleux S, Bastholt L, Krause T, et al. Vandetanib in locally advanced or metastatic differentiated thyroid cancer: a randomised, double-blind, phase 2 trial. Lancet Oncol 2012;13(9):897–905.
74. Bortezomib in treating patients with metastatic thyroid cancer that did not respond to radioactive iodine therapy. Available at: ClinicalTrials.gov.
75. Cediranib maleate with or without lenalidomide in treating patients with thyroid cancer. Available at: ClinicalTrials.gov.
76. Ain KB, Lee C, Williams KD. Phase II trial of thalidomide for therapy of radioiodine-unresponsive and rapidly progressive thyroid carcinomas. Thyroid 2007;17(7):663–70.
77. Thalidomide in treating patients with thyroid cancer. Available at: ClinicalTrials.gov.
78. Mrozek E, Kloos RT, Ringel MD, et al. Phase II study of celecoxib in metastatic differentiated thyroid carcinoma. J Clin Endocrinol Metab 2006;91(6):2201–4.
79. Piekarz R, Luchenko L, Draper D, et al. Phase I trial of romidepsin, a histone deacetylase inhibitor, given on days one, three and five in patients with thyroid and other advanced cancers. J Clin Oncol 2008;26(15S):3571.
80. Amiri-Kordestani L, Luchenko V, Peer CJ, et al. Phase I trial of a new schedule of romidepsin in patients with advanced cancers. Clin Cancer Res 2013;19(16):4499–507.
81. Sherman EJ, Su YB, Lyall A, et al. Evaluation of romidepsin for clinical activity and radioactive iodine reuptake in radioactive iodine-refractory thyroid carcinoma. Thyroid 2013;23(5):593–9.
82. Romidepsin in treating patients with recurrent and/or metastatic thyroid cancer that has not responded to radioactive iodine. Available at: ClinicalTrials.gov.

83. A phase II trial of valproic acid in patients with advanced thyroid cancers of follicular cell origin. Available at: ClinicalTrials.gov.
84. Woyach JA, Kloos RT, Ringel MD, et al. Lack of therapeutic effect of the histone deacetylase inhibitor vorinostat in patients with metastatic radioiodine-refractory thyroid carcinoma. J Clin Endocrinol Metab 2009;94(1):164–70.
85. Azacitidine to restore thyroid function in patients with persistent or metastatic thyroid cancer. Available at: ClinicalTrials.gov.
86. Decitabine in treating patients with metastatic papillary thyroid cancer or follicular thyroid cancer unresponsive to iodine I 131. Available at: ClinicalTrials.gov.
87. SOM230 alone or in combination with RAD001 in patients with medullary thyroid cancer. Available at: ClinicalTrials.gov.
88. Kurzrock R, Sherman SI, Ball DW, et al. Activity of XL184 (cabozantinib), an oral tyrosine kinase inhibitor, in patients with medullary thyroid cancer. J Clin Oncol 2011;29(19):2660–6.
89. Schoffski P, Elisei R, Muller S, et al. An international, double-blind, randomized, placebo-controlled Phase III trial (EXAM) of cabozantinib (XL184) in medullary thyroid carcinoma (MTC) patients (pts) with documented RECIST progression at baseline. J Clin Oncol 2012;30S:5508.
90. Frank-Raue K, Fabel M, Delorme S, et al. Efficacy of imatinib mesylate in advanced medullary thyroid carcinoma. Eur J Endocrinol 2007;157(2):215–20.
91. Imatinib in combination with dacarbazine and capecitabine in medullary thyroid carcinoma. Available at: ClinicalTrials.gov.
92. Schlumberger M. A phase II trial of the multitargeted kinase inhibitor lenvatinib (E7080) in advanced medullary thyroid cancer (MTC). J Clin Oncol 2012;30S [abstract: 5591].
93. Schlumberger MJ, Elisei R, Bastholt L, et al. Phase II study of safety and efficacy of motesanib in patients with progressive or symptomatic, advanced or metastatic medullary thyroid cancer. J Clin Oncol 2009;27(23):3794–801.
94. Ponatinib for advanced medullary thyroid cancer. Available at: ClinicalTrials.gov.
95. Lam ET, Ringel MD, Kloos RT, et al. Phase II clinical trial of sorafenib in metastatic medullary thyroid cancer. J Clin Oncol 2010;28(14):2323–30.
96. Sorafenib tosylate in treating patients with metastatic, locally advanced, or recurrent medullary thyroid cancer. Available at: ClinicalTrials.gov.
97. Robinson BG, Paz-Ares L, Krebs A, et al. Vandetanib (100 mg) in patients with locally advanced or metastatic hereditary medullary thyroid cancer. J Clin Endocrinol Metab 2010;95(6):2664–71.
98. Wells SA Jr, Robinson BG, Gagel RF, et al. Vandetanib in patients with locally advanced or metastatic medullary thyroid cancer: a randomized, double-blind phase III trial. J Clin Oncol 2012;30(2):134–41.
99. To compare the effects of two doses of vandetanib in patients with advanced medullary thyroid cancer. Available at: ClinicalTrials.gov.
100. Ha HT, Lee JS, Urba S, et al. A phase II study of imatinib in patients with advanced anaplastic thyroid cancer. Thyroid 2010;20(9):975–80.
101. Savvides P, Nagaiah G, Lavertu P, et al. Phase II trial of sorafenib in patients with advanced anaplastic carcinoma of the thyroid. Thyroid 2013;23(5):600–4.
102. Nagaiah G, Fu P, Wasman JK, et al. Phase II trial of sorafenib (bay 43-9006) in patients with advanced anaplastic carcinoma of the thyroid (ATC). J Clin Oncol 2009;27(Suppl 15). [abstract 6058].
103. Combretastatin A4 phosphate in treating patients with advanced anaplastic thyroid cancer. Available at: ClinicalTrials.gov.

104. Cooney MM, Savvides P, Agarwala S. Phase II study of combretastatin A4 phosphate (CA4P) in patients with advanced anaplastic thyroid carcinoma (ATC). J Clin Oncol 2006;24(18S):5580.

105. A phase i/ii trial of crolibulin (EPC2407) plus cisplatin in adults with solid tumors with a focus on anaplastic thyroid cancer (ATC). Available at: ClinicalTrials.gov.

106. Mooney CJ, Nagaiah G, Fu P, et al. A phase II trial of fosbretabulin in advanced anaplastic thyroid carcinoma and correlation of baseline serum-soluble intracellular adhesion molecule-1 with outcome. Thyroid 2009;19(3):233–40.

107. Fosbretabulin or placebo in combination with carboplatin/paclitaxel in anaplastic thyroid cancer (FACT2). Available at: ClinicalTrials.gov.

108. Sosa JA, Elisei R, Jarzab B, et al. Randomized safety and efficacy study of fosbretabulin with paclitaxel/carboplatin against anaplastic thyroid carcinoma. Thyroid 2014;24(2):232–40.

Controversy Over Radioiodine Ablation In Thyroid Cancer: Who Benefits?

Don C. Yoo, MD[a],*, Richard B. Noto, MD[a], Peter J. Mazzaglia, MD[b]

KEYWORDS

- Thyroid cancer • Radioiodine ablation • RIA • Risk stratification • Overdiagnosis

KEY POINTS

- Since the early 1970s, the incidence of thyroid cancer, mainly papillary, in the United States has almost tripled with unchanged mortality.
- The extent of surgery performed for small thyroid cancers is controversial but only patients who have undergone total thyroidectomy are candidates for radioiodine ablation (RIA).
- RIA in low-risk patients has not been shown to decrease mortality and may not be indicated.
- Intermediate-risk patients may benefit from selective administration of RIA.
- Retrospective data support the use of iodine-131 (I-131) in high-risk patients, resulting in decreased recurrence and improved mortality.
- Lower doses of I-131 have been proven effective for RIA of remnant thyroid tissue after thyroidectomy.

INTRODUCTION

In the United States, the first use of radioactive iodine therapy as an alternative to surgery for toxic goiter was in 1943. Its subsequent use in the treatment of thyroid cancer was documented in 1948 in a patient with hyperthyroidism due to pulmonary metastases.[1] In the 1950s and 1960s, the ability of neoplastic thyroid tissue to concentrate radioactive iodine and cause subsequent destruction was elucidated. Soon there were reports of improved survival in patients suffering with metastatic thyroid cancer who were treated with radioiodine ablation (RIA).[2] Over the last 70 years, the use of RIA in well-differentiated thyroid cancer has evolved and become the standard of care in many cases. The concept of thyroid remnant ablation was introduced in the 1970s[3]

[a] Department of Diagnostic Imaging, Rhode Island Hospital, The Warren Alpert Medical School of Brown University, 593 Eddy Street, Providence, RI 02903, USA; [b] Department of General Surgery, Rhode Island Hospital, The Warren Alpert Medical School of Brown University, 593 Eddy Street, Providence, RI 02903, USA
* Corresponding author.
E-mail address: dyoo@lifespan.org

Surg Clin N Am 94 (2014) 573–586
http://dx.doi.org/10.1016/j.suc.2014.03.004
0039-6109/14/$ – see front matter © 2014 Elsevier Inc. All rights reserved.

and, in an effort to eradicate thyroglobulin production, is now cited as one of the main goals of therapy.[4]

Currently, about 50% of patients diagnosed with thyroid cancer will receive adjuvant RIA.[5] However, there is still considerable controversy about the appropriate role of RIA in thyroid cancer. In the United States, recommendations for appropriate use of RIA come from the organizations American Thyroid Association (ATA) and National Comprehensive Cancer Network (NCCN), with consensus guidelines predominantly based on retrospective cohort studies.[4,6] Until recently, large prospective randomized studies evaluating the use of RIA had not been published. The controversy concerning RIA is complicated by the ever-increasing numbers of small, low-risk thyroid cancers being diagnosed. To better understand some of the controversies, the evolving epidemiology of the disease must be examined.

EPIDEMIOLOGY

The incidence of thyroid cancer in the United States has almost tripled since the early 1970s and nearly doubled during the last decade, especially in women. Thyroid cancer is now the fifth most common cancer in women in the United States.[7] Despite this continued increase in incidence, the mortality rate from thyroid cancer has not significantly changed.[7] The 2013 US statistics for thyroid cancer estimate 60,220 new cases (45,310 women and 14,910 men). However, the number of deaths estimated are only 1850 (1040 women and 810 men).[8]

The reasons for such a steep increase in thyroid cancer incidence were not well understood until recently. The study by Chen and colleagues[9] investigated the increasing incidence of differentiated thyroid cancer in the United States from 1988 to 2005 and found the highest rate of increase was for small, localized thyroid cancers. It suggested that the increase was partly due to better cancer detection by ultrasonography and other imaging techniques. They also found an increased incidence across all tumor sizes and suggested that increased diagnostic scrutiny is not the sole explanation. Other possible causes, including environmental influences, should be considered.

Another study by Nikiforov[10] hypothesized that increased exposure to ionizing radiation, a known risk factor, especially for papillary thyroid cancer (PTC), may be playing a role. Historically, increased incidence of papillary thyroid carcinomas have occurred in areas of high radiation exposure. Specific examples include children in the Marshall Islands after atomic bomb testing and in the Ukraine after the Chernobyl nuclear accident.[11,12]

However, ionizing radiation is an unlikely explanation for the marked increase in incidence of thyroid cancer in the United States,[13] where the highest amount of radiation is from background exposure to radon, followed by medical radiation, including CT scans.[13,14] Although there has been increasing attention paid to rising levels of medical radiation, the attributable cancer risk from medical imaging is relatively low and certainly would not be expected to account for a significant component of the rising thyroid cancer incidence.

Another explanation for the explosion of thyroid cancer diagnoses is increased detection during pathologic evaluation of surgical specimens. In a 40-year retrospective study of 2260 thyroidectomies for retrosternal goiter without known history of thyroid cancer, Grodski and colleagues[15] showed that the percentage of thyroid cancer increased from 3.6% to 7.5% over time ($P<.05$). However, once papillary thyroid microcarcinomas (PTMCs), which are defined as small PTCs less than 1 cm by the World Health Organization,[16] were excluded, there was no increase in cancer incidence. The increased incidence of subcentimeter thyroid cancers was attributed to better pathologic evaluation techniques, raising the possibility that the current epidemic of thyroid cancer may be largely manmade.

OVERDIAGNOSIS

Recent studies by Morris and colleagues,[13] Udelsman,[17] and Davies and Welch[5] have proposed that overdiagnosis is probably the principal cause of the increased incidence of thyroid cancer. Morris and colleagues[13] believe that the rapidly rising incidence of PTC is due to overdiagnosis of a reservoir of subclinical disease. This large reservoir of subclinical disease is supported by two independent autopsy studies in normal-appearing thyroid glands that showed that occult PTCs were identified in 33.3% and 35.6% of subjects in Finland and Turkey, respectively.[18,19] Using these prevalence rates, the investigators estimate that between 25 to 100 million Americans currently have occult PTC. If this trend continues, many more occult thyroid cancers will be detected, resulting in many more treatments. Morris and colleagues[13] concluded that the additional treatments resulting from overdiagnosis of these occult thyroid cancers are of no benefit and are potentially harmful. This makes thyroid cancer overdiagnosis a growing public health concern, especially in older Medicare patients where access to health care is abundant.

Udelsman and Zhang[20] report that this epidemic of thyroid cancer is a classic example of "cancer overdiagnosis" in which the diagnosis is made in a silent disease reservoir and treatment is initiated for individuals who are unlikely to develop symptoms or have their life-spans shortened. They evaluated thyroid cancer incidence rates and the densities of endocrinologists, general surgeons, and primary care physicians, as well as the frequencies of neck ultrasonography and thyroid biopsy. They found that the incidence of thyroid cancer correlated with the densities of endocrinologists and surgeons. No significant association between primary care physicians and the incidence rates of thyroid cancer was seen. An association with the frequency of thyroid ultrasounds ordered and thyroid cancer incidence rates was also seen. The study concludes that the growing epidemic of thyroid cancer is due to increased detection of a reservoir of previously occult disease, which results in therapeutic interventions, including surgery and radioactive iodine treatment, that may be of limited benefit.

Davies and Welch[5] also report that the epidemic of thyroid cancer is due to an epidemic of overdiagnosis of PTC, especially PTMC. They report that from 1988 to 1989, when Surveillance, Epidemiology and End Results (SEER) first began collecting data on tumor size, 25% of detected thyroid cancers were PTMCs. However, in the most recent SEER data (2008–2009), 39% were PTMCs. They conclude that the time has come to address the problem of PTC overdiagnosis and overtreatment.

The rapid rise in the number of new cases of thyroid cancer, especially PTMC, is a problem without an easy solution. In 2005, the Society of Radiologists in Ultrasound consensus panel,[21] consisting of specialists in radiology, endocrinology, cytopathology, and surgery, released a statement to help address this issue. One of their main goals was to limit the unnecessary biopsy of small, benign-appearing thyroid nodules. These guidelines evaluated important features of thyroid nodules, such as size, presence of microcalcifications, and solid versus cystic nature. These are summarized in (**Box 1**).

However, when these recommendations were made in 2005, statistics estimated that in the United States 25,690 new cases of thyroid cancer were diagnosed with a mortality of 1460 patients compared with current data that estimate more than 60,000 new cases in 2013.[8,22] Interestingly, in the United States, the incidence of

> **Box 1**
> **Summary of management of thyroid nodules detected at US: Society of Radiologists in Ultrasound consensus conference statement**
>
> 1 cm or larger, highly suspicious nodules with microcalcifications should have biopsy
>
> 1.5 cm or larger, solid nodules or nodules with coarse calcifications should have biopsy
>
> 2 cm or larger, less suspicious mixed, solid, and cystic nodules or cystic nodules with a mural component should have biopsy
>
> Rapidly growing nodules should have biopsy
>
> Routine biopsy of less than 1 cm nodules is not recommended

PTMC is increasing in all age groups but disproportionally so in patients older than 45 years. In fact, in this age group most papillary cancers are less than 1 cm at the time of discovery.[23] This suggests that the nationally published biopsy guidelines are not being routinely followed and that many of these diagnoses are probably made postoperatively.[4,6,21]

EXTENT OF SURGERY

Successful administration of radioiodine requires a total thyroidectomy, which is presently the standard of care for patients with well-differentiated thyroid cancer. However, patients who have undergone either diagnostic or therapeutic thyroid lobectomy, whose pathologic evaluation reveals PTMC, are not required to undergo completion thyroidectomy because it does not improve survival.[24] Therefore, these patients are not candidates for RIA. Attempting to achieve completion thyroidectomy by administering radioactive iodine in patients with lobectomy for thyroid cancer is not recommended[4] because no data exists demonstrating satisfactory long-term outcomes and may result in large, unnecessary radiation doses to the lower neck.

Current statistics show that most patients who are diagnosed with thyroid cancer have total thyroidectomy even for small thyroid cancers. However, lobectomy for PTMC in a low-risk patient carries no additional risk of recurrence or mortality.[25] Unfortunately, the widespread adoption of RIA, despite evidence of its lack of benefit for low-risk patients, has been used as part of the argument to continue to perform total thyroidectomy in these patients.

Some investigators advocate that total thyroidectomy be performed in all patients with thyroid cancer regardless of the tumor size or risk stratification. Advocates for total thyroidectomy argue that PTMC is often multifocal and seen routinely in autopsy studies, putting the patient at risk for developing a contralateral cancer. In one retrospective review of 539 subjects who had total thyroidectomy for PTC (311 PTMC and 228 PTC >1 cm), equal rates of multifocality, 35% in each group, were reported. They also found cervical lymph node metastases in 19.7% of cancers greater than 1 cm and 9.7% of PTMCs.[26] Total thyroidectomy also allows for the option of RIA and easier surveillance with neck ultrasounds and thyroglobulin.

Other investigators argue that, because most studies do not show a survival benefit for total thyroidectomy in low-risk patients, lobectomy should be sufficient. The largest retrospective review of total thyroidectomy versus lobectomy was performed by Bilimoria and colleagues.[25] They evaluated 52,173 patients (43,227 had total thyroidectomy and 8946 had lobectomy) from the National Cancer Data Base who underwent surgery for PTC in the United States from 1985 to 1998. For patients with tumors less than 1.0 cm, there was no difference in recurrence or survival between total thyroidectomy and lobectomy. However, for patients with tumors greater than 1.0 cm, lobectomy was associated with a 15% higher risk of recurrence and 31% higher risk of death. They concluded that total thyroidectomy improved survival in thyroid cancers greater than 1 cm but the survival benefit was unchanged in patients with tumors less than 1 cm.

Hay and colleagues,[27] in a retrospective review of 900 cases of PTMC observed over 60 years, reported that the extent of thyroid surgery (total or near-total thyroidectomy vs unilateral lobectomy) did not affect recurrence rates. The recurrence rates at 10, 15, and 20 years in patients who had lobectomy was 5.7%, 5.7%, and 9.8%, respectively, compared with recurrence rates of 4.5%, 4.7%, and 5.5%, respectively, in patients who had total or near-total thyroidectomy.[24]

There are no current published studies in the United States comparing long-term follow-up of patients with PTMC who are observed instead of immediately having surgery. However, in Japan, Ito and colleagues[28] followed 340 patients with PTMC who chose to be observed instead of having immediate surgery at time of thyroid cancer diagnosis. The proportions of patients whose PTMC showed enlargement by 3 mm or more were 6.4% at 5-year follow-up and 15.9% on 10-year follow-up. Of these, 109 patients ended up having surgery after observation primarily due to tumor enlargement. None of these patients showed tumor recurrence after surgery on follow-up (average follow-up was 76 months). The investigators concluded observation can be a viable option instead of surgery for PTMC without unfavorable features.

In light of these ongoing questions into whether or not a total thyroidectomy is necessary for small PTC, it is logical to question the indications for RIA in most patients at low-risk for thyroid cancer who have excellent long-term disease-free survival.

ADVANTAGES OF RADIOIODINE TREATMENT

In 2014, most patients with thyroid cancer will undergo total thyroidectomy and at least 50% will undergo adjuvant RIA.[5] The traditional arguments for postoperative administration of radioiodine have been (1) to decrease the risks for cancer recurrence and mortality; (2) to potentially diagnose and treat possible additional sites of microscopic tumor in the remnant thyroid tissue, cervical lymph nodes, and distant sites; and (3) to facilitate surveillance with thyroglobulin monitoring by ablating any viable remnant thyroid tissue in the thyroid bed.[29] Thyroglobulin is more sensitive than a diagnostic iodine scan to detect residual or recurrent disease.[30]

However, when considering these arguments, one must not forget the excellent prognosis for most patients with PTC. The disease-specific mortality in well-differentiated, low-risk PTC ranges from 0.4% to 1.7%.[31,32] In the series published by Memorial Sloan Kettering in 1994, looking at 1038 patients, there was 99% 20-year survival and 4% recurrence for low-risk patients treated with lobectomy and isthmusectomy, and long-term hormonal suppression.[33] In light of these data, the justifications for RIA deserve reexamination.

RECENT GUIDELINES

Currently, there are numerous published sets of guidelines for risk stratification and determination of which patients should or should not receive RIA. Lang and colleagues[34] showed that as many as 16 different staging systems for thyroid cancer have been proposed. The most widely used guidelines are from the NCCN (2012) and ATA (2009). They differ slightly and the ATA is scheduled to publish new guidelines in June, 2014. As of this writing, the ATA guidelines state that a large number of retrospective studies show significant reductions in disease recurrence rates and cause-specific mortality, in support of RIA.[4] However, subgroup analyses have shown these advantages to be limited to higher risk patients.

Previously, the traditional staging systems AMES (age, metastases, extent, size), AGES (age, grade, extent, size), and MACIS (metastases, age, completeness of resection, invasion, size),[35–37] classified low-risk patients as younger patients with histologically classic or follicular-variant PTC, without extrathyroidal extension or distant metastases.

Notably, none of these staging systems included the presence of lymph node metastases as a prognostic factor. These low-risk patients have typically comprised 70% to 85% of diagnosed thyroid cancer.[4] However, this percentage has grown given the disproportionate increase in the detection of smaller thyroid malignancies.[5]

Most pathologists and clinicians are now using the more universal TNM (tumor, nodes, metastases) staging system published by the American Joint Committee on Cancer (AJCC). The TNM staging for thyroid cancer is unique because patients who are younger than 45 years old are limited to stage I unless they have distant metastases, whereas those 45 years or older are classified in the more traditional TNM method of staging (AJCC 2002). Based on the available data in 2009, the ATA recommended RIA for a broad group of patients, including all stage III and IV, virtually all stage II, and selected stage I patients. These stage I patients are described as "those with multifocal disease, nodal metastases, extrathyroidal or vascular invasion, and/or more aggressive histologies."[4]

The NCCN guidelines updated in 2013 also recommend that a large proportion of patients with PTC receive RIA. Essentially, all patients are recommended for RIA unless they meet all of the following criteria: primary tumor less than 1 cm, classic PTC, no extrathyroidal extension, no vascular invasion, postoperative stimulated thyroglobulin less than 1 ng/mL, and no clinical lymph node or distant metastases.[6]

As a consequence of the broadly described categories of patients who may benefit from and are, therefore, candidates for RIA, in both publications there has been little motivation to curb the use of RIA. This is despite scant data supporting its use in low-risk patients who have had a complete tumor resection and who make up most current new thyroid cancer diagnoses.

WHO BENEFITS?
High-Risk Patients

Currently, there is little argument that RIA benefits patients at high risk for thyroid cancer recurrence. Known predictors of recurrence and metastasis include tumor size greater than 4 cm, extrathyroidal extension, residual tumor, gross lymph node metastases, as well as thyroglobulinemia out of proportion to what is seen on the posttreatment scan.[4] Numerous studies have shown a benefit of RIA in these patients. Age of the patient is not an absolute indication for whether a patient should receive I-131; however, patients who are younger and older usually receive higher risk stratification. Tuttle and colleagues[38] stratify patients younger than 20 years or older than 60 years as high-risk. Other investigators stratify patients older than 45 years as high-risk and may not define younger patients as being high-risk.[39]

In the meta-analysis by Sacks and colleagues,[40] examining 79 studies published from 1966 to 2008 that compared radioiodine treatment versus no treatment for thyroid cancer, high-risk patients had significantly reduced recurrence rates and improved survival after treatment with RIA.

One of the earlier and most quoted studies is by Mazzaferri and Jhiang.[41] They demonstrated a 30% relative risk for thyroid cancer recurrence rates in 1355 subjects treated with RIA and thyrotropin suppression with mean follow-up of 15.7 years. Similar retrospective studies published in the early 1990s by DeGroot and colleagues,[42] and Samaan and colleagues,[43] strongly supported the use of RIA. Accordingly, both the NCCN and ATA guidelines recommend RIA for all such patients.[4,6] NCCN also recommends radioiodine treatment of all patients with gross residual disease after surgery.[6] However, in all of these studies, the benefits were restricted to subjects with tumors greater than 1.5 cm or with residual disease.

Lack of Benefit for Low-risk Patients

One of today's primary goals for the administration of radioactive iodine is ablation of the very small amount of thyroid tissue that surgeons may leave behind in cases when it is necessary for recurrent laryngeal nerve protection. However, several investigators have questioned the legitimacy of the claim that ablation of very small normal remnant tissue will decrease recurrences. They have also challenged the necessity of mandating an undetectable postoperative thyroglobulin versus accepting a low level that can be followed.[27]

The following studies have shown no benefit for RIA in low-risk subjects. Hay and colleagues,[24] reviewing long-term outcomes in 2444 subjects treated over 60 years, showed that RIA did not change local recurrence or disease specific mortality in subjects with MACIS scores lower than 6, regardless of lymph node status. In a 2004 Lahey Clinic study, RIA added no survival benefit in 727 subjects stratified by AMES as 585 low-risk and 142 high-risk. The 20-year survival in low-risk, younger high-risk, and older high-risk patients receiving RIA versus no RIA was 100% versus 97.6% ($P = .24$), 64.2% versus 73.2% ($P = .53$), and 44.7% versus 44.4% ($P = .53$), respectively.[44] In a case control study using the Swedish Cancer Registry, Lundgren and colleagues[45] compared 595 subjects dying of thyroid cancer with 595 matched controls and found that the administration of I-131 was associated with poorer survival, even in early-stage disease. The most important prognostic factor was complete tumor removal.

The meta-analysis by Sawka and colleagues[46] examined studies for a benefit of RIA in low-risk subjects, for either recurrence or disease-specific survival. Incremental benefit was unclear and improved survival could not be established. A meta-analysis by Sacks and colleagues,[40] looking at 79 studies, found the preponderance of evidence suggests that RIA is not associated with improved survival in subjects with low-risk thyroid cancer. None of the studies used a randomized controlled trial design and overwhelmingly used a retrospective cohort design.

Neither the NCCN nor the ATA recommend RIA for patients with either unifocal or multifocal papillary microcarcinomas (<1 cm) confined to the thyroid. In a study of more than 900 PTMCs, there was no difference in recurrence rates at local ($P = .34$) or distant sites ($P = .84$) in the 758 subjects who had total or near-total thyroidectomy but did not receive RIA (84%) compared with the subjects that did (16%).[24] However, in clinical practice, use of radioiodine in many such low-risk patients still occurs.

Patients Who May Benefit from Radioiodine Treatment: Intermediate-Risk

The ATA defines TNM stage I patients as low-risk if they have none of the following: regional metastases, extrathyroidal extension, aggressive pathologic condition, and I-131 uptake outside the thyroid bed. Presence of any of these place the patient into an intermediate-risk category, whereas the presence of distant metastases, macroscopic extrathyroidal extension, or incomplete surgical resection are all considered high-risk.

Both NCCN and ATA address intermediate-risk patients in the following manner. NCCN guidelines recommend RIA in selected patients without gross residual disease who are at higher risk for recurrence, including histologic features associated with a higher risk for recurrence, elevated postoperative thyroglobulin, vascular invasion, and cervical lymph node metastases.[6] ATA guidelines recommend RIA in selected patients with 1-cm to 4-cm cancers that are confined to the thyroid who have documented lymph node metastases, or when the combination of the patients' age, tumor size, lymph node status, and histology put the patient at intermediate or higher risk of recurrence or mortality.[4] In actuality, except for patients with unifocal or multifocal papillary microcarcinoma, current ATA guidelines still recommend considering postoperative RIA treatment of all thyroid cancer patients.

When considering both ATA and NCCN guidelines as they pertain to a large group of thyroid cancer patients, much is left to the practitioner's interpretation. Often, out of a need to believe that everything possible is being done to minimize the risk of cancer recurrence, in the minds of both physician and patient, I-131 is likely being administered more frequently than justified.

Even in patients with thyroid cancer greater than 1 cm but less than 4 cm without additional high-risk findings, some studies have not shown a survival benefit with RIA. In a retrospective study by Schvartz and colleagues[47] of patients with thyroid cancers from 1 cm to 4 cm with no high-risk findings, no survival benefit was seen at 10 years. In a meta-analysis published in 2008, Sawka and colleagues[46] examined 12 prognostically adjusted studies looking at thyroid cancer recurrence and survival. Only two showed a survival benefit of RIA. They could not confirm a significant, consistent benefit of RIA in decreasing cause-specific mortality or recurrence in early-stage well-differentiated thyroid cancer. RIA was associated with a significantly decreased risk of distant metastases; however, this was rare in PTC.

In an effort to better illuminate the outcomes for patients in intermediate-risk categories when RIA is not administered, Nixon and colleagues[48] published a retrospective study focusing on such patients treated at Memorial Sloan Kettering. They reviewed 1129 cases of total thyroidectomy. RIA was administered selectively to 691 patients (61%). Recurrence rates were based on palpable disease, not rising thyroglobulin or ultrasound. For patients with T1 or T2, N0 disease, RIA provided no benefit. Surprisingly for patients with T1 or T2, N1 disease, there was no benefit to RIA at 5 years. Even in patients with T3 and T4 disease, RIA did not improve regional or distant recurrence-free survival. Their discussion emphasized the critical role of excellent surgical technique in removing all thyroid tissue and any gross lymph node metastases at the time of operation. They suggested that young patients with T1 and T2, N1 disease with less than 5 nodal metastases may not require RIA. The patients who did well were noted to have small (<1 cm) lymph node metastases.

CHANGING APPROACHES TO RADIOIODINE THERAPY

In the past, RIA was more difficult for patients to prepare for because they required thyroid hormone withdrawal, which decreased their quality of life. In 2007, thyrotropin alfa (Thyrogen), was approved for use in the United States by the Food and Drug Administration for combination use with radioiodine to ablate the remaining thyroid tissue in patients who have had surgery for differentiated thyroid cancer. Thyrotropin alfa has advantages over thyroid hormone withdrawal, including prevention of symptoms and risks of hypothyroidism, improved quality of life, and decrease in whole-body radiation exposure due to more rapid clearance of I-131 with thyrotropin alfa.[49]

There have been many studies comparing thyrotropin alfa to thyroid hormone withdrawal. Hugo and colleagues[50] showed in a retrospective study of 586 subjects (many of whom were considered to be intermediate-risk or high-risk patients) that the 9-year clinical outcomes of thyrotropin alfa–stimulated RIA were similar to thyroid hormone withdrawal with similar recurrence rates (1.5% for thyrotropin alfa vs 1.2% for thyroid hormone withdrawal). Rosario and colleagues[51] also showed that thyrotropin alfa is as effective as thyroid hormone withdrawal in subjects at intermediate and high risk in a prospective, consecutive, nonrandomized trial of subjects treated with 100 to 150 mCi of I-131. The subjects with both thyrotropin alfa and thyroid hormone withdrawal RIA had equivalent ablation success rates of 80% at 5 years, using stimulated thyroglobulin less than 1 ng/mL, negative diagnostic whole-body scan, and negative neck ultrasonography to determine treatment success.

Until recently, there were no large randomized prospective controlled trials evaluating the completeness of RIA remnant ablation. In the past, if radioiodine was given for remnant ablation, the typical dose was 3.7 gigabecquerels (GBq; 100 mCi) of I-131. Currently, the RIA dose necessary for successful remnant ablation has shown to be much less than previously thought.

Two separate, large, prospective randomized multi-institutional trials by Mallick and colleagues[52] (438 subjects) and Schlumberger and colleagues[53] (752 subjects) were published studying the efficacy of RIA in low-risk subjects comparing low-dose and high-dose I-131 treatments: 1.1 GBq (30 mCi) versus 3.7 GBq (100 mCi), and thyrotropin alfa versus thyroid hormone withdrawal. A two-by-two design of each dosage level with each method was used in both studies. Schlumberger and colleagues[53] had a complete ablation success rate of 91.7% with thyrotropin alfa and 92.9% with thyroid hormone withdrawal, which did not meet statistical significance. Both studies showed that ablative success rates were independent of dosage or treatment technique. Therefore, a 1.1 GBq (30 mCi) dose with thyrotropin alfa was noninferior to a 3.7 GBq (100 mCi) with thyroid hormone withdrawal. They both proposed that the quality of life and whole-body radiation was improved with thyrotropin alfa compared with thyroid hormone withdrawal. Therefore, giving a low-dose radioiodine treatment with thyrotropin alfa is an effective and convenient treatment method, providing significant advantages in patients needing remnant ablation.

Examining these two studies, Onitilo and Doi[54] cautioned that many of the subjects had small tumors and were low risk without evidence of nodal metastases. They were likely to have low chance of ablation failure, regardless of the dose or method of RIA. Therefore, the results pertaining to this population cannot be generalized to patients with thyroid cancer with a baseline risk that is different from that of these subjects and certainly does not imply that patients with iodine-avid recurrent or metastatic disease should be treated with lower doses of I-131.

THE ROLE OF PREABLATION, DIAGNOSTIC WHOLE-BODY SCANS

Obtaining diagnostic radioiodine scans before I-131 therapy is an area of controversy. The ATA guidelines do not recommend routinely obtaining a diagnostic iodine scan but state that it has value in selected patients. The ATA recommends against the routine use of a pretherapy I-131 scan because of its low impact on the decision to ablate and because of the possibility of the diagnostic I-131 scan causing stunning of normal thyroid remnants and distant metastases.[4]

The NCCN guidelines recommend the routine use of diagnostic radioiodine scans before RIA but it is not a unanimous recommendation. The arguments for diagnostic I-131 scanning are that it can alter therapy when unsuspected metastases or an unexpectedly large remnant is identified. Such a remnant may require additional surgery or a reduction in radioiodine dosage to avoid substantial radiation thyroiditis. Reducing the dose of I-131 to 2 to 3 mCi reduces the risk of stunning. Stunning is not an issue if the diagnostic scan is performed with I-123 instead of I-131 because I-123 does not have beta emissions, which are necessary for stunning to occur.[6]

SIDE EFFECTS AND RISK OF SECONDARY MALIGNANCY

Lower RIA doses will probably mean that low-risk patients will have decreased risks of secondary radiation and side effects. However, this may also translate to more low-risk patients being treated. The advantages of radioiodine treatment in low-risk patients should be weighed against the potential side effects, the increased risk of second primary cancers from exposure to radiation, and the additional medical costs.[55]

Acute side effects, such as nausea and sialadenitis, are relatively common after treatment with large doses of I-131 but they are usually mild and resolve rapidly. Men may have a transient reduction in spermatogenesis and women may have transient ovarian failure. There is an increased frequency of miscarriages in women treated with I-131 during the year preceding the conception. Therefore, it is recommended that conception be postponed for 1 year after treatment with I-131.[56]

Radiation-associated thyroiditis is usually minimal; however, if the thyroid remnant is large, patients may develop inflammation and have severe pain if the dose of I-131 is too high. In patients who have large thyroid remnants, which can be seen on diagnostic iodine studies with I-131 or I-123, repeat surgery should be considered before RIA. If I-131 ablation is performed in a patient with a large remnant, the ablation dose should be decreased.

The overall relative risk of secondary carcinoma or leukemia is increased when patients are given a high cumulative dose of I-131 of 18.5 GBq (500 mCi) or more.[4] Rubino and colleagues[57] found a linear dose-response relationship with I-131 administration for all cancers combined and for leukemia. In addition, they identified a relationship between the cumulative activity of I-131 and risk of bone and soft-tissue cancer, colorectal cancer, and salivary gland cancer.

SUMMARY

Lively debate continues concerning the management of small thyroid cancers in patients considered to be low-risk and intermediate-risk for recurrent disease. For patients and tumors in the high-risk category, there is near consensus in the literature for a beneficial effect of RIA following total thyroidectomy. Traditional guidelines also agree that small cancers less than 1 cm that lack any aggressive features do not benefit from RIA and should not be treated with I-131.

For patients in the intermediate-risk group, the role of RIA is evolving. The studies are conflicting and there is little convincing evidence to steer decision-making in patients with thyroid cancers between 1 and 4 cm, with or without limited nodal disease, who do not have distant metastases or gross extrathyroidal extension. Currently, most of these patients undergo total thyroidectomy and possible level VI lymph node dissection, followed by RIA.

Certainly, as a consequence of the dramatically increasing incidence of disease, more low and intermediate-risk patients are being referred for RIA. Instead of continuing to follow current management guidelines based on retrospective data dating back to 50 years, it is time to consider performing a multicenter prospective randomized trial evaluating the benefits of RIA in this patient population.

REFERENCES

1. Seidlin SM, Marinelli LD, Oshry E. Radioactive iodine therapy; effect on functioning metastases of adenocarcinoma of the thyroid. J Am Med Assoc 1946; 132(14):838–47.
2. Coliez R, Tubiana M, Dutreix J, et al. Results of examination of 85 cases of cancer of the thyroid with radioactive iodine. J Radiol Electrol Arch Electr Medicale 1951;32(11–12):881–95 [in Undetermined Language].
3. Mazzaferri EL, Young RL. Papillary thyroid carcinoma: a 10 year follow-up report of the impact of therapy in 576 patients. Am J Med 1981;70(3):511–8.
4. Cooper DS, Doherty GM, Haugen BR, et al. Revised American Thyroid Association management guidelines for patients with thyroid nodules and differentiated thyroid cancer. Thyroid 2009;19(11):1167–214.
5. Davies L, Welch HG. Current Thyroid Cancer Trends in the United States. JAMA Otolaryngol Head Neck Surg 2014. [Epub ahead of print].
6. Tuttle RM, Ball DW, Byrd D, et al. NCCN Clinical Practice Guidelines in Oncology (NCCN Guidelines) Thyroid Carcinoma version 2.2012 NCCN.org. 2012. Available at: http://www.nccn.org/professionals/physician_gls/pdf/thyroid.pdf.
7. Howlader N, Noone AM, Krapcho M, et al, editors. SEER Cancer statistics review, 1975-2010. Bethesda (MD): National Cancer Institute; 2012. Available at: http://seer.cancer.gov/csr/1975_2010/. Based on November 2012 SEER data submission, posted to the SEER web site, April 2013.
8. Siegel R, Naishadham D, Jemal A. Cancer statistics, 2013. CA Cancer J Clin 2013;63(1):11–30.
9. Chen AY, Jemal A, Ward EM. Increasing incidence of differentiated thyroid cancer in the United States, 1988-2005. Cancer 2009;115(16):3801–7.
10. Nikiforov YE. Is ionizing radiation responsible for the increasing incidence of thyroid cancer? Cancer 2010;116(7):1626–8.
11. Dobyns BM, Hyrmer BA. The surgical management of benign and malignant thyroid neoplasms in Marshall Islanders exposed to hydrogen bomb fallout. World J Surg 1992;16(1):126–39 [discussion: 139–40].
12. Kazakov VS, Demidchik EP, Astakhova LN. Thyroid cancer after Chernobyl. Nature 1992;359(6390):21.
13. Morris LG, Sikora AG, Tosteson TD, et al. The increasing incidence of thyroid cancer: the influence of access to care. Thyroid 2013;23(7):885–91.
14. Sinnott B, Ron E, Schneider AB. Exposing the thyroid to radiation: a review of its current extent, risks, and implications. Endocr Rev 2010;31(5):756–73.
15. Grodski S, Brown T, Sidhu S, et al. Increasing incidence of thyroid cancer is due to increased pathologic detection. Surgery 2008;144(6):1038–43 [discussion: 1043].
16. Hedinger C, Williams E, Sobin LD, editors. Histological typing of thyroid tumours. International Histological Classification of Tumours, vol. 11. Geneva (Switzerland): World Health Organization; 1988. p. 1–18.
17. Udelsman R. Is total thyroidectomy the procedure of choice for papillary thyroid cancer? Nat Clin Pract Oncol 2008;5(4):184–5.
18. Harach HR, Franssila KO, Wasenius VM. Occult papillary carcinoma of the thyroid. A "normal" finding in Finland. A systematic autopsy study. Cancer 1985; 56(3):531–8.
19. Tanriover O, Comunoglu N, Eren B, et al. Occult papillary thyroid carcinoma: prevalence at autopsy in Turkish people. Eur J Cancer Prev 2011;20(4): 308–12.

20. Udelsman R, Zhang Y. The epidemic of thyroid cancer in the United States: the role of endocrinologists and ultrasounds. Thyroid 2014;24(3):472–9.
21. Frates MC, Benson CB, Charboneau JW, et al. Management of thyroid nodules detected at US: Society of Radiologists in Ultrasound consensus conference statement. Ultrasound Q 2006;22(4):231–8 [discussion: 239–40].
22. Jemal A, Murray T, Ward E, et al. Cancer statistics, 2005. CA Cancer J Clin 2005; 55(1):10–30.
23. Hughes DT, Haymart MR, Miller BS, et al. The most commonly occurring papillary thyroid cancer in the United States is now a microcarcinoma in a patient older than 45 years. Thyroid 2011;21(3):231–6.
24. Hay ID, Hutchinson ME, Gonzalez-Losada T, et al. Papillary thyroid microcarcinoma: a study of 900 cases observed in a 60-year period. Surgery 2008;144(6): 980–7 [discussion: 987–8].
25. Bilimoria KY, Bentrem DJ, Ko CY, et al. Extent of surgery affects survival for papillary thyroid cancer. Ann Surg 2007;246(3):375–81 [discussion: 381–4].
26. Karatzas T, Vasileiadis I, Kapetanakis S, et al. Risk factors contributing to the difference in prognosis for papillary versus micropapillary thyroid carcinoma. Am J Surg 2013;206(4):586–93.
27. Hay ID, McDougall IR, Sisson JC. Perspective: the case against radioiodine remnant ablation in patients with well-differentiated thyroid carcinoma. J Nucl Med 2008;49(8):1395–7.
28. Ito Y, Miyauchi A, Inoue H, et al. An observational trial for papillary thyroid microcarcinoma in Japanese patients. World J Surg 2010;34(1):28–35.
29. Sosa JA, Udelsman R. Total thyroidectomy for differentiated thyroid cancer. J Surg Oncol 2006;94(8):701–7.
30. Elisei R, Schlumberger M, Driedger A, et al. Follow-up of low-risk differentiated thyroid cancer patients who underwent radioiodine ablation of postsurgical thyroid remnants after either recombinant human thyrotropin or thyroid hormone withdrawal. J Clin Endocrinol Metab 2009;94(11):4171–9.
31. Hay ID, McConahey WM, Goellner JR. Managing patients with papillary thyroid carcinoma: insights gained from the Mayo Clinic's experience of treating 2,512 consecutive patients during 1940 through 2000. Trans Am Clin Climatol Assoc 2002;113:241–60.
32. Sawka AM, Thephamongkhol K, Brouwers M, et al. Clinical review 170: a systematic review and metaanalysis of the effectiveness of radioactive iodine remnant ablation for well-differentiated thyroid cancer. J Clin Endocrinol Metab 2004;89(8):3668–76.
33. Shaha AR, Loree TR, Shah JP. Intermediate-risk group for differentiated carcinoma of thyroid. Surgery 1994;116(6):1036–40 [discussion: 1040–1].
34. Lang BH, Lo CY, Chan WF, et al. Staging systems for papillary thyroid carcinoma: a review and comparison. Ann Surg 2007;245(3):366–78.
35. Hay ID, Bergstralh EJ, Goellner JR, et al. Predicting outcome in papillary thyroid carcinoma: development of a reliable prognostic scoring system in a cohort of 1779 patients surgically treated at one institution during 1940 through 1989. Surgery 1993;114(6):1050–7 [discussion: 1057–8].
36. Hay ID, Grant CS, Taylor WF, et al. Ipsilateral lobectomy versus bilateral lobar resection in papillary thyroid carcinoma: a retrospective analysis of surgical outcome using a novel prognostic scoring system. Surgery 1987;102(6): 1088–95.
37. Cady B, Rossi R. An expanded view of risk-group definition in differentiated thyroid carcinoma. Surgery 1988;104(6):947–53.

38. Tuttle RM, Rondeau G, Lee NY. A risk-adapted approach to the use of radioactive iodine and external beam radiation in the treatment of well-differentiated thyroid cancer. Cancer Control 2011;18(2):89–95.

39. Onitilo AA, Engel JM, Lundgren CI, et al. Simplifying the TNM system for clinical use in differentiated thyroid cancer. J Clin Oncol 2009;27(11):1872–8.

40. Sacks W, Fung CH, Chang JT, et al. The effectiveness of radioactive iodine for treatment of low-risk thyroid cancer: a systematic analysis of the peer-reviewed literature from 1966 to April 2008. Thyroid 2010;20(11):1235–45.

41. Mazzaferri EL, Jhiang SM. Long-term impact of initial surgical and medical therapy on papillary and follicular thyroid cancer. Am J Med 1994;97(5):418–28.

42. DeGroot LJ, Kaplan EL, McCormick M, et al. Natural history, treatment, and course of papillary thyroid carcinoma. J Clin Endocrinol Metab 1990;71(2):414–24.

43. Samaan NA, Schultz PN, Hickey RC, et al. The results of various modalities of treatment of well differentiated thyroid carcinomas: a retrospective review of 1599 patients. J Clin Endocrinol Metab 1992;75(3):714–20.

44. Kim S, Wei JP, Braveman JM, et al. Predicting outcome and directing therapy for papillary thyroid carcinoma. Arch Surg 2004;139(4):390–4 [discussion: 393–4].

45. Lundgren CI, Hall P, Dickman PW, et al. Influence of surgical and postoperative treatment on survival in differentiated thyroid cancer. Br J Surg 2007;94(5):571–7.

46. Sawka AM, Brierley JD, Tsang RW, et al. An updated systematic review and commentary examining the effectiveness of radioactive iodine remnant ablation in well-differentiated thyroid cancer. Endocrinol Metab Clin North Am 2008;37(2):457–80, x.

47. Schvartz C, Bonnetain F, Dabakuyo S, et al. Impact on overall survival of radioactive iodine in low-risk differentiated thyroid cancer patients. J Clin Endocrinol Metab 2012;97(5):1526–35.

48. Nixon IJ, Patel SG, Palmer FL, et al. Selective use of radioactive iodine in intermediate-risk papillary thyroid cancer. Arch Otolaryngol Head Neck Surg 2012;138(12):1141–6.

49. Rosario PW, Xavier AC, Calsolari MR. Recombinant human thyrotropin in thyroid remnant ablation with 131-iodine in high-risk patients. Thyroid 2010;20(11):1247–52.

50. Hugo J, Robenshtok E, Grewal R, et al. Recombinant human thyroid stimulating hormone-assisted radioactive iodine remnant ablation in thyroid cancer patients at intermediate to high risk of recurrence. Thyroid 2012;22(10):1007–15.

51. Rosario PW, Mineiro Filho AF, Lacerda RX, et al. Long-term follow-up of at least five years after recombinant human thyrotropin compared to levothyroxine withdrawal for thyroid remnant ablation with radioactive iodine. Thyroid 2012;22(3):332–3.

52. Mallick U, Harmer C, Yap B, et al. Ablation with low-dose radioiodine and thyrotropin alfa in thyroid cancer. N Engl J Med 2012;366(18):1674–85.

53. Schlumberger M, Catargi B, Borget I, et al. Strategies of radioiodine ablation in patients with low-risk thyroid cancer. N Engl J Med 2012;366(18):1663–73.

54. Onitilo AA, Doi SA. Recent data regarding low versus high 131I activity for remnant ablation in differentiated thyroid cancer are not generalizable beyond eligibility criteria. Nucl Med Commun 2012;33(11):1217–8.

55. Iyer NG, Morris LG, Tuttle RM, et al. Rising incidence of second cancers in patients with low-risk (T1N0) thyroid cancer who receive radioactive iodine therapy. Cancer 2011;117(19):4439–46.

56. Carballo M, Quiros RM. To treat or not to treat: the role of adjuvant radioiodine therapy in thyroid cancer patients. J Oncol 2012;2012:707156.
57. Rubino C, de Vathaire F, Dottorini ME, et al. Second primary malignancies in thyroid cancer patients. Br J Cancer 2003;89(9):1638–44.

Minimizing Cost and Maximizing Success in the Preoperative Localization Strategy for Primary Hyperparathyroidism

Carmen C. Solorzano, MD[a],*, Denise Carneiro-Pla, MD[b]

KEYWORDS

- Hyperparathyroidism • Parathyroidectomy • Ultrasonography • Localization
- Sestamibi scan • Four-dimensional computed tomography • Cost-effectiveness

KEY POINTS

- Ultrasonography of the thyroid, parathyroid, and soft tissues of the neck should always be performed before parathyroidectomy.
- Ultrasonography performed by an experienced surgeon or radiologist has similar sensitivity to sestamibi scan in localizing eutopic parathyroid adenomas.
- Ultrasonography is the least expensive localization study.
- The most cost-effective localization strategies seem to be ultrasonography followed by four-dimensional computed tomography (4DCT) or ultrasonography followed by sestamibi ± 4DCT. These localization strategies are highly dependent on the quality of imaging (sensitivities are variable).
- Surgeons should critically evaluate the imaging and operative data at their own institution to determine the best preoperative localization strategy before parathyroidectomy.
- Surgeons should communicate with the referring physicians about the best localization algorithms in the local area and become the decision maker as to when to obtain them.

INTRODUCTION

Bilateral neck exploration (BNE) for the treatment of sporadic primary hyperparathyroidism (SPHPT) has a success rate ranging from 94% to 98% when performed by experienced surgeons.[1–3] Minimally invasive parathyroidectomy, with its advantages

a Division of Surgical Oncology and Endocrine Surgery, Vanderbilt University Medical Center, 597 PRB, 2220 Pierce Avenue, Nashville, TN 37232, USA; b Division of Oncologic and Endocrine Surgery, Medical University of South Carolina, 25 Courtenay Drive, 7008, Charleston, SC 29414, USA
* Corresponding author.
E-mail address: Carmen.solorzano@vanderbilt.edu

Surg Clin N Am 94 (2014) 587–605
http://dx.doi.org/10.1016/j.suc.2014.02.006   surgical.theclinics.com
0039-6109/14/$ – see front matter Published by Elsevier Inc.

of smaller incisions, lesser dissection, eligibility for outpatient surgery, and cost savings, has become the preferred surgical approach to SPHPT.[3] To allow a focused dissection and maintain the same success rate as the gold standard operation, minimally invasive parathyroidectomy has required advances in preoperative imaging and development of intraoperative adjuncts.

Although imaging studies guide the surgeon to the precise location of the abnormal parathyroid gland, intraoperative parathyroid hormone monitoring (IPM) assures the surgeon that all the hyperfunctioning tissue has been removed before the patient leaves the operating room.[4] Localization studies should not be used to diagnose hyperparathyroidism or to indicate operative intervention. Rather, once the patient has a secure biochemical diagnosis, the surgeon depends on accurate localization solely to allow a focused approach. Most experienced endocrine surgeons are proponents of localization studies, with the most commonly used method being a combination of ultrasonography (US) and technetium 99m (Tc 99m) sestamibi scintigraphy (MIBI). Four-dimensional computed tomography (4DCT) is usually reserved for reoperative cases; however, some surgeons are now using this methodology as the primary localization study. This review focuses on the most commonly used localization studies in SPHPT (US, MIBI, and 4DCT) and emphasizes their clinical effectiveness and cost-effectiveness.

Parathyroid Embryology and Anatomy As It Relates to Imaging Interpretation

Ideally, the reporting radiologist and the operating surgeon should have a thorough understanding of parathyroid embryology and anatomy. Most patients have 4 parathyroid glands (2 superior and 2 inferior), although supernumerary glands can be encountered in 2% to 13% of cases.[5,6] Understanding the eutopic and ectopic locations of the parathyroid glands is of utmost importance in the interpretation of imaging studies as they relate to the surgical procedure. The surgeon should always review the radiologic images when planning the operative approach and never rely on the radiology report alone. The superior glands are derived from the fourth branchial pouch along with the lateral lobes of the thyroid. The inferior glands arise from the third pouch along with the thymus.

Superior parathyroid anatomic and imaging location

The superior parathyroids are usually located in a posterior plane when compared with the inferior glands. The possible location of the superior parathyroid is posterior to the midportion of the superior thyroid lobe near the crycothyroid junction (>90%), posterior to the midthyroid lobe (4%), superior to the thyroid lobe (3%), in the retropharyngeal/retroesophageal location (1%), or intrathyroidal (0.2%).[5-7] A superior gland that has fallen down because of growth and gravity into the tracheoesophageal groove or paraesophageal area can be imaged in a relatively low cervical location.[8] The inexperienced radiologist or surgeon may interpret this finding as an inferior gland when it is an ectopic superior gland low in the neck.[9] One of the most common locations of a missed parathyroid during a previous failed parathyroidectomy is a superior gland in the posterior and low paraesophageal area.[10] The posterior location of the superior gland can be confirmed on US, CT or single-photon emission computed tomography (SPECT) MIBI images, or the oblique images of a planar MIBI scan. A retropharyngeal/retroesophageal superior gland may not be apparent on US, and 4DCT and MIBI with SPECT or MIBI-SPECT/CT are more suitable to image such posterior locations. An intrathyroidal parathyroid gland can be localized with MIBI scans; however, US is ideal in assisting the surgeon to determine if the abnormality is parathyroid tissue (**Fig. 1**).

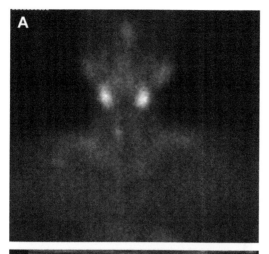

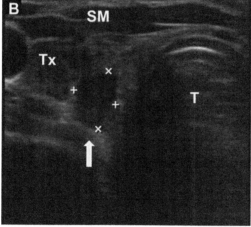

Fig. 1. (*A*) Planar sestamibi image of a superior parathyroid. (*B*) Intrathyroidal location of the same superior parathyroid (*arrow*) in a patient with Hashimoto thyroiditis. SM, strap muscles; T, trachea; Tx, thyroid.

Inferior parathyroid anatomic and imaging location

The possible locations of the inferior parathyroid are caudad, posterior, or lateral to the lower thyroid pole (69%), in the thyrothymic ligament or thymic tongue (26%), superior to the superior parathyroid gland as an undescended inferior parathyroid, in the mediastinal thymus or in the mediastinum outside the thymus (2%).[5–7] An inferior gland is usually located in a lower and generally more anterior cervical location when compared with a superior gland. Often, it seems to protrude out of the lower pole of the thyroid (**Fig. 2**). A rare deep mediastinal parathyroid is impossible to image with US, but 4DCT and SPECT MIBI or SPECT/CT MIBI are usually successful.

US

We believe that all patients should have surgeon-performed US (SUS) or a radiologist-performed US before parathyroidectomy. The information provided by preoperative

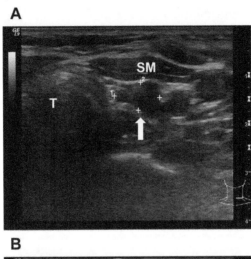

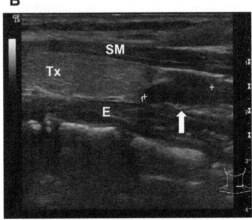

Fig. 2. (*A*) Transverse view of a left inferior parathyroid adenoma and (*B*) longitudinal view of the same gland protruding from the lower pole of the thyroid. *Arrows* point to the parathyroid. E, esophagus; SM, strap muscles; T, trachea; Tx, thyroid.

US is essential in patients with hyperparathyroidism.[11] This method of parathyroid gland localization is convenient, does not involve radiation exposure, is noninvasive, provides the surgeon with excellent detailed topographic information, identifies concomitant thyroid disease, and is the least costly parathyroid localization method.[12,13] In many centers, US may be the only localization study needed to plan a minimally invasive parathyroidectomy guided by IPM.[13–19] Any thyroid disease should be identified and addressed preoperatively, modifying the surgical procedure accordingly. Another advantage of US is that it can frequently identify an intrathyroidal or cystic parathyroid gland not easily identified by other modalities (see **Fig. 1**). Furthermore, US can be used to guide fine-needle aspiration (FNA) of intrathyroidal lesions when parathyroid origin is unclear. A portion of the aspirate can be sent for cytology, and another can be diluted in 1 mL of saline solution to measure parathyroid hormone (PTH). FNA of parathyroid glands should be used only when absolutely necessary, because it creates a local inflammatory reaction, making the operation more challenging.[20]

Typical US Appearance and Location of Parathyroid Adenomas

The typical US appearance of a parathyroid adenoma located in the inferior position is depicted in **Fig. 2**. On gray-scale imaging, parathyroid adenomas are nearly always homogenous and hypoechoic when compared with the thyroid (**Box 1**). In most patients, the 3 most common locations for the inferior parathyroid can be imaged by US. Ultrasonographers should always scan posterior to the clavicle by angling the US probe under it and asking the patient to swallow. This maneuver is helpful in localization of thymic or thoracic inlet parathyroid glands. When US fails to show an abnormal parathyroid in its eutopic location, the lateral neck, particularly the area medial to the carotid artery (level II lymph node basin) should be carefully scanned, looking for a rare ectopic or undescended gland.

The location of the superior parathyroid is less variable, yet its posterior position can be challenging to visualize with US, particularly in obese patients, those with goiters, or in the presence of thyroiditis (**Fig. 3**).

Accuracy of US

A contemporary meta-analysis[21] evaluated the accuracy of common preoperative localization techniques in patients with primary hyperparathyroidism against the gold standard of intraoperative visualization and histology. The pooled sensitivity and positive predictive value of US was 76.1% (57%–89%) and 93.2% (85%–100%), respectively. Ruda and colleagues[22] reviewed the literature from 1995 to 2003 and reported US sensitivity of 79% in localizing abnormal parathyroid glands. As mentioned earlier, the results of US are operator dependent and can be negatively influenced by the presence of thyroid nodular disease, increased body mass index, presence of multiglandular/ectopic parathyroid disease, and small parathyroid size.[23] Posterior thyroid nodules and cysts can be mistaken for a parathyroid adenoma and vice versa. US is less sensitive when parathyroids are located behind the trachea, esophagus, in the superior mediastinum, and in patients with thyroiditis. Even when performed by surgeons or expert radiologists, US has limitations, and surgeons

---

Box 1
US characteristics of a parathyroid adenoma

Typical features

- Solid
- Bean-shaped or oval
- Hypoechoic
- Homogenous
- Smooth border
- Polar vessel forming arc or rim of peripheral vascularity

Atypical features

- Partially cystic
- Lobular
- Hyperechoic
- Heterogeneous
- Calcified

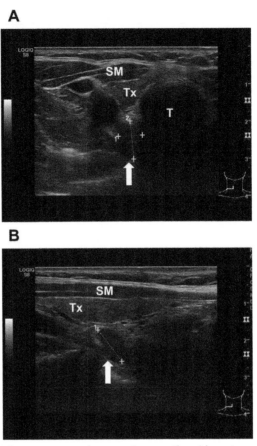

Fig. 3. (*A*) Typical US appearance of a superior parathyroid on transverse view and (*B*) Longitudinal view of the same gland. *Arrows* point to the parathyroid. SM, strap muscles; T, trachea; Tx, thyroid.

should evaluate their institutional results before relying exclusively on this imaging method.

Cost-Effectiveness of US

Wang and colleagues[13] reported on a cost-utility analysis to optimize preoperative imaging for SPHPT. A decision tree was constructed to determine the incremental cost-utility ratio of 5 localization strategies: (1) US; (2) MIBI-SPECT; (3) 4DCT; (4) MIBI-SPECT and US; and (5) MIBI-SPECT and US ± 4DCT (4DCT added when MIBI and US were discordant). The investigators concluded that US is the least expensive imaging modality. However, the most cost-effective strategy involved the use of US combined with MIBI-SPECT and, if needed, 4DCT. This strategy costs less and accrued more utility (a measure of quality of life) mostly because BNE was avoided, hence decreasing the overall cost of parathyroidectomy. Using MIBI-SPECT as the sole localization study was the least cost-effective strategy.

In another economic analysis of preoperative localization strategies for primary hyperparathyroidism, Lubitz and colleagues[12] constructed a decision-analytical model to evaluate 8 different localization strategies, as shown in **Table 1**. The investigators

Table 1		
Cost by localization strategy		
Localization Strategy	**Cost ($)**	**Increasing Costs Compared with US Followed by 4DCT Strategy**
US followed by 4DCT[a]	5901	
US	6028	127
4DCT	6110	209
Sestamibi followed by 4DCT[a]	6266	365
US and sestamibi followed by 4DCT[a]	6319	418
US and sestamibi	6329	428
Sestamibi	6374	473
BNE	6824	923

[a] Followed by the next test only when the first test is indeterminate or negative.
Data from Lubitz CC, Stephen AE, Hodin RA, et al. Preoperative localization strategies for primary hyperparathyroidism: an economic analysis. Ann Surg Oncol 2012;19(13):4202–9.

concluded that US, followed by 4DCT when the US results were indeterminate, was the least costly strategy. Differences in cost were largely based on improved sensitivity for detecting single gland disease and, therefore, on the proportion of patients able to undergo minimally invasive procedures with shorter operating time and same-day discharge.

Both studies mentioned earlier concluded that the cost of BNE without localization was always higher, even when the sensitivity of localizations studies was lowest (ie, localization studies were least useful). Most cost-effectiveness studies assume that most patients undergoing BNE require longer operating times and overnight stays in the hospital, therefore driving the costs of parathyroidectomy higher. An increasing number of high-volume parathyroid surgeons who perform BNE via small incisions discharge their patients the same day, possibly neutralizing the cost of this approach when compared with minimally invasive procedures.[24]

We use SUS in all patients with SPHPT who are scheduled for parathyroidectomy. When a clear parathyroid adenoma is localized by SUS, patients are explored using US as the only localization study.[14–18] However, we always use IPM to guide the extent of resection and avoid missing multiple gland disease. Recently, Untch and colleagues[15] confirmed previous findings that SUS has the same sensitivity as MIBI scans and can be used as the only localization study, resulting in excellent operative success when parathyroidectomy is guided by IPM.

MIBI

Introduced by Coakley and colleagues[25] in 1989, sestamibi parathyroid scintigraphy is the most widely used preoperative localization technique. MIBI scans are believed to be more sensitive and less operator dependent when compared with US. On the other hand, the performance of MIBI can vary widely depending on the imaging technique used, the weight and size of the parathyroid gland, and who is interpreting the images (**Table 2**).[7,9,21,26–28] Hyperactive parathyroid adenomas uptake and retain the sestamibi isotope for longer periods when compared with the thyroid gland. Dual-phase imaging takes advantage of this differential uptake, consisting of early (5 or 15 minutes) and delayed phase images (2 hours). The delayed images allow for sestamibi to wash out from the thyroid, enhancing the detection of parathyroid adenomas (**Fig. 4**).

Table 2
Scintigraphic localization sensitivities for smaller versus larger parathyroid lesions

	Early Images (%)	Late Images (%)	Subtraction Images (%)	SPECT (%)	Early and Late Images (%)	Planar Images (%)	All Images (%)
All Lesions							
<600 mg	58[a]	69[a]	74[a]	77[a]	77[a]	83[a]	86[a]
>600 mg	76	90	88	90	91	94	94
SGD							
<600 mg	68[a]	78[a]	83[a]	86[a]	86[a]	93[a]	96
>600 mg	80	95	92	94	95	99	99
MGD							
<600 mg	39	52	53	55	59	61	62
>600 mg	42	49	56	64	63	66	69

Abbreviations: MGD, multiple gland disease; SGD, single gland disease.
[a] *P*<.05 for comparison <600 mg versus >600 mg groups.
Data from Nichols KJ, Tomas MB, Tronco GG, et al. Preoperative parathyroid scintigraphic lesion localization: accuracy of various types of readings. Radiology 2008;248(1):221–32.

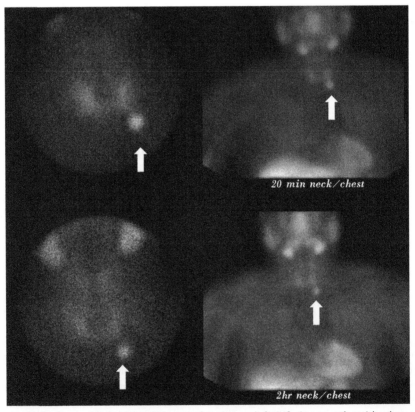

Fig. 4. Dual-phase planar sestamibi scan showing a left inferior parathyroid adenoma. *Arrows* point to the parathyroid.

Multiple imaging techniques and protocols have been described since the introduction of MIBI scans. Techniques can vary in the timing: single or dual phase, and extent of imaging: planar, oblique views, three-dimensional images with SPECT or fusion of SPECT with CT images (SPECT/CT) (**Fig. 5**). Other approaches use the fusion of

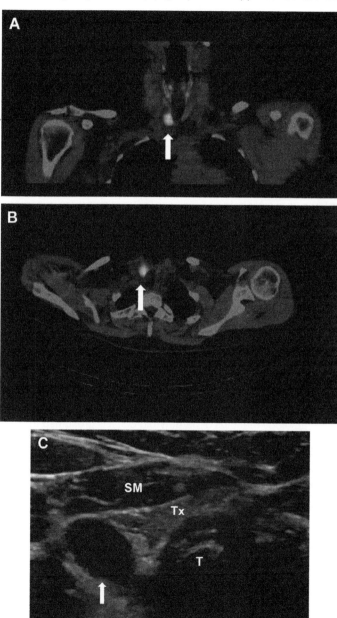

Fig. 5. (*A*) Coronal view of an right inferior parathyroid gland imaged by SPECT fused with CT scan, and (*B*) transverse view of the same inferior parathyroid adenoma showing its anterior position. (*C*) US of the same gland adjacent to the lower pole of the right thyroid lobe. *Arrows* point to the parathyroid. SM, strap muscles; T, trachea; Tx, thyroid.

thyroid imaging with Tc 99m-pertechnetate or ^{123}I-sodium iodide concomitantly with MIBI planar images. Using computer techniques, the thyroid can be subtracted from the MIBI images, therefore providing potentially better visualization of the hyperfunctioning parathyroid gland.

Choosing the Appropriate Scintigraphy Study

The best scintigraphic methodology to image the parathyroid continues to be debatable. Sharma and colleagues[28] evaluated 4 different MIBI scintigraphic modalities among 833 patients undergoing parathyroidectomy. There were 138 planar MIBI scans, 165 SPECT scans, 350 MIBI-SPECT scans with ^{123}I thyroid subtraction and 180 MIBI-SPECT/CT included in the analysis. After correlating imaging results with intraoperative findings, these investigators concluded that multiplanar MIBI-SPECT-based imaging offered three-dimensional localization and improved detection when compared with planar scans; however, the difference in results was not statistically significant (85% vs 77% for single adenoma). Subtraction techniques have not been shown to be superior to nonsubtracted techniques in localizing abnormal parathyroid glands.

In another large study, Nichols and colleagues[27] evaluated the accuracy of various parathyroid scintigraphy readings for single gland disease and multiglandular disease in primary hyperparathyroidism (see **Table 2**). Among 462 patients, a total of 534 parathyroid lesions were excised. The investigators found that reading all the MIBI images together was more accurate (89%) than was reading early (79%), late (85%), subtraction (86%), and MIBI-SPECT images (88%) separately; however, it was not significantly more accurate than reading planar MIBI images (88%) or early and late images together (87%). Furthermore, the result of reading all images was significantly affected by the gland weight (>600 mg 94% vs <600 mg 86%).

It seems that the contribution of SPECT/CT over and above SPECT alone is greatest in terms of localization when the abnormal gland is ectopic.[29] The role of SPECT/CT in eutopic tumors remains controversial, given their extra imaging time and radiation exposure (see **Fig. 5**; the same gland is clearly imaged on US). Joint reporting and reading of MIBI scans by the radiologist and surgeon have been shown to significantly improve localization rates.[9] Similar to previous studies showing that SUS improves the accuracy of the radiology readings of parathyroid US, it is presumed that the cause of the increased accuracy of MIBI scan localization is the surgeon's increased knowledge of neck anatomy and clinical history.[30]

Accuracy and Cost-Effectiveness of Scintigraphy

A recent meta-analysis (2004–2012)[22] reported the pooled sensitivity and positive predictive value of MIBI-SPECT scan to be 79% (49%–91%) and 91% (84%–96%), respectively. This study concluded that SPECT MIBI scans and US are comparable with regards to their ability to preoperatively localize parathyroid adenomas in patients undergoing a first operation for hyperparathyroidism. A meta-analysis from Ruda and colleagues[22] reported a sensitivity of 88% for MIBI scans, whereas Gotthardt and colleagues[31] described a sensitivity of 45% at their center and 72% (39%–92%) in the meta-analysis portion of the study. The investigators concluded that the value of MIBI scans may be overestimated and that some of the differences in sensitivities could be explained by the definitions of what constitutes a true positive result and who is interpreting the images. Both studies included patients with persistent disease and secondary hyperparathyroidism, conditions associated with multiglandular disease or ectopic glands.

Two cost-effectiveness analyses[12,13] evaluated different strategies for preoperative localization of parathyroid adenomas in primary hyperparathyroidism and found that using MIBI scans alone was the most costly localization strategy (see **Table 1** and cost-effective discussion in US section). The only other strategy more costly than using MIBI scans as the only localization study was performing a BNE without using preoperative localization studies (even when IPM was not included) (see **Table 1**).[12]

4DCT

4DCT is a multiphase multidetector CT examination similar to CT angiography. Multi-detector CT provides rapid volumetric acquisition and spatial resolution of 1 mm or better, allowing exquisitely detailed images of the cervical area and parathyroid glands.[8] The name is derived from three-dimensional CT scanning, with an added dimension from the changes in perfusion of contrast over time (uptake and washout of parathyroid glands) (**Fig. 6**). 4DCT is believed to provide both anatomic and functional information and hence overcomes the limitations of US and MIBI scan, both of which can miss deep-seeded glands or may fail to provide clear anatomic resolution.

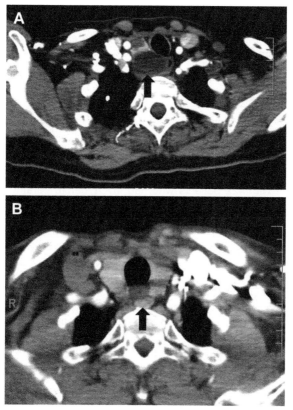

Fig. 6. (*A*) 4DCT scan showing a large solid and cystic retrotracheal parathyroid gland in a patient with a failed parathyroidectomy, and (*B*) hypervascular retroesophageal parathyroid also missed at initial exploration. *Arrows* point to the parathyroid.

Accuracy of 4DCT

In 2006, Rodgers and colleagues[8] reported their experience using 4DCT in 75 patients with SPHPT. All patients underwent localization with radiology performed US, MIBI-SPECT/CT, and 4DCT. 4DCT had greater sensitivity (88%) when compared with US (57%) and MIBI-SPECT/CT (65%). The investigators also observed that 4DCT was superior not only at lateralizing the parathyroid to 1 side of the neck (left or right) but also to pinpoint their superior or inferior location (correct quadrant identified in 70% 4DCT vs 30% MIBI). In addition, 4DCT tended to perform better than other modalities in patients with larger glands and with multiglandular disease. The investigators concluded that 4DCT plays an important role in localization before both initial and reoperative parathyroidectomy.

In their meta-analysis of localization studies used in hyperparathyroidism, Cheung and colleagues[21] commented that although there were an insufficient number of homogenous studies examining 4DCT, the accuracy was improved when this method was used as the primary imaging technique. The weighted average of 2 studies yielded a sensitivity and positive predictive value of 89% and 93.5%, respectively. Preliminary results suggest that 4DCT may be more effective than both US and SPECT MIBI scan.[8,32] Other investigators[31–34] have suggested the routine use of 4DCT as the initial localization study in patients with mild hypercalcemia and smaller glands, because of its superior sensitivity when compared with US and MIBI scans. Many experienced parathyroid surgeons who operate on patients with persistent or recurrent hyperparathyroidism obtain a 4DCT to aid in the localization of the missing gland.[35] It remains to be proved whether 4DCT will supersede MIBI scan as the preferred and most used localization study in patients with SPHPT.

Cost-Effectiveness of 4DCT

Cost-effective analyses including 4DCT find it to be cost-effective when US is negative or when the combination of US and MIBI scan is negative or discordant. The cost-effectiveness of this approach is mainly derived by the avoidance of BNE, with its associated longer operative times and hospital stays (see **Table 1** and US cost-effectiveness section). Abbott and colleagues[36] recently reported a single institution experience with 422 patients who had 4DCT before parathyroidectomy and compared outcomes with a group of patients who did not have 4DCT in their preoperative localization strategy. The study evaluated whether outcomes were better in terms of operative time, hospital length of stay, and overall cost for patients who had 4DCT. In this study, 4DCT did not seem to shorten operating room time or decrease failure rates. However, preoperative 4DCT was associated with shorter hospital stays and improved rates of minimally invasive parathyroidectomy. Despite this finding, the cost of routine use of 4DCT was higher than US and MIBI scan alone. These investigators proposed, as others did before, that 4DCT could be used selectively in cases in which US and MIBI scans are negative/equivocal or have limitations because of patient disease.[12,13,33,36,37] **Table 3** provides current charges at the institution of one the authors of this article as well as the national payment from the Centers for Medicare and Medicaid Services for the localization studies discussed earlier.

Other Considerations Regarding 4DCT

Traditional CT scans of the neck or chest do not use thin sections or multiphase acquisition when compared with 4DCT, and thus, the surgeon should be aware

Table 3			
Current charges at 1 institution			
National Payment from Centers for Medicare Medicaid Services			
Study Type/CPT Code	Medicare Reimbursement ($)[a]	Physician Fee + Technical Charge ($)	National Payment ($)
US 76536	123	24.15–163.18	124
CT 70491	250	59.30–353.89	271
Planar sestamibi 78070	280	33.50–407.52	306
SPECT sestamibi 78071	331	50.56–477.52	361
Sample of Current Charges at 1 Institution			
Study Type/CPT Code		Physician Fee/Technical Fee ($)	
US 76536		105/334	
CT 70491		297/943	
Planar sestamibi 78070		156/418	
SPECT sestamibi 78071		215/971	

Abbreviation: CPT, current procedure terminology.

ᵃ http://www.cms.gov/apps/physician-fee-schedule/search/search-criteria.aspx; https://ocm.ama-assn.org/OCM/CPTRelativeValueSearch.do?submitbutton=accept.

that ordering a CT scan of the parathyroid glands, without the proper imaging protocol and multidisciplinary collaboration, fails to deliver the desired results.

Disadvantages of 4DCT include increased radiation exposure and the need for iodinated contrast injection, which limits its use in renal failure and in patients with contrast allergy. A recent study calculated the amount of radiation delivered by 4DCT compared with SPECT MIBI (10.4 mSv vs 7.8 mSv, respectively). This finding is in contrast to an annual background radiation exposure of approximately 3 mSv. The dose of radiation to the thyroid with 4DCT was 57 times higher (92 vs 1.6 mGy) when compared with MIBI scans, which amounted to a calculated risk of 4DCT-related thyroid cancer of 0.1%.[38] The investigators concluded that this modality should be used judiciously in young patients. Others contend that most patients with hyperparathyroidism are cured at their first operation and require only 1-time localization studies. The radiation exposure of SPECT MIBI and 4DCT ranges from 6 to 11 mSv and 10 to 24 mSv, respectively, yet the lifetime attributed risk of cancer incidence and death remains low.[12]

DIFFERENTIAL JUGULAR VENOUS SAMPLING

Although historically, differential jugular venous sampling (DJVS) was performed either by interventional radiology or intraoperatively by the surgeon using IPM to measure PTH levels obtained from each jugular vein, this method of lateralization/localization has recently been described to be accurate as an office-based procedure.[39–41] In this procedure, the surgeon uses US to guide the internal jugular venous sampling as low in the neck as possible (**Fig. 7**). Whole blood is collected from each internal jugular vein and sent to the laboratory for PTH measurement. If the jugular venous PTH level on 1 side of the neck is 10% higher than the opposite side, DJVS is considered positive. This test is correct in lateralizing the abnormal parathyroid glands in 71% to

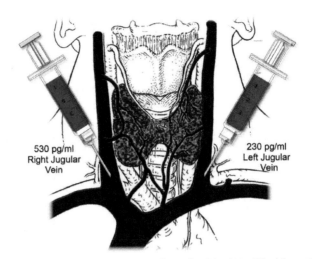

530 pg/ml
Right Jugular
Vein

230 pg/ml
Left Jugular
Vein

Fig. 7. Representation of a positive DJVS on the right side. (*Modified from* Carneiro–Pla D, Pellitteri PK. Intraoperative PTH monitoring during parathyroid surgery. In: Rudolph G, editor. Surgery of the thyroid and parathyroid glands. 2nd edition. Philadelphia: Elsevier; 2012. p. 605–12; with permission.)

81% of patients and has been suggested to be suitable as the second localization study when SUS is equivocal or negative.[39,41]

There are no data available regarding the cost-effectiveness of DJVS. Some surgeons use DJVS before making an incision in an attempt to avoid BNE (when the MIBI and US are negative or equivocal) or intraoperatively when they realize that the abnormal gland is not where the preoperative imaging initially suggested (false-positive result).[17]

SUMMARY AND RECOMMENDATIONS

Most parathyroid surgeons use localization studies and perform focused, directed, or minimally invasive parathyroidectomies. Moreover, even surgeons performing routine BNE almost always use localization studies. Regardless of which parathyroidectomy approach is planned, we believe that all patients should undergo preoperative US, not only to localize the abnormal parathyroid gland but also to properly address the frequently coexisting thyroid disease. Drawing from our own experience and from reviewing the literature, US is the least expensive localization study in patients with SPHPT. When the surgeon can rely on accurate and clear US results to localize the parathyroid gland, they should proceed with parathyroidectomy solely guided by the US results and intraoperative PTH. When the parathyroid gland is not clearly identified or the images are equivocal, an additional study such as MIBI scan, 4DCT, or office-based US-guided DJVS should be obtained. The choice of which additional localization study to obtain depends on local expertise, surgeon comfort level with such study, and experience. Our algorithm for parathyroid localization is shown in **Fig. 8.**

In our clinical practice, patients with negative or equivocal studies (US and MIBI scans) do not routinely undergo 4DCT. Instead, 4DCT is used selectively for reoperative or difficult cases. Even when the images studies are read as negative, the surgeons' review of the images could give a clue as to where to start the exploration (**Fig. 9**).[42] The side of the neck most likely to contain the abnormal parathyroid is

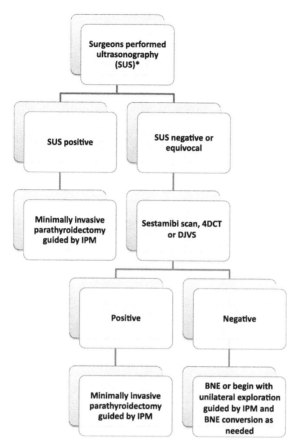

Fig. 8. Suggested algorithm for parathyroid gland localization in patients with sporadic primary hyperparathyroidism. * US can also be performed by expert radiologist; # Please see text for details on using DJVS. BNE, bilateral neck exploration; DJVS, differential jugular venous sampling; IPM, Intraoperative Parathyroid Hormone Monitoring; MIBI, Tc 99m sestamibi scan; 4DCT, four-dimensional computed tomography.

explored first, and if a large gland is found, with the help of IPM, unilateral neck exploration is possible in most patients. BNE is performed when multiglandular disease is suspected, no dominant gland is found on the initially explored side of the neck, or when the intraoperative PTH levels fail to drop after excision of a clearly abnormal gland (multiple gland disease).

Although the abnormal parathyroid gland can often be localized with US, many patients referred for surgical evaluation have already had 1 or more usually negative MIBI scans. To contain cost and improve patient management, the parathyroid surgeon, not the primary care physician or endocrinologist, should determine which localization study is best suited and has the best sensitivity in their local environment. Furthermore, localization studies should never be used to select patients for surgical referral. Collaboration with the referring physicians is important to establish the best algorithm for parathyroid localization and improve cost-effectiveness.

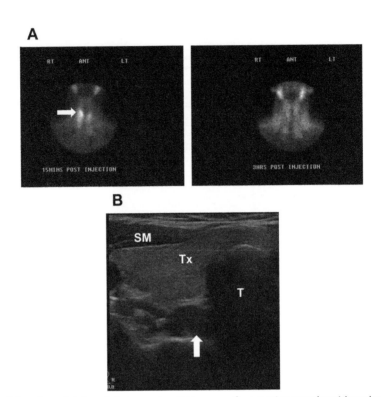

Fig. 9. (*A*) Early and delayed planar sestamibi images of a superior parathyroid read as negative by the radiologist but interpreted as positive by the surgeon. (*B*) Office-based SUS confirming a superior parathyroid correlating well with the sestamibi early images. SM, strap muscles; T, trachea; Tx, thyroid.

REFERENCES

1. Siperstein A, Berber E, Barbosa GF, et al. Predicting the success of limited exploration for primary hyperparathyroidism using ultrasound, sestamibi, and intraoperative parathyroid hormone: analysis of 1158 cases. Ann Surg 2008;248(3): 420–8.
2. Bergenfelz A, Jansson S, Martensson H, et al. Scandinavian Quality Register for Thyroid and Parathyroid Surgery: audit of surgery for primary hyperparathyroidism. Langenbecks Arch Surg 2007;392(4):445–51.
3. Irvin GL 3rd, Carneiro DM, Solorzano CC. Progress in the operative management of sporadic primary hyperparathyroidism over 34 years. Ann Surg 2004;239(5): 704–8 [discussion: 708–11].
4. Irvin GL 3rd, Solorzano CC, Carneiro DM. Quick intraoperative parathyroid hormone assay: surgical adjunct to allow limited parathyroidectomy, improve success rate, and predict outcome. World J Surg 2004;28(12):1287–92.
5. Wang C. The anatomic basis of parathyroid surgery. Ann Surg 1976;183(3):271–5.
6. Akerstrom G, Malmaeus J, Bergstrom R. Surgical anatomy of human parathyroid glands. Surgery 1984;95(1):14–21.
7. Johnson NA, Tublin ME, Ogilvie JB. Parathyroid imaging: technique and role in the preoperative evaluation of primary hyperparathyroidism. AJR Am J Roentgenol 2007;188(6):1706–15.

8. Rodgers SE, Hunter GJ, Hamberg LM, et al. Improved preoperative planning for directed parathyroidectomy with 4-dimensional computed tomography. Surgery 2006;140(6):932–40 [discussion: 940–1].

9. Melton GB, Somervell H, Friedman KP, et al. Interpretation of 99mTc sestamibi parathyroid SPECT scan is improved when read by the surgeon and nuclear medicine physician together. Nucl Med Commun 2005;26(7):633–8.

10. Udelsman R, Donovan PI. Remedial parathyroid surgery: changing trends in 130 consecutive cases. Ann Surg 2006;244(3):471–9.

11. Milas M, Mensah A, Alghoul M, et al. The impact of office neck ultrasonography on reducing unnecessary thyroid surgery in patients undergoing parathyroidectomy. Thyroid 2005;15(9):1055–9.

12. Lubitz CC, Stephen AE, Hodin RA, et al. Preoperative localization strategies for primary hyperparathyroidism: an economic analysis. Ann Surg Oncol 2012; 19(13):4202–9.

13. Wang TS, Cheung K, Farrokhyar F, et al. Would scan, but which scan? A cost-utility analysis to optimize preoperative imaging for primary hyperparathyroidism. Surgery 2011;150(6):1286–94.

14. Deutmeyer C, Weingarten M, Doyle M, et al. Case series of targeted parathyroidectomy with surgeon-performed ultrasonography as the only preoperative imaging study. Surgery 2011;150(6):1153–60.

15. Untch BR, Adam MA, Scheri RP, et al. Surgeon-performed ultrasound is superior to 99Tc-sestamibi scanning to localize parathyroid adenomas in patients with primary hyperparathyroidism: results in 516 patients over 10 years. J Am Coll Surg 2011;212(4):522–9 [discussion: 529–31].

16. Jabiev AA, Lew JI, Solorzano CC. Surgeon-performed ultrasound: a single institution experience in parathyroid localization. Surgery 2009;146(4):569–75 [discussion: 575–7].

17. Solorzano CC, Lee TM, Ramirez MC, et al. Surgeon-performed ultrasound improves localization of abnormal parathyroid glands. Am Surg 2005;71(7): 557–62 [discussion: 562–3].

18. Solorzano CC, Carneiro-Pla DM, Irvin GL 3rd. Surgeon-performed ultrasonography as the initial and only localizing study in sporadic primary hyperparathyroidism. J Am Coll Surg 2006;202(1):18–24.

19. Tublin ME, Pryma DA, Yim JH, et al. Localization of parathyroid adenomas by sonography and technetium Tc 99m sestamibi single-photon emission computed tomography before minimally invasive parathyroidectomy: are both studies really needed? J Ultrasound Med 2009;28(2):183–90.

20. Norman J, Politz D, Browarsky I. Diagnostic aspiration of parathyroid adenomas causes severe fibrosis complicating surgery and final histologic diagnosis. Thyroid 2007;17(12):1251–5.

21. Cheung K, Wang TS, Farrokhyar F, et al. A meta-analysis of preoperative localization techniques for patients with primary hyperparathyroidism. Ann Surg Oncol 2012;19(2):577–83.

22. Ruda JM, Hollenbeak CS, Stack BC Jr. A systematic review of the diagnosis and treatment of primary hyperparathyroidism from 1995 to 2003. Otolaryngol Head Neck Surg 2005;132(3):359–72.

23. Berber E, Parikh RT, Ballem N, et al. Factors contributing to negative parathyroid localization: an analysis of 1000 patients. Surgery 2008;144(1):74–9.

24. Greene AB, Butler RS, McIntyre S, et al. National trends in parathyroid surgery from 1998 to 2008: a decade of change. J Am Coll Surg 2009;209(3): 332–43.

25. Coakley AJ, Kettle AG, Wells CP, et al. 99Tcm sestamibi–a new agent for parathyroid imaging. Nucl Med Commun 1989;10(11):791–4.

26. Lavely WC, Goetze S, Friedman KP, et al. Comparison of SPECT/CT, SPECT, and planar imaging with single- and dual-phase (99m)Tc-sestamibi parathyroid scintigraphy. J Nucl Med 2007;48(7):1084–9.

27. Nichols KJ, Tomas MB, Tronco GG, et al. Preoperative parathyroid scintigraphic lesion localization: accuracy of various types of readings. Radiology 2008;248(1): 221–32.

28. Sharma J, Mazzaglia P, Milas M, et al. Radionuclide imaging for hyperparathyroidism (HPT): which is the best technetium-99m sestamibi modality? Surgery 2006;140(6):856–63 [discussion: 863–5].

29. Dasgupta DJ, Navalkissoor S, Ganatra R, et al. The role of single-photon emission computed tomography/computed tomography in localizing parathyroid adenoma. Nucl Med Commun 2013;34(7):621–6.

30. Van Husen R, Kim LT. Accuracy of surgeon-performed ultrasound in parathyroid localization. World J Surg 2004;28(11):1122–6.

31. Gotthardt M, Lohmann B, Behr TM, et al. Clinical value of parathyroid scintigraphy with technetium-99m methoxyisobutylisonitrile: discrepancies in clinical data and a systematic metaanalysis of the literature. World J Surg 2004; 28(1):100–7.

32. Starker LF, Mahajan A, Bjorklund P, et al. 4D parathyroid CT as the initial localization study for patients with de novo primary hyperparathyroidism. Ann Surg Oncol 2011;18(6):1723–8.

33. Lubitz CC, Hunter GJ, Hamberg LM, et al. Accuracy of 4-dimensional computed tomography in poorly localized patients with primary hyperparathyroidism. Surgery 2010;148(6):1129–37 [discussion: 1137–8].

34. Eichhorn–Wharry LI, Carlin AM, Talpos GB. Mild hypercalcemia: an indication to select 4-dimensional computed tomography scan for preoperative localization of parathyroid adenomas. Am J Surg 2011;201(3):334–8 [discussion: 338].

35. Mortenson MM, Evans DB, Lee JE, et al. Parathyroid exploration in the reoperative neck: improved preoperative localization with 4D-computed tomography. J Am Coll Surg 2008;206(5):888–95 [discussion: 895–6].

36. Abbott DE, Cantor SB, Grubbs EG, et al. Outcomes and economic analysis of routine preoperative 4-dimensional CT for surgical intervention in de novo primary hyperparathyroidism: does clinical benefit justify the cost? J Am Coll Surg 2012; 214(4):629–37 [discussion: 637–9].

37. Harari A, Zarnegar R, Lee J, et al. Computed tomography can guide focused exploration in select patients with primary hyperparathyroidism and negative sestamibi scanning. Surgery 2008;144(6):970–6 [discussion: 976–9].

38. Mahajan A, Starker LF, Ghita M, et al. Parathyroid four-dimensional computed tomography: evaluation of radiation dose exposure during preoperative localization of parathyroid tumors in primary hyperparathyroidism. World J Surg 2012;36(6): 1335–9.

39. Carneiro–Pla D. Effectiveness of "office"-based, ultrasound-guided differential jugular venous sampling (DJVS) of parathormone in patients with primary hyperparathyroidism. Surgery 2009;146(6):1014–20.

40. Carneiro–Pla DM, Solorzano CC, Irvin GL 3rd. Consequences of targeted parathyroidectomy guided by localization studies without intraoperative parathyroid hormone monitoring. J Am Coll Surg 2006;202(5):715–22.

41. Ito F, Sippel R, Lederman J, et al. The utility of intraoperative bilateral internal jugular venous sampling with rapid parathyroid hormone testing. Ann Surg 2007; 245(6):959–63.
42. Neychev VK, Kouniavsky G, Shiue Z, et al. Chasing "shadows": discovering the subtleties of sestamibi scans to facilitate minimally invasive parathyroidectomy. World J Surg 2011;35(1):140–6.

Operative Treatment of Primary Hyperparathyroidism
Balancing Cost-effectiveness with Successful Outcomes

Dina Elaraj, MD, Cord Sturgeon, MD, MS*

KEYWORDS

- Parathyroidectomy • Hyperparathyroidism • Cost-effectiveness • Outcomes

KEY POINTS

- Randomized prospective trials have shown no difference in cure rate between focused parathyroidectomy and bilateral exploration.
- Costs of the two techniques differ depending on the preoperative and intraoperative localization used, speed of the operation, ability to discharge the patient on the same day as the operation, cure rate, and complications.
- There is considerable controversy about how to balance cost-effectiveness with successful outcomes. Although several studies have suggested that there is lower cost with the focused approach, it may be less costly and more effective to use a policy of routine 4-gland exploration without the use of preoperative or intraoperative localization studies.
- Although most surgeons consider the measurement of intraoperative parathyroid hormone (IOPTH) to be essential during focused parathyroidectomy, several studies have suggested that measuring IOPTH kinetics does not improve the cure rate for those patients with clear preoperative localization studies.
- Parathyroidectomy has been shown to be more cost-effective than observation or pharmacologic therapy for the treatment of primary hyperparathyroidism (PHPT). Despite these findings and the establishment of expert guidelines that favor surgical treatment, only approximately 1 in 4 patients with PHPT is referred for surgery.
- Because of the increasing prevalence of PHPT and the negative economic impact of untreated disease, one of the broad goals for endocrine surgeons should be to deliver the message that, from a societal perspective, parathyroidectomy is the preferred treatment strategy.

Section of Endocrine Surgery, Department of Surgery, Feinberg School of Medicine, Northwestern University, 676 North Saint Clair Street, Chicago, IL 60611, USA
* Corresponding author. Department of Surgery, Northwestern University, 676 North Saint Clair Street, Suite 650, Chicago, IL 60611.
E-mail address: csturgeo@nmh.org

Surg Clin N Am 94 (2014) 607–623
http://dx.doi.org/10.1016/j.suc.2014.02.011
0039-6109/14/$ – see front matter © 2014 Elsevier Inc. All rights reserved.

INTRODUCTION

Primary hyperparathyroidism (PHPT) is a common disease affecting approximately 0.25% to 0.66% of the population.[1] Women are affected more often than men by a ratio of nearly 3:1. Incidence increases with age, and rises dramatically after 50 years of age.[1] In addition, the prevalence of the disease seems to be increasing.[1] This may partially be caused by PHPT being either under-recognized or undertreated. When untreated, PHPT may lead to a broad range of symptoms and comorbidities such as nephrolithiasis and decreased bone mineral density that reduce the quality of life and increase the cost of health care.[2–4] Parathyroidectomy has been shown to be more cost-effective than observation or pharmacologic therapy for the treatment of PHPT.[5–7]

Parathyroidectomy for PHPT has a success rate greater than 95% in the hands of experienced surgeons, which is independent of preoperative localization or surgical technique used.[8–13] The gold-standard operation for PHPT is a 4-gland parathyroid exploration, in which all 4 parathyroid glands are exposed and the abnormal gland or glands are resected.[14] The safety and efficacy of all other parathyroidectomy techniques are compared with those of the 4-gland exploration. In the past, preoperative localization studies were considered unnecessary for an index parathyroid exploration.[15,16] Because of the development of high-fidelity preoperative parathyroid imaging and rapid intraoperative measurement of parathyroid hormone (PTH), the focused removal of diseased parathyroid glands without disturbing the normal glands became possible[17,18] and by 2003 had become the favored approach by many surgeons.[16,19,20] Focused parathyroidectomy is now commonly performed in the outpatient setting at many specialized centers across the United States.[18,21–28] In some centers, focused parathyroidectomy is even performed under local or regional anesthesia and sedation, and patients are discharged home the same day as the operation.[18,26]

Both approaches are safe and effective, and consequently 4-gland exploration and focused parathyroidectomy are both acceptable surgical options in patients with sporadic PHPT.[29] However, over the last decade there has been considerable controversy about the relative effectiveness of each surgical technique. Some investigators have cautioned that multigland disease may be missed by focused parathyroidectomy in approximately 15% to 25% of cases, and argue in favor of 4-gland exploration in all cases.[30–32] Supporting this view is the observation that the probability of detecting multigland disease seems to depend on the surgical technique used for parathyroidectomy.[8,32,33] One early report indicated that the rates of multigland disease identified via 4-gland exploration and focused parathyroidectomy were 20.6% and 5.3% respectively.[33] A multi-institution report of 800 parathyroid operations found multigland disease in 16.5% of patients undergoing routine 4-gland exploration, and in only 11.1% of patients undergoing focused parathyroidectomy.[8] A single-institution series reported finding multigland disease 24.7% of the time with 4-gland exploration and only 3.1% of the time with unilateral exploration.[32] Some experts point to the difference in the rate of multigland disease depending on the surgical technique used, and warn that focused parathyroidectomy is missing additional abnormal glands that may someday cause recurrent or persistent hyperparathyroidism. In contrast, some experts hypothesize that the additional enlarged glands that are found on bilateral exploration may not be biologically significant (ie, overactive).[34] This hypothesis is supported by many findings that focused parathyroidectomy with use of intraoperative PTH (IOPTH) has a long-term success rate that is equivalent to 4-gland exploration.[8,11,34,35]

The economy of health care delivery in the United States has become highly scrutinized and politicized in the past several decades and attention has now been focused on maximizing value and safety. The results of comparative effectiveness studies show that parathyroidectomy delivers the greatest value to most patients with PHPT, even those considered asymptomatic.[5–7] As the economic demands for health care delivery continue to increase, even greater pressure will be applied to physicians to manage disease in the most effective and least costly manner. Surgeons will not be immune to this pressure, and will likewise be expected to conduct their operations with both costs and outcomes in mind. This article discusses the competing surgical techniques of routine 4-gland exploration and focused parathyroidectomy with the use of preoperative localization studies and intraoperative confirmation of cure.

THE ARGUMENTS IN FAVOR OF ROUTINE 4-GLAND EXPLORATION
Learn from History or Be Doomed to Repeat It

American philosopher George Santayana[36] wrote that "those who cannot remember the past are condemned to repeat it." Studying the history of parathyroid surgery teaches valuable lessons regarding not only the various manifestations and natural history of PHPT but also the results of unilateral and bilateral exploration. The arguments in favor of routine 4-gland exploration should therefore begin with a reminder that the first successful parathyroidectomy conducted for PHPT was a 4-gland exploration. In contrast, the first attempted parathyroidectomy in the United States was a unilateral exploration that failed to cure the patient. Examination of these historical cases illuminates the key tenets of parathyroid surgery. First, the capsule of the parathyroid should not be violated or ruptured. Second, the index operation offers the highest chance for cure. Third, never resect normal glands. Fourth, parathyroid tumors are not always in eutopic locations. In addition, the early experiences with parathyroid surgery led to an era of routine 4-gland exploration that lasted more than half a century and yielded excellent results.

Recurrent and persistent PHPT has been called the bête noire of the endocrine surgeon.[37] Surgeons have been haunted by this nefarious disease from the time that Dr Felix Mandl performed the first parathyroidectomy for PHPT on July 30, 1925, in Vienna on Herr Albert Jahne, a 38-year-old streetcar conductor with incapacitating osteitis fibrosa cystica.[38] This first operation was a bilateral exploration performed under local anesthesia. One abnormal and 3 normal glands were found. The abnormal gland was a 2.5-cm left-sided gland that was greyish white and adherent to the recurrent laryngeal nerve.[38,39] Dr Mandl had to use sharp dissection to free the tumor from the trachea and recurrent nerve. Despite a good recovery in the short term, Albert Jahne had a recurrence of hyperparathyroidism from what many believe was parathyroid carcinoma. Four years after surgery in 1929, hypercalcemia and hypercalciuria returned, followed by kidney stones in 1932. By 1933, he was again incapacitated by the disease. Reexploration did not identify a second abnormal parathyroid, but multiple microscopic foci of parathyroid tissue were found on pathologic examination of the tissues surrounding the thyroid. This finding is the basis of the suspicion that Jahne had either parathyroid carcinoma or parathyromatosis. Jahne ultimately died of uremia in 1936 at age 49 and his autopsy revealed many of the end-organ effects of PHPT, including decalcified vertebra, multiple fractures, and nephrocalcinosis. The original pathologic slides have not been reexamined in the modern era, thus the diagnosis of parathyroid cancer cannot be confirmed. Parathyromatosis is also a plausible explanation. The risk of tumor capsule violation must have been high, considering that sharp dissection was required to separate the parathyroid tumor from the trachea and recurrent nerve in an awake patient.

One of the most infamous cases of persistent PHPT is that of the first case diagnosed in the United States. In 1926, Charles Martell, a 38-year-old merchant sea captain, suffered persistent PHPT following a unilateral neck exploration at the Massachusetts General Hospital by Dr Elliot Richardson in which only a normal parathyroid was removed. He subsequently underwent 5 more unsuccessful cervical operations in Boston and New York in which additional normal glands were removed. After researching his own disease extensively in the Harvard Medical Library, Martell himself advised his surgeons to perform a mediastinal exploration.[40] In 1932, Edward Churchill and Oliver Cope obliged him and via sternotomy identified and subtotally resected a 3-cm mediastinal tumor.[41] However, 3 days following this seventh operation Martell developed tetany and then, 6 weeks later, at age 43 years, died of laryngospasm following a procedure to relieve ureteral obstruction.[41]

The biology of PHPT has not dramatically changed in the last century. The pitfalls and challenges faced by modern surgeons recapitulate those from 90 years ago. The first successful parathyroidectomy was a 4-gland operation performed by Felix Mandl, but, because of the biology of the tumor, the disease recurred. Oliver Cope performed multiple unilateral operations on Charles Martell to satisfy himself that there was no eutopic parathyroid adenoma. Had Richardson performed a 4-gland exploration on Charles Martell at the index operation, and left normal parathyroid tissue intact, it might have saved Martell from some of his subsequent negative cervical explorations and perhaps reduced the severity of hypocalcemia after his seventh exploration.

Four-gland Exploration May Yield the Highest Long-term Cure Rate

Four-gland exploration has had a 95% success rate in the hands of experienced parathyroid surgeons for more than half a century independent of preoperative localization or surgical technique used.[8–12,42–44] During that time it was widely thought that approximately 15% to 20% of patients with PHPT had multigland disease, and that unilateral exploration would result in failure to cure these individuals. The availability of high-resolution preoperative parathyroid imaging and rapid intraoperative measurement of PTH in the 1990s allowed a shift to unilateral or focused exploration for most patients.[16–20] Since then, surgical series of focused parathyroidectomy have revealed an approximately 5% to 10% rate of multigland disease.[8,34,45] The reason for the 2-fold to 4-fold difference in rate of multiglandular disease between series of focused and bilateral exploration is not clear. The failure to cure PHPT is frequently due to the inability to discriminate multigland disease from single-gland disease.[46] Several contemporary investigators contend that preoperative localization and intraoperative PTH are insensitive for multigland disease, and therefore 4-gland exploration offers the best chance of cure.[30–32,47,48] One large series reported a recurrence rate 11-fold higher for unilateral exploration than bilateral exploration.[32] A series of routine 4-gland explorations from the Cleveland Clinic revealed unsuspected multigland disease in 15% of patients with concordant sestamibi and ultrasonography results and curative drop in PTH.[30] Another Cleveland Clinic series reported unsuspected multiglandular disease in approximately 20% of patients who had concordant preoperative localization followed by 4-gland exploration.[31] The use of intraoperative PTH reduced unsuspected multigland disease to 16% in this series. Although there is some debate over whether the additional abnormal glands in these series were hypersecretory, these investigators concluded that a routine 4-gland exploration offers the best opportunity for long-term cure.

Four-gland Exploration Is a Low-risk, Safe Operation

The overall complication rate for a first-time 4-gland exploration is approximately 3% to 10%.[11,49] The rate of temporary recurrent nerve injury is approximately 2% to 7%.[49,50] The rate of permanent recurrent nerve injury is less than 1%.[11,49–51] Temporary postoperative hypocalcemia is common, and occurs approximately 3% to 10% of the time following subtotal parathyroidectomy and up to 25% or 30% of the time following total parathyroidectomy with autotransplantation, depending on the patient comorbidities and the surgical technique used.[51–54] The rate of permanent hypoparathyroidism is approximately 1%.[51,55]

In a randomized prospective trial of unilateral versus bilateral parathyroid exploration, in 44 patients who underwent bilateral exploration there were 3 patients with postoperative hypoparathyroidism (6.8%), 1 of which was permanent (1.1%).[49] One patient had temporary recurrent nerve paresis (2.3%) and no patients had permanent recurrent nerve paresis. One patient underwent reoperation for bleeding. In a series of 379 patients who underwent an index 4-gland exploration at the Mayo Clinic there were 4 wound infections (1%), 11 cases of temporary hypoparathyroidism (3%), and 1 case of permanent hypoparathyroidism (0.3%). Six cases of recurrent nerve paresis (2.4%) were identified in the postoperative period, but only 2 cases were permanent (0.8%).[51] Other expert surgeon series have shown similar low permanent complication rates for 4-gland exploration.[11,22]

Reoperation Has a Lower Cure Rate and Higher Complication Rate Than Initial Surgery

The optimal surgical approach for PHPT should yield the highest cure rate with the lowest complication rate. Furthermore, the new overarching goal for health delivery systems and health care policy is to deliver the greatest value to patients. Value in health care is defined as the heath outcome achieved per dollar spent.[56] Given this framework and that the cure rate for 4-gland exploration is high (95% or more), and the permanent complication rate is low (approximately 1%), it can be argued that routine 4-gland exploration should be the preferred approach. One method to decrease cure rate and simultaneously increase complication rate and costs is to have a high number of failed index operations that leads to a reoperative parathyroidectomy. The success rate of remedial parathyroidectomy by expert surgeons exceeds 90%; however, the optimal time to cure the patient is during the first operation, when the likelihood of cure without surgical complications is greatest.[57–59] There is a higher risk of complications such as recurrent nerve injury (4%–10%) or hypoparathyroidism (10%–20%) after reoperative surgery.[57,58,60–64] Furthermore, the results of reoperative parathyroid surgery are usually not as satisfactory as those of an index operation for PHPT. Cure rates have been reported to be as high as 95% in expert centers,[57,65] but most investigators report that the success rate for reoperative surgery is only approximately 90%.[60–62,64,66–68] In addition, because of mandatory localization studies, longer operative times, higher complication rates, and higher technical fees, reoperative surgery must be considerably more costly than a first-time operation for PHPT.

Four-gland Exploration Is Mandatory in Patients with High Risk of Multigland Disease

Four-gland exploration is mandatory in patients with a high risk of multiglandular disease.[14] Patients with multiple endocrine neoplasia type 1 (MEN-1) and multiple endocrine neoplasia type 2a (MEN-2a) almost always have an asymmetric 4-gland hyperplasia.[69,70] Although some clinicians contend that focused parathyroidectomy is an acceptable approach in some patients with MEN-2a,[71] guideline statements indicate that focused parathyroidectomy is not recommended in MEN-1 and MEN-2a.[72,73] Patients with secondary and tertiary hyperparathyroidism caused by renal failure have enlargement of all parathyroid tissue and should undergo routine bilateral exploration. Radiation exposure at a young age, prolonged lithium exposure, and hyperparathyroidism jaw tumor syndrome all are associated with a higher risk of multigland disease and should be managed with a 4-gland exploration. Nonlocalized patients should undergo 4-gland exploration because the risk of multigland disease is high. Patients with nonlocalizing sestamibi studies have a risk of multigland disease of approximately 25%.[74] In addition, the risk factors for multigland disease are not always known at the time of surgery, and unsuspected MEN-1 may be found in up to 18% of patients with PHPT.[72]

Preoperative Localization Studies and Their Costs Are Not Necessary Before 4-Gland Exploration

Preoperative localization studies are not necessary when planning a 4-gland exploration. In the past, preoperative localization studies were not performed before an initial parathyroid exploration.[13,15,16] The guiding principle for the first half century of parathyroid surgery was summarized by the aphorism from the late John Doppman: "the only localization that a patient needs who has primary hyperparathyroidism is the localization of an experienced surgeon."[75] Preoperative localization studies are expensive and some contemporary studies suggest that they may not significantly improve the cure rate.[8,76] Furthermore, high-quality localization studies are not universally available. In addition, when available, localization studies are not uniformly reliable. For example, parathyroid ultrasonography is highly operator dependent. Localization studies may also be misleading in cases of inherited or acquired hyperparathyroidism, particularly MEN-1. Only approximately two-thirds of patients are candidates for a focused parathyroidectomy given the limitations of localization,[47] and, when localization studies are negative, a 4-gland exploration should be performed.[14] One randomized controlled trial of preoperative localization showed that routine preoperative localization was not cost-effective if the intention was to offer focused parathyroidectomy to only those patients who have 2 concordant localization studies.[77] Another study revealed that routine 4-gland exploration without the use of preoperative or intraoperative localization or confirmation studies is less costly than attempting sestamibi scan–directed parathyroidectomy in all patients.[78]

Intraoperative Adjuncts, Including IOPTH, Are Not Necessary in 4-Gland Exploration

Intraoperative PTH is not necessary when performing 4-gland exploration. IOPTH adds cost to the operation, is not universally available, and several studies suggest that it may not add significantly to the cure rate even in focused parathyroidectomy.[79–82] IOPTH may also be unreliable in patients with multigland disease or with kidney or liver disease.[47,48,83] Many criteria exist for the interpretation of PTH kinetics; consequently, the PTH data may be misinterpreted leading to either premature discontinuation or unnecessary extension of the operation.[84] At the Cleveland Clinic clinicians have shown that, even with the use of IOPTH, additional abnormal parathyroid glands are found in 15% of patients by 4-gland exploration.[30]

Depending on the Time Required for IOPTH, 4-Gland Exploration May Be Faster

Drawing blood for IOPTH and waiting for the results before converting to a 4-gland exploration adds time to the operation. Depending on how quickly blood can be drawn and transported to the laboratory, and the turnaround time for the assay, it may be faster to do a bilateral exploration at some institutions. If this is the case, it may be less costly to perform a bilateral exploration because it may save operating room time as well as the costs of preoperative localization studies and IOPTH assays. In one large series, 4-gland exploration took only 6 minutes longer than unilateral exploration.[32] Most IOPTH assays have a turnaround time of 15 to 20 minutes and are not drawn until 5 or 10 minutes following parathyroid resection. This combined time of 20 to 30 minutes is sufficient to perform a contralateral exploration in most patients.

Summary of the arguments in favor of routine 4-gland exploration

A greater number of abnormal glands are found during bilateral exploration than during focused parathyroidectomy. This high rate of unsuspected abnormal glands raises a legitimate concern about the long-term durability of cure from focused parathyroidectomy in approximately 15% of patients. Furthermore, unsuspected MEN-1 may be the underlying cause of PHPT in up to 18% of patients with apparently sporadic disease. Because the underlying biology of disease is asymmetric 4-gland hyperplasia, focused parathyroidectomy does not adequately address parathyroid disease in MEN-1. It must be more cost-effective to have a higher cure rate at initial exploration than to rely on a reoperation for persistent disease. In order for a focused approach to be of greater economic value, the added time and cost expenditure of preoperative localization and intraoperative confirmation of curative reduction in PTH should be associated with fewer complications and a higher cure rate than routine 4-gland exploration without preoperative localization and intraoperative adjuncts. Furthermore, those added costs must be considered reasonable for the incremental benefit that is gained.

THE ARGUMENTS IN FAVOR OF FOCUSED PARATHYROIDECTOMY
Focused Parathyroidectomy and 4-Gland Exploration Have Similar Cure Rates

Multiple studies have shown that focused parathyroidectomy has a cure rate similar to that of traditional 4-gland exploration (**Table 1**).[11,34,36,81,85–87] A prospective study of 91 Swedish patients randomized to unilateral versus bilateral neck exploration found no differences between the two groups with respect to ionized calcium, PTH, or rates of persistent or recurrent hyperparathyroidism either in the short term or with 5 years of follow-up.[35,49] A similar, smaller, randomized trial of 48 Lithuanian patients also found no difference between the two groups with respect to serum calcium or PTH at 6 months of follow-up.[81] In a prospective randomized trial of preoperative localization

Table 1
Arguments in favor of routine 4-gland exploration and arguments in favor of focused parathyroidectomy

Arguments in Favor of Routine 4-gland Exploration	Arguments in Favor of Focused Parathyroidectomy
A greater number of abnormal glands are found	Lower complication rate
May have higher cure rate	Cure rate identical to 4-gland exploration
Reoperation is less effective and higher risk	No unnecessary dissection risks
Four-gland exploration is mandatory for some patients (eg, MEN)	Less patient discomfort
Localization studies and IOPTH unnecessary	Most patients can be localized
May be faster	May be faster
May be less costly	May be less costly

in 100 patients with PHPT, 50 patients were randomized to routine bilateral exploration without localization studies and 50 were randomized to undergo preoperative localization and focused parathyroidectomy if the studies were positive (criteria satisfied in only 23 of 50). The routine bilateral exploration group had a cure rate of 94%, and the preoperative localization group had a cure rate of 96%.[77] Larger, nonrandomized experiences have reported similar findings. The Mayo Clinic group published their results of 1361 consecutive patients who underwent surgery for PHPT with a mean follow-up of 25 months, 734 (54%) of whom underwent conventional 4-gland exploration, 601 (44%) of whom underwent focused parathyroidectomy, and 26 (2%) of whom had conversion of focused parathyroidectomy to a 4-gland exploration.[85] Cure rates and rates of persistent and recurrent hyperparathyroidism were similar between the groups. A single-surgeon, 2-institution experience of 1650 consecutive patients, 613 of whom underwent conventional 4-gland exploration and 1037 of whom underwent focused parathyroidectomy, with a mean follow-up of 15 to 37 months, showed slightly higher but statistically significant cure rates in the focused parathyroidectomy group versus the 4-gland exploration group (99% vs 97%).[86] A 2-institution study of routine 4-gland exploration versus focused parathyroidectomy with IOPTH in 800 consecutive patients found no statistically significant difference in the cure rates between the two approaches (96.3% vs 97.7%).[8] In addition, 1 study of lateral approach parathyroidectomy without the use of IOPTH in 500 localized patients revealed a cure rate comparable with 4-gland exploration of 97.4%.[87]

Focused Parathyroidectomy Is Less Costly Than 4-Gland Exploration

Focused parathyroidectomy has been shown to be cost saving in multiple studies (both theoretic and outcomes based), primarily because of reduced operative charges and same-day hospital discharge.[11,22,25] In these studies the addition of preoperative imaging and/or the use of the IOPTH assay during parathyroidectomy was not associated with increased cost. A cost-benefit analysis modeling a nondirected 4-gland exploration versus focused parathyroidectomy with preoperative 99 m technetium sestamibi scintigraphy, IOPTH assay, or intraoperative radioguidance found that the use of any localizing strategy reduced total charges, the risk of persistent hyperparathyroidism, and the cumulative risk of recurrent laryngeal nerve injury compared with a nondirected 4-gland exploration.[88] A cost-utility analysis comparing 5 different preoperative localization strategies and focused-approach parathyroidectomy when the preoperative imaging was correct and IOPTH criteria were met (and 4-gland exploration if the preoperative localization was incorrect based on IOPTH criteria or intraoperative findings) found that 4-gland exploration was less cost-effective than any combination of preoperative imaging strategies.[89]

Outcomes of surgical series have shown either equivalent costs or cost savings associated with focused-approach parathyroidectomy. One study comparing 401 bilateral explorations with 255 focused operations revealed that focused parathyroidectomy had an approximately 50% reduction in operating time, a 7-fold reduction in length of hospital stay, and a mean cost saving of US$2693 per procedure.[11] The investigators concluded that focused parathyroidectomy resulted in an almost 50% reduction in total hospital charges. A prospective study of 91 Swedish patients randomized to unilateral versus bilateral neck exploration found no differences between the two groups with respect to costs (US$2258 ± $509 vs US$2097 ± $505, respectively).[49] A single-surgeon, 2-institution experience of 1650 consecutive patients who underwent surgery for PHPT found that focused parathyroidectomy had decreased total hospital charges compared with traditional 4-gland exploration, with a mean cost saving of US$1471 per case.[86]

Focused Parathyroidectomy May Have Lower Complication Rates Than 4-Gland Exploration

Focused parathyroidectomy may have a lower complication rate than 4-gland exploration.[11,49] It is intuitive that an operation associated with limited dissection should have lower complication rates than an operation associated with more extensive dissection. However, this comparison is difficult to study because complication rates are so low, particularly with experienced parathyroid surgeons. In several publications the rate of temporary hypoparathyroidism has been higher in 4-gland exploration,[90] especially if routine parathyroid biopsy is performed.[91,92] In a randomized trial of unilateral versus bilateral exploration the complication rate was lower (4% vs 11% respectively) with unilateral exploration.[49] A prospective randomized study found that patients who underwent the bilateral approach experienced a higher rate of transient postoperative hypocalcemia and consumed more oral calcium than those in the unilateral exploration group.[49] A series of 1650 consecutive patients found that focused parathyroidectomy was associated with a statistically significantly lower overall complication rate compared with 4-gland exploration (1.45% vs 3.10%), although rates of hypocalcemia and rates of recurrent laryngeal nerve injury were less than 1% for both groups.[86]

Focused Parathyroidectomy Should Be Faster Than 4-Gland Exploration

Because it is not necessary to mobilize both lobes of the thyroid gland and identify all 4 parathyroid glands, focused parathyroidectomy should take less time. Several reports indicate that focused parathyroidectomy takes less time than a 4-gland exploration.[11,22,80] In a single-surgeon series of 656 consecutive parathyroid operations, the focused approach was significantly faster (1.3 hours) than conventional 4-gland exploration (2.4 hours).[11] In another series of 100 patients the mean operative time for unilateral exploration was 42 minutes compared with 76 minutes for bilateral exploration.[80] In a series of 81 patients who underwent conventional parathyroidectomy compared with 76 patients who underwent a focused technique the operative times were statistically significantly shorter for the focused technique: 29 versus 62 minutes.[93] It is clear from these three examples that there is a time cost to bilateral exploration. However, the time required is substantially different in each example (range approximately 33–66 minutes). The time required for IOPTH measurement and processing may or may not be offset by the time required to perform exploration of the contralateral central neck. Several studies report a high cure rate (90%–98%) for focused parathyroidectomy without the use of IOPTH in localized patients,[79,80,87,94–96] which raises the question of whether the time and cost of IOPTH is necessary in all cases.

Focused Parathyroidectomy Is Associated with Less Patient Discomfort

Many investigators have indicated that focused parathyroidectomy should be associated with less patient discomfort.[18,22,81,97,98] The rationale for this is primarily that the operation can usually be performed through a smaller incision, using less dissection, and endotracheal intubation may not be necessary. Parathyroid operations performed under cervical block and intravenous sedation are well tolerated. In a report from 1996 of bilateral superficial cervical block and intravenous sedation for thyroid and parathyroid surgery, only 1 patient in a series of 21 required conversion to endotracheal anesthesia, and 2 patients required supplemental inhaled anesthetic.[99] In a report from 1999 of 33 patients undergoing parathyroidectomy via cervical block and intravenous sedation, only 1 patient required conversion to general anesthesia because of discomfort.[18] In a single-surgeon series of 441 patients undergoing focused parathyroidectomy under superficial cervical block and monitored anesthesia care, only 5 required conversion because of patient discomfort (1.1%).[100] Together, these data suggest that a minority of patients experience intraoperative discomfort that alters the anesthetic plan. The advantages of avoiding general anesthesia include less throat discomfort from intubation and a reduced need for postoperative antiemetic administration. In a series of 89 patients who underwent focused parathyroidectomy under local anesthesia, only 3 (3.3%) required antiemetic medication; however, 29% of patients who had general anesthesia required antiemetic medication.[98] In a series of 81 patients who underwent conventional parathyroidectomy compared with 76 patients who underwent a focused technique, there was statistically significantly less pain reported by visual analog scale at both 1 hour and 24 hours after the operation by the patients having focused parathyroidectomy.[93] In a prospective randomized trial of focused parathyroidectomy under either regional or general anesthesia, less postoperative pain was reported by patients in the regional anesthesia group.[101] In a prospective, randomized, blinded trial comparing 23 patients who underwent bilateral exploration with 24 patients who underwent focused parathyroidectomy, the patients in the focused parathyroidectomy arm reported less postoperative pain and had fewer requests for analgesics, lower analgesic consumption, shorter scar length, and a better cosmetic satisfaction rate in the immediate postoperative period.[81] Despite postoperative pain, nausea, and discomfort being difficult to quantify, these reports suggest that focused parathyroidectomy is well tolerated and results in less overall postoperative discomfort.

A Policy of Routine Bilateral Exploration Is Equivalent to Performing Unnecessary Dissection 95% of the Time

Focused parathyroidectomy with the use of IOPTH has a cure rate of 95% or higher.[8,11,24,26,34,35,49,81,85,86,102] The long-term cure rate of 4-gland exploration and focused parathyroidectomy are statistically equivalent in most studies.[8,49,77,85] Regardless, if the superior cure rate with 4-gland exploration is statistically real and meaningful, then subjecting all patients to a 4-gland exploration would be tantamount to performing unnecessary dissection in at least 95% of patients to achieve an improved long-term cure in less than 5% of patients. Surgeons must keep in mind that bilateral exploration exposes both recurrent nerves and all 4 parathyroid glands to risk of injury, and that prospective studies have indicated that there are higher complication rates with bilateral exploration. These higher rates of complications must be substantially outweighed by the increased probability of cure offered with a bilateral exploration in order for a policy of routine 4-gland exploration to meet the scrutiny of a simple risk-benefit analysis. For most surgeons, the added risks of routine 4-gland exploration are not outweighed by the potential benefits in a small percentage of patients.

Summary of the arguments in favor of focused parathyroid exploration

Between 80% and 85% of cases of PHPT are caused by a single overactive parathyroid adenoma, and approximately 15% are caused by multigland disease. It stands to reason that when such a large percentage of patients have only a single abnormal gland, if these patients could be identified preoperatively, they could be selected for a more minimally invasive procedure targeting just the parathyroid adenoma. The development of high-fidelity preoperative localization studies and the ability to rapidly measure PTH during surgery have been the two breakthroughs that have allowed the widespread adoption of minimally invasive techniques for parathyroid surgery.[16–20] When ultrasonography and sestamibi are concordant the sensitivity for single-gland disease at that location is approximately 96%.[16] Most patients (approximately 60%) with PHPT have concordant imaging studies when they are performed at high-volume centers.[30,31,77] Because of the reliability of preoperative localization and intraoperative PTH measurement, focused parathyroidectomy has become the favored approach by many surgeons.[16,19,20] A focused operation based on preoperative localization (or even just lateralization) would be more expeditious and potentially safer and less painful because of the smaller dissection field. Faster operative procedures should be associated with lower costs for operating room and anesthesia time. In addition, low-risk minimally invasive procedures with a low level of patient discomfort can be performed in the outpatient setting, which has multiple facets of cost savings including fewer inpatient beds occupied, lower opportunity cost, and fewer perioperative analgesic and antiemetic agents consumed. Most studies have revealed a similar cure rate between focused parathyroidectomy and 4-gland exploration. In addition, several studies have found the focused approach to be less costly, faster, and associated with fewer complications than bilateral exploration. In addition, because of the excellent cure rate from focused parathyroidectomy in localized patients, it does not make sense to expose patients to additional surgical risk by dissecting in the region of both recurrent nerves and all 4 parathyroid glands when it is unnecessary to do so.

SUMMARY

Randomized prospective trials have shown no difference in cure rate between focused parathyroidectomy and bilateral exploration.[35,49,77,81] Costs of the two techniques differ depending on the preoperative and intraoperative localization used, speed of the operation, ability to discharge the patient on the same day as the operation, cure rate, and complications. There is considerable controversy about how to balance cost-effectiveness with successful outcomes. Although several studies have suggested that there is lower cost with the focused approach,[11,22,25,88,89] it may be less costly and more effective to use a policy of routine 4-gland exploration without the use of preoperative or intraoperative localization studies.[78] Although most surgeons consider the measurement of IOPTH to be essential during focused parathyroidectomy,[103] several studies have suggested that measuring IOPTH kinetics does not improve the cure rate for those patients with clear preoperative localization studies.[79,80,87,94–96] This raises a question about the necessity and value of IOPTH for localized patients. Other studies indicate that sestamibi may not be necessary when surgeon-performed ultrasonography and IOPTH measurement are combined.[103–105] Despite the controversy surrounding this topic,[106] little attention has been paid to linking the costs and outcomes of the various approaches. The potential economic impact and the expected outcome of the various strategies should be evaluated through formal cost-effectiveness analysis from the societal perspective.

Parathyroidectomy has been shown to be more cost-effective than observation or pharmacologic therapy for the treatment of PHPT.[5–7] Despite these findings and the establishment of expert guidelines that favor surgical treatment,[29] only approximately 1 in 4 patients with PHPT is referred for surgery.[107,108] Because of the increasing prevalence of PHPT and the negative economic impact of untreated disease, one of the broad goals for endocrine surgeons should be to deliver the message that, from a societal perspective, parathyroidectomy is the preferred treatment strategy. Clinicians should also be focused on delivering the highest value to patients undergoing parathyroidectomy.

REFERENCES

1. Yeh MW, Ituarte PH, Zhou HC, et al. Incidence and prevalence of primary hyperparathyroidism in a racially mixed population. J Clin Endocrinol Metab 2013; 98(3):1122–9.
2. Sheldon DG, Lee FT, Neil NJ, et al. Surgical treatment of hyperparathyroidism improves health-related quality of life. Arch Surg 2002;137(9):1022–6 [discussion: 1026–8].
3. Burney RE, Jones KR, Christy B, et al. Health status improvement after surgical correction of primary hyperparathyroidism in patients with high and low preoperative calcium levels. Surgery 1999;125(6):608–14.
4. Quiros RM, Alef MJ, Wilhelm SM, et al. Health-related quality of life in hyperparathyroidism measurably improves after parathyroidectomy. Surgery 2003;134(4): 675–81 [discussion: 681–3].
5. Sejean K, Calmus S, Durand-Zaleski I, et al. Surgery versus medical follow-up in patients with asymptomatic primary hyperparathyroidism: a decision analysis. Eur J Endocrinol 2005;153(6):915–27.
6. Zanocco K, Angelos P, Sturgeon C. Cost-effectiveness analysis of parathyroidectomy for asymptomatic primary hyperparathyroidism. Surgery 2006;140(6): 874–81 [discussion: 881–2].
7. Zanocco K, Sturgeon C. How should age at diagnosis impact treatment strategy in asymptomatic primary hyperparathyroidism? A cost-effectiveness analysis. Surgery 2008;144(2):290–8.
8. McGill J, Sturgeon C, Kaplan SP, et al. How does the operative strategy for primary hyperparathyroidism impact the findings and cure rate? A comparison of 800 parathyroidectomies. J Am Coll Surg 2008;207(2):246–9.
9. Clark OH. Symposium: parathyroid disease - Part 1. Contemp Surg 1998;52(2): 137–52.
10. Richmond BK, Eads K, Flaherty S, et al. Complications of thyroidectomy and parathyroidectomy in the rural community hospital setting. Am Surg 2007; 73(4):332–6.
11. Udelsman R. Six hundred fifty-six consecutive explorations for primary hyperparathyroidism. Ann Surg 2002;235(5):665–70 [discussion: 670–2].
12. Miura D, Wada N, Arici C, et al. Does intraoperative quick parathyroid hormone assay improve the results of parathyroidectomy? World J Surg 2002;26(8):926–30.
13. Oertli D, Richter M, Kraenzlin M, et al. Parathyroidectomy in primary hyperparathyroidism: preoperative localization and routine biopsy of unaltered glands are not necessary. Surgery 1995;117(4):392–6.
14. Ogilvie JB, Clark OH. Parathyroid surgery: we still need traditional and selective approaches. J Endocrinol Invest 2005;28(6):566–9.
15. Doppman JL, Miller DL. Localization of parathyroid tumors in patients with asymptomatic hyperparathyroidism and no previous surgery. J Bone Miner Res 1991;6(Suppl 2):S153–8 [discussion: S159].
16. Arici C, Cheah WK, Ituarte PH, et al. Can localization studies be used to direct focused parathyroid operations? Surgery 2001;129(6):720–9.
17. Irvin GL 3rd, Prudhomme DL, Deriso GT, et al. A new approach to parathyroidectomy. Ann Surg 1994;219(5):574–9 [discussion: 579–81].
18. Chen H, Sokoll LJ, Udelsman R. Outpatient minimally invasive parathyroidectomy: a combination of sestamibi-SPECT localization, cervical block anesthesia, and intraoperative parathyroid hormone assay. Surgery 1999;126(6):1016–21 [discussion: 1021–2].

19. Inabnet WB 3rd, Dakin GF, Haber RS, et al. Targeted parathyroidectomy in the era of intraoperative parathormone monitoring. World J Surg 2002;26(8): 921–5.
20. Burkey SH, Snyder WH 3rd, Nwariaku F, et al. Directed parathyroidectomy: feasibility and performance in 100 consecutive patients with primary hyperparathyroidism. Arch Surg 2003;138(6):604–8 [discussion: 608–9].
21. Burkey SH, Van Heerden JA, Farley DR, et al. Will directed parathyroidectomy utilizing the gamma probe or intraoperative parathyroid hormone assay replace bilateral cervical exploration as the preferred operation for primary hyperparathyroidism? World J Surg 2002;26(8):914–20.
22. Udelsman R, Donovan PI. Open minimally invasive parathyroid surgery. World J Surg 2004;28(12):1224–6.
23. Sosa JA, Udelsman R. Minimally invasive parathyroidectomy. Surg Oncol 2003; 12(2):125–34.
24. Dillavou ED, Cohn HE. Minimally invasive parathyroidectomy: 101 consecutive cases from a single surgeon. J Am Coll Surg 2003;197(1):1–7.
25. Udelsman R. Surgery in primary hyperparathyroidism: the patient without previous neck surgery. J Bone Miner Res 2002;17(Suppl 2):N126–32.
26. Udelsman R, Donovan PI, Sokoll LJ. One hundred consecutive minimally invasive parathyroid explorations. Ann Surg 2000;232(3):331–9.
27. Irvin GL 3rd, Sfakianakis G, Yeung L, et al. Ambulatory parathyroidectomy for primary hyperparathyroidism. Arch Surg 1996;131(10):1074–8.
28. Greene AB, Butler RS, McIntyre S, et al. National trends in parathyroid surgery from 1998 to 2008: a decade of change. J Am Coll Surg 2009;209(3):332–43.
29. Udelsman R, Pasieka JL, Sturgeon C, et al. Surgery for asymptomatic primary hyperparathyroidism: proceedings of the third international workshop. J Clin Endocrinol Metab 2009;94(2):366–72.
30. Siperstein A, Berber E, Mackey R, et al. Prospective evaluation of sestamibi scan, ultrasonography, and rapid PTH to predict the success of limited exploration for sporadic primary hyperparathyroidism. Surgery 2004;136(4):872–80.
31. Siperstein A, Berber E, Barbosa GF, et al. Predicting the success of limited exploration for primary hyperparathyroidism using ultrasound, sestamibi, and intraoperative parathyroid hormone: analysis of 1158 cases. Ann Surg 2008; 248(3):420–8.
32. Norman J, Lopez J, Politz D. Abandoning unilateral parathyroidectomy: why we reversed our position after 15,000 parathyroid operations. J Am Coll Surg 2012; 214(3):260–9.
33. Lee NC, Norton JA. Multiple-gland disease in primary hyperparathyroidism: a function of operative approach? Arch Surg 2002;137(8):896–9 [discussion: 899–900].
34. Lew JI, Irvin GL 3rd. Focused parathyroidectomy guided by intra-operative parathormone monitoring does not miss multiglandular disease in patients with sporadic primary hyperparathyroidism: a 10-year outcome. Surgery 2009; 146(6):1021–7.
35. Westerdahl J, Bergenfelz A. Unilateral versus bilateral neck exploration for primary hyperparathyroidism: five-year follow-up of a randomized controlled trial. Ann Surg 2007;246(6):976–80 [discussion: 980–1].
36. Santayana G. Reason in common sense. The life of reason. London: Archibald Constable; 1906. p. 284.
37. Caron N, Sturgeon C, Clark OH. Persistent and recurrent hyperparathyroidism. Curr Treat Options Oncol 2004;5:335–45.

38. Holt S, van Heerden J, Niederle B. Herr Albert Jahne: renowned streetcar conductor. In: Zeiger MA, Shen W, Felger E, editors. The supreme triumph of the surgeon's art. A narrative history of endocrine surgery. Berkeley (CA): University of California Medical Humanities Press; 2013. p. 75–85.

39. Niederle BE, Schmidt G, Organ CH, et al. Albert J and his surgeon: a historical reevaluation of the first parathyroidectomy. J Am Coll Surg 2006;202(1):181–90.

40. Clark OH. Captain Charles Martell. America's first parathyroid patient. In: Zeiger MA, Shen W, Felger E, editors. The supreme triumph of the surgeon's art. A narrative history of endocrine surgery. Berkeley (CA): University of California Medical Humanities Press; 2013. p. 86–97.

41. Organ CH Jr. The history of parathyroid surgery, 1850-1996: the Excelsior Surgical Society 1998 Edward D Churchill Lecture. J Am Coll Surg 2000;191(3):284–99.

42. Cope O. Hyperparathyroidism: diagnosis and management. Am J Surg 1960; 99:394–403.

43. Hellstrom J. Reminiscence: observations on hyperparathyroidism. Rev Surg 1965;22(6):381–96.

44. McGeown MG, Morrison E. Hyperparathyroidism. Postgrad Med J 1959; 35(404):330–7.

45. Chapuis Y, Fulla Y, Bonnichon P, et al. Values of ultrasonography, sestamibi scintigraphy, and intraoperative measurement of 1-84 PTH for unilateral neck exploration of primary hyperparathyroidism. World J Surg 1996;20(7):835–9 [discussion: 839–40].

46. Bagul A, Patel HP, Chadwick D, et al. Primary hyperparathyroidism: an analysis of failure of parathyroidectomy. World J Surg 2014;38:534–41.

47. Perrier ND, Ituarte PH, Morita E, et al. Parathyroid surgery: separating promise from reality. J Clin Endocrinol Metab 2002;87(3):1024–9.

48. Gauger PG, Agarwal G, England BG, et al. Intraoperative parathyroid hormone monitoring fails to detect double parathyroid adenomas: a 2-institution experience. Surgery 2001;130(6):1005–10.

49. Bergenfelz A, Lindblom P, Tibblin S, et al. Unilateral versus bilateral neck exploration for primary hyperparathyroidism: a prospective randomized controlled trial. Ann Surg 2002;236(5):543–51.

50. Landerholm K, Wasner AM, Jarhult J. Incidence and risk factors for injuries to the recurrent laryngeal nerve during neck surgery in the moderate-volume setting. Langenbecks Arch Surg 2014. [Epub ahead of print].

51. van Heerden JA, Grant CS. Surgical treatment of primary hyperparathyroidism: an institutional perspective. World J Surg 1991;15(6):688–92.

52. Kraimps JL, Duh QY, Demeure M, et al. Hyperparathyroidism in multiple endocrine neoplasia syndrome. Surgery 1992;112(6):1080–6 [discussion: 1086–8].

53. Castleman B, Schantz A, Roth S. Parathyroid hyperplasia in primary hyperparathyroidism: a review of 85 cases. Cancer 1976;38(4):1668–75.

54. Alveryd A, El-Zawahry MD, Herlitz P, et al. Primary hyperplasia of the parathyroids. Acta Chir Scand 1975;141(1):24–30.

55. Rudberg C, Akerstrom G, Palmer M, et al. Late results of operation for primary hyperparathyroidism in 441 patients. Surgery 1986;99(6):643–51.

56. Porter ME. What is value in health care? N Engl J Med 2010;363(26):2477–81.

57. Shen W, Duren M, Morita E, et al. Reoperation for persistent or recurrent primary hyperparathyroidism. Arch Surg 1996;131(8):861–7 [discussion: 867–9].

58. Jaskowiak N, Norton JA, Alexander HR, et al. A prospective trial evaluating a standard approach to reoperation for missed parathyroid adenoma. Ann Surg 1996;224(3):308–20 [discussion: 320–1].

59. Prescott JD, Udelsman R. Remedial operation for primary hyperparathyroidism. World J Surg 2009;33(11):2324–34.
60. Akerstrom G, Rudberg C, Grimelius L, et al. Causes of failed primary exploration and technical aspects of re-operation in primary hyperparathyroidism. World J Surg 1992;16(4):562–8 [discussion: 568–9].
61. Gaz RD. Revision parathyroid surgery. In: Randolph GW, editor. Surgery of the thyroid and parathyroid glands. Philadelphia: WB Saunders; 2003. p. 564–70.
62. Wang CA. Parathyroid re-exploration. A clinical and pathological study of 112 cases. Ann Surg 1977;186(2):140–5.
63. Mariette C, Pellissier L, Combemale F, et al. Reoperation for persistent or recurrent primary hyperparathyroidism. Langenbecks Arch Surg 1998;383(2): 174–9.
64. Brennan MF, Norton JA. Reoperation for persistent and recurrent hyperparathyroidism. Ann Surg 1985;201(1):40–4.
65. Carty SE, Norton JA. Management of patients with persistent or recurrent primary hyperparathyroidism. World J Surg 1991;15(6):716–23.
66. Lo CY, van Heerden JA. Parathyroid reoperations. In: Clark OH, Duh QY, editors. Textbook of endocrine surgery. 1st edition. Philadelphia: WB Saunders; 1997. p. 411–7.
67. Levin KE, Clark OH. The reasons for failure in parathyroid operations. Arch Surg 1989;124(8):911–4 [discussion: 914–5].
68. Grant CS, van Heerden JA, Charboneau JW, et al. Clinical management of persistent and/or recurrent primary hyperparathyroidism. World J Surg 1986; 10(4):555–65.
69. Thakker RV, Newey PJ, Walls GV, et al. Clinical practice guidelines for multiple endocrine neoplasia type 1 (MEN1). J Clin Endocrinol Metab 2012;97(9): 2990–3011.
70. Wells SA Jr, Pacini F, Robinson BG, et al. Multiple endocrine neoplasia type 2 and familial medullary thyroid carcinoma: an update. J Clin Endocrinol Metab 2013;98(8):3149–64.
71. Scholten A, Schreinemakers JM, Pieterman CR, et al. Evolution of surgical treatment of primary hyperparathyroidism in patients with multiple endocrine neoplasia type 2A. Endocr Pract 2011;17(1):7–15.
72. Thakker RV. Multiple Endocrine Neoplasia Type 1 (MEN1). In: Robertson R, Thakker RV, editors. Translat Endocrinol Metab 2. Chevy Chase (MD): The Endocrine Society; 2011. p. 13–44.
73. Brandi ML, Gagel RF, Angeli A, et al. Guidelines for diagnosis and therapy of MEN type 1 and type 2. J Clin Endocrinol Metab 2001;86(12):5658–71.
74. Chiu B, Sturgeon C, Angelos P. What is the link between nonlocalizing sestamibi scans, multigland disease, and persistent hypercalcemia? A study of 401 consecutive patients undergoing parathyroidectomy. Surgery 2006;140(3): 418–22.
75. Brennan MF. Lessons learned. Ann Surg Oncol 2006;13(10):1322–8.
76. Roe SM, Burns RP, Graham LD, et al. Cost-effectiveness of preoperative localization studies in primary hyperparathyroid disease. Ann Surg 1994;219(5): 582–6.
77. Aarum S, Nordenstrom J, Reihner E, et al. Operation for primary hyperparathyroidism: the new versus the old order. A randomised controlled trial of preoperative localisation. Scand J Surg 2007;96(1):26–30.
78. Mihai R, Weisters M, Stechman MJ, et al. Cost-effectiveness of scan-directed parathyroidectomy. Langenbecks Arch Surg 2008;393(5):739–43.

79. Mihai R, Palazzo FF, Gleeson FV, et al. Minimally invasive parathyroidectomy without intraoperative parathyroid hormone monitoring in patients with primary hyperparathyroidism. Br J Surg 2007;94(1):42–7.

80. Wong W, Foo FJ, Lau MI, et al. Simplified minimally invasive parathyroidectomy: a series of 100 cases and review of the literature. Ann R Coll Surg Engl 2011; 93(4):290–3.

81. Slepavicius A, Beisa V, Janusonis V, et al. Focused versus conventional parathyroidectomy for primary hyperparathyroidism: a prospective, randomized, blinded trial. Langenbecks Arch Surg 2008;393(5):659–66.

82. Haciyanli M, Genc H, Damburaci N, et al. Minimally invasive focused parathyroidectomy without using intraoperative parathyroid hormone monitoring or gamma probe. J Postgrad Med 2009;55(4):242–6.

83. Habener JF, Rosenblatt M, Potts JT Jr. Parathyroid hormone: biochemical aspects of biosynthesis, secretion, action, and metabolism. Physiol Rev 1984; 64(3):985–1053.

84. Chiu B, Sturgeon C, Angelos P. Which intraoperative parathyroid hormone assay criterion best predicts operative success? A study of 352 consecutive patients. Arch Surg 2006;141(5):483–7 [discussion: 487–8].

85. Grant CS, Thompson G, Farley D, et al. Primary hyperparathyroidism surgical management since the introduction of minimally invasive parathyroidectomy: Mayo Clinic experience. Arch Surg 2005;140(5):472–8 [discussion: 478–9].

86. Udelsman R, Lin Z, Donovan P. The superiority of minimally invasive parathyroidectomy based on 1650 consecutive patients with primary hyperparathyroidism. Ann Surg 2011;253(3):585–91.

87. Pang T, Stalberg P, Sidhu S, et al. Minimally invasive parathyroidectomy using the lateral focused mini-incision technique without intraoperative parathyroid hormone monitoring. Br J Surg 2007;94(3):315–9.

88. Fahy BN, Bold RJ, Beckett L, et al. Modern parathyroid surgery: a cost-benefit analysis of localizing strategies. Arch Surg 2002;137(8):917–22 [discussion: 922–3].

89. Wang TS, Cheung K, Farrokhyar F, et al. Would scan, but which scan? A cost-utility analysis to optimize preoperative imaging for primary hyperparathyroidism. Surgery 2011;150(6):1286–94.

90. Lorenz K, Nguyen-Thanh P, Dralle H. Unilateral open and minimally invasive procedures for primary hyperparathyroidism: a review of selective approaches. Langenbecks Arch Surg 2000;385(2):106–17.

91. Kaplan EL, Bartlett S, Sugimoto J, et al. Relation of postoperative hypocalcemia to operative techniques: deleterious effect of excessive use of parathyroid biopsy. Surgery 1982;92(5):827–34.

92. Edis AJ, Beahrs OH, van Heerden JA, et al. Conservative versus liberal approach to parathyroid neck exploration. Surgery 1977;82(4):466–73.

93. Rio PD, Vicente D, Maestroni U, et al. A comparison of minimally invasive video-assisted parathyroidectomy and traditional parathyroidectomy for parathyroid adenoma. J Cancer 2013;4(6):458–63.

94. Sprouse LR 2nd, Roe SM, Kaufman HJ, et al. Minimally invasive parathyroidectomy without intraoperative localization. Am Surg 2001;67(11):1022–9.

95. Gil-Cardenas A, Gamino R, Reza A, et al. Is intraoperative parathyroid hormone assay mandatory for the success of targeted parathyroidectomy? J Am Coll Surg 2007;204(2):286–90.

96. Barczynski M, Konturek A, Cichon S, et al. Intraoperative parathyroid hormone assay improves outcomes of minimally invasive parathyroidectomy mainly in

patients with a presumed solitary parathyroid adenoma and missing concordance of preoperative imaging. Clin Endocrinol 2007;66(6):878–85.

97. Dralle H, Lorenz K, Nguyen-Thanh P. Minimally invasive video-assisted parathyroidectomy–selective approach to localized single gland adenoma. Langenbecks Arch Surg 1999;384(6):556–62.

98. Monchik JM, Barellini L, Langer P, et al. Minimally invasive parathyroid surgery in 103 patients with local/regional anesthesia, without exclusion criteria. Surgery 2002;131(5):502–8.

99. Kulkarni RS, Braverman LE, Patwardhan NA. Bilateral cervical plexus block for thyroidectomy and parathyroidectomy in healthy and high risk patients. J Endocrinol Invest 1996;19(11):714–8.

100. Carling T, Donovan P, Rinder C, et al. Minimally invasive parathyroidectomy using cervical block: reasons for conversion to general anesthesia. Arch Surg 2006;141(4):401–4 [discussion: 404].

101. Miccoli P, Barellini L, Monchik JM, et al. Randomized clinical trial comparing regional and general anaesthesia in minimally invasive video-assisted parathyroidectomy. Br J Surg 2005;92(7):814–8.

102. Cohen MS, Finkelstein SE, Brunt LM, et al. Outpatient minimally invasive parathyroidectomy using local/regional anesthesia: a safe and effective operative approach for selected patients. Surgery 2005;138(4):681–7 [discussion: 687–9].

103. Deutmeyer C, Weingarten M, Doyle M, et al. Case series of targeted parathyroidectomy with surgeon-performed ultrasonography as the only preoperative imaging study. Surgery 2011;150(6):1153–60.

104. Solorzano CC, Carneiro-Pla DM, Irvin GL 3rd. Surgeon-performed ultrasonography as the initial and only localizing study in sporadic primary hyperparathyroidism. J Am Coll Surg 2006;202(1):18–24.

105. Arora S, Balash PR, Yoo J, et al. Benefits of surgeon-performed ultrasound for primary hyperparathyroidism. Langenbecks Arch Surg 2009;394(5):861–7.

106. Hodin R, Angelos P, Carty S, et al. No need to abandon unilateral parathyroid surgery. J Am Coll Surg 2012;215(2):297 [author reply: 297–300].

107. Yeh MW, Wiseman JE, Ituarte PH, et al. Surgery for primary hyperparathyroidism: are the consensus guidelines being followed? Ann Surg 2012;255(6): 1179–83.

108. Wermers RA, Khosla S, Atkinson EJ, et al. Incidence of primary hyperparathyroidism in Rochester, Minnesota, 1993-2001: an update on the changing epidemiology of the disease. J Bone Miner Res 2006;21(1):171–7.

Radiographic Evaluation of Nonfunctioning Adrenal Neoplasms

Peter J. Mazzaglia, MD

KEYWORDS

- Adrenal neoplasm • Incidentaloma • Adrenocortical cancer • CT • MRI • PET

KEY POINTS

- Incidental adrenal neoplasms are usually nonfunctioning benign adenomas.
- After hormonal production has been assessed, the nonsecreting lesions must be evaluated for the possibility of malignancy.
- As radiologic technology advances, a lesion's malignant potential can more accurately be determined, thereby allowing physicians to make more informed treatment recommendations.

ADRENAL INCIDENTALOMA AND RATES OF ADRENOCORTICAL CARCINOMA

Adrenal neoplasms are being discovered more than ever before because of the widespread use of abdominal imaging with CT, MRI, and positron emission tomography (PET). The overall prevalence is 5%, with rates less than 1% in the young and up to 7% in patients more than 70 years of age.[1] The increased identification of these patients mandates the institution of appropriate diagnostic and therapeutic protocols that efficiently and accurately determine which neoplasms are nonfunctioning and benign and which are functioning and/or harbor malignant potential. When lesions are characterized as nonfunctional and benign, they can safely be observed, whereas most functioning and potentially malignant lesions must be excised.

The assessment of incidentally discovered adrenal neoplasms for biochemical function is usually straightforward and has been described in detail elsewhere.[2] However, the radiographic characterization of biochemically inactive adrenal lesions can often be indeterminate. Many findings on CT or MRI are known to predict the benign nature of an adrenal lesion with high accuracy. However, the ability of radiography to confidently assess a lesion's malignant potential is still evolving. This article

Department of General Surgery, The Warren Alpert School of Medicine, Brown University, 593 Eddy Street, APC 4, Providence, RI 02905, USA
E-mail address: peterjmazzaglia@gmail.com

Surg Clin N Am 94 (2014) 625–642
http://dx.doi.org/10.1016/j.suc.2014.03.002
0039-6109/14/$ – see front matter © 2014 Elsevier Inc. All rights reserved.
surgical.theclinics.com

primarily focuses on the radiographic characteristics used to describe adrenal neoplasms, specifically as they relate to the neoplasm's malignant potential.

To appreciate the sheer number of newly identified adrenal neoplasms that will require assessment of malignant potential, one needs to understand the epidemiology of the disease. Historically, autopsy studies document the prevalence of asymptomatic benign adrenal neoplasms ranging anywhere from 2% to 20%,[3] so the number of people with unrecognized adrenal neoplasms is large. Based on a cutoff of 1 cm or larger as defining an adrenal incidentaloma, the prevalence ranges from less than 1% in people younger than 30 years of age up to 7% in those age 70 and older.[4] Fortunately, adrenocortical carcinoma (ACC) accounts for only 0.2% of cancer deaths and has an estimated incidence of 1 to 2 per million.[5]

Traditionally accepted percentages for the most commonly diagnosed conditions associated with adrenal neoplasms are 82% benign adenoma, 5.3% subclinical Cushing syndrome, 5.1% pheochromocytoma, 4.7% ACC, 2.5% metastatic disease, and 1.0% aldosteronoma.[6] Other infrequent diagnoses include adrenal cyst, hemorrhage, lymphoma, sarcoma, and neuroganglioma. However, the true risk of an adrenal incidentaloma being an ACC is estimated as low as 1 in 4000.[7]

Given the rarity of this malignancy, it is paramount to the evaluation and treatment of patients harboring these lesions to proceed judiciously. Even though laparoscopic adrenalectomy allows for the safe removal of adrenal incidentalomas, this does not necessarily justify its frequent use as a diagnostic tool. Since the introduction of laparoscopic adrenalectomy in 1992, there is reasonable evidence that the size threshold for recommending adrenalectomy has decreased.[8] Obviously laparoscopic adrenalectomy is a tremendous advance compared with the open approach and it has revolutionized the care of patients with functioning adrenal neoplasms.[9–11] However, it is still not an acceptable means of resecting ACC, despite literature suggesting it may be.[12] The risks of tumor breakage and inadequate tumor margin, along with higher recurrence rates, make laparoscopic adrenalectomy for ACC unacceptable.[13]

The problem at hand is that approximately 85% of adrenal incidentalomas are nonfunctional and asymptomatic. Most are benign adenomas. The roughly 70% that are lipid-rich are easily characterized. However, the 30% that are lipid-poor are difficult to distinguish from ACC.[14] Epidemiologic statistics overwhelmingly indicate that most of these lipid-poor adrenal incidentalomas are also benign. Cawood and colleagues[15] investigated the true incidence of malignancy in patients with adrenal incidentaloma by performing a literature review excluding surgical and oncological series, which would be expected to bias the results. They reviewed nine series including 1804 subjects and found the incidence of adrenal carcinoma was 1.9% versus the more traditional 5% value that is often reported. Also, metastatic lesions accounted for only 0.7% versus 2.3%. Their study also recognized that mean incidentaloma size decreased with later date of publication, attributed to better imaging quality. These smaller lesions are more likely benign. The development of malignancy during follow-up was only 0.2%. Their review suggests that the false-positive rate for functional or malignant adrenal lesions is initially five times greater than the true positive rate and 50 times greater during follow-up imaging.[15]

Contrary to traditionally quoted rates of ACC, which approached 5%,[6] the likelihood of this diagnosis is less than 1% for all patients with incidentaloma. This discrepancy stems from the previously reported prevalence that was usually based on skewed surgical series, which did not account for the complete denominator of total number of incidentalomas.[15] Current guidelines issued by the National Institutes of Health (NIH) regarding nonfunctioning incidentalomas suggest resection of lesions larger than or equal to 4 cm.[7] Based on these guidelines and the prevalence of ACC, most laparoscopic adrenalectomies performed for biochemically silent lesions show benign adrenal adenomas. The National Italian Study Group on Adrenal Tumors found that a 4 cm adrenal lesion had a 93% sensitivity but only 24% specificity for ACC.[16]

INITIAL RADIOGRAPHIC PRESENTATION

The problem has been, and it continues to be, distinguishing lipid-poor adenomas from malignancies. Thus, the question arises, how to capitalize on the knowledge gained over the last two decades regarding the radiographic signature of benign versus malignant adrenal lesions. Using that information, physicians can learn to properly assign patients to open adrenalectomy for probable ACC, diagnostic laparoscopic adrenalectomy, or observation with a follow-up radiologic study.

In most cases, a patient initially presents after CT or MRI has revealed an adrenal neoplasm. Because the indication for imaging is rarely to investigate adrenal disease, the CT or MRI techniques often contain limited information about the adrenal lesion. Frequently, there are sufficient data to characterize the lesion as benign. Following is a discussion of the radiographic findings in adrenal neoplasms that are used to characterize them as benign or possibly malignant. In roughly 30% of cases, on initial CT or MRI, the neoplasm is characterized as indeterminate for malignancy. This usually prompts either additional focused scanning or adrenalectomy (see later discussion).

Features common to CT and MRI used to distinguish benign from malignant neoplasms include size, contour, heterogeneity, and change in size over time (**Table 1**).

Occasionally some of these attributes will be grossly abnormal and, therefore, strongly suggest malignancy; however, the lack of classic features of carcinoma does not uniformly rule out the diagnosis. In addition, the specificity of some of these findings is low. For instance, in studies looking at a 4 cm cutoff, there was 90% sensitivity but only 24% specificity for ACC.[16,17] In addition, although heterogeneity is common to ACC, the uniformly benign myelolipoma can often appear very heterogeneous. Other features that are not helpful but are present in benign and malignant neoplasms include calcifications and hypervascularity.

Benign adrenocortical adenomas typically contain increased amounts of intracytoplasmic fat in the form of cholesterol, fatty acids, and neutral fat, which serve as precursors for hormone synthesis.[14] However, some malignant lesions, especially adrenal metastases, appear similar to nonfunctional adenomas on unenhanced CT.[18] Song and colleagues[19] studied 973 subjects without history of malignancy but with 1049 adrenal incidentalomas. Follow-up consisted of imaging at 1 year or at least 2 years of clinical follow-up. Of these, 75% of the lesions were adenomas and 78% were lipid-rich.

Table 1		
Imaging features used in CT and MRI to distinguish benign from malignant adrenal neoplasms		
	Benign	**Malignant**
Size	<4 cm	>6 cm
Contour	Smooth, planes between adjacent organs respected	Irregular, planes between adjacent organs indistinct
Density	Homogeneous	Heterogeneous
Change in size over time	Stable	>5–10 mm growth over time

ADRENAL CT

Since the 1990s, the presence of intracytoplasmic fat has reliably predicted benign adrenal adenomas. This determination is made on unenhanced CT by measuring the lesion's Hounsfield unit (HU) density. The region of interest is placed over an area that comprises one-half to two-thirds of the adrenal lesion. The early studies reported that a HU density of 0 provided 47% sensitivity but 100% specificity for adenoma.[18] A 1998 meta-analysis published by Boland and colleagues[20] reported that using a cut-off of 10 HU improved the sensitivity for adenoma to 71% with a minimal decrease in specificity of 98%. This became the standard by which HU less than or equal to 10 on noncontrast-enhanced CT was accepted as diagnostic of a benign process (**Fig. 1**). In such cases, the administration of contrast can usually be avoided. Lesions with noncontrast HU from 10 to 40 must undergo further evaluation. Lesions with noncontrast HU greater than 40 are considered suspicious for malignancy.[21]

ADRENAL MRI

MRI has earned a prominent place in the characterization of adrenal neoplasms. In general, adenomas are homogeneously enhancing and are isointense or hypointense compared with normal adrenal tissue. Because malignant adrenal lesions contain more water and less fat than benign adenomas, they have higher signal intensity on T2-weighted images (**Fig. 2**). However, there is a large area of overlap and approximately one-third of adrenal neoplasms are indeterminate.[22,23]

The use of gadolinium enhancement on the T1 images improves characterization.[24,25] Adenomas will typically have homogeneous or ring enhancement, whereas malignancies appear heterogeneous.[26] As with the T2-weighted images, gadolinium-enhanced T1-weighted imaging is not specific enough to be accurately used for many adrenal neoplasms.[27]

MRI uses a technique known as chemical shift imaging (CSI) that depends on differing resonance frequencies of hydrogen atoms in fat and water. Images are obtained in two phases: in-phase (IP) and opposed-phase (OP). In-phase imaging

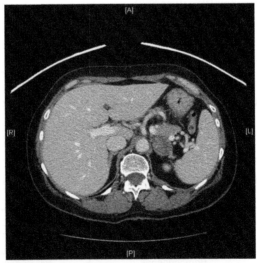

Fig. 1. Benign adrenal adenoma appears hypointense relative to normal adrenal tissue (HU<10).

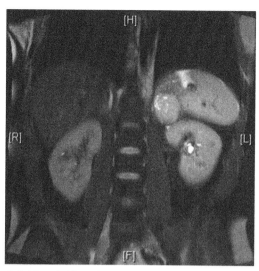

Fig. 2. ACC appears bright on T2 imaging.

uses an echo time that aligns the fat and water proton signals, making them additive. Opposed-phase imaging uses an echo time that causes the fat and water proton signals to be opposed 180°, thus canceling each other and causing a drop in signal. Using this technique, masses that have either fat or water in a single voxel will not show cancellation, whereas masses with both will.[14] Therefore, an adrenal lesion relatively high in fat will show near complete signal loss, whereas a lesion with little fat relative to water will still display high signal intensity on opposed-phase imaging (**Fig. 3**). Using CSI, studies report sensitivities for adenoma ranging from 81% to 100% and specificities ranging from 94% to 100%.[28,29]

With current technology, the in-phase and out-of-phase imaging can be obtained simultaneously with a single breath hold. The loss of signal assessment is sometimes made by the radiologist qualitatively but can also be quantitatively measured, which is more reproducible. This is accomplished in several ways. An internal reference called

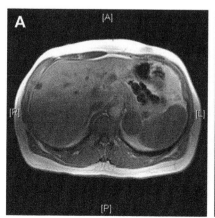
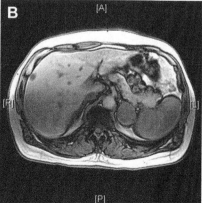

Fig. 3. ACC on MRI (*A*) in-phase and (*B*) out-of-phase.

the adrenal-to-spleen chemical shift ratio is used. The spleen has been chosen because of its relative homogeneity and because it is not susceptible to fatty infiltration like the liver. This is calculated by dividing the lesion-to-spleen signal intensity ratio on opposed-phase sequences by the lesion-to-spleen signal intensity ratio on the in-phase sequences. Using this quantitative technique, McNicholas and colleagues[30] showed all adrenal adenomas have an adrenal-to-spleen ratio less than or equal to 70. However, specificity is poor and many metastatic tumors also have indices in this range.[31]

Another quantitative measure of CSI is the signal intensity index (SI-i). It is calculated using the formula [(IP-OP)/IP] × 100. Fujiyoshi and colleagues[31] looked at 102 adrenal neoplasms and found no adenomas if the result was less than 16.5%. Accuracy was greatest between 11.2% and 16.5%. Another study that compared the chemical shift ratio to the SI-i in 41 adrenal masses, including 27 adenomas and 14 metastases, found the SI-i to be more accurate. All adenomas had an SI-i greater than or equal to 20%.[32]

There is no consensus as to which modality, unenhanced CT or MRI with CSI, is more useful. However, when lesions have indeterminate, unenhanced HU in the range of 10 to 30, performing chemical shift MRI is often helpful. Studies have shown that in these instances, MRI with CSI was 89% sensitive and 100% specific for a small number of adenomas.[33]

CT WASHOUT TECHNIQUES

For the 30% of benign adrenal adenomas that are lipid-poor, neither noncontrast CT nor CSI are very helpful. However, a technique that was developed to look at contrast enhancement and washout on CT has become a standard tool in the armamentarium to diagnose these lesions. The neovascularization that occurs with malignancies leads to increased and prolonged contrast accumulation.[34] In general, contrast washes out of adenomas, both lipid-rich and lipid-poor, faster than malignant neoplasms and pheochromocytomas (**Figs. 4** and **5**). The most reliable way to measure this phenomenon is to calculate a washout ratio.[21] A noteworthy caveat is that washout values can only reliably be calculated in relatively homogeneous adrenal masses, thus excluding lesions with significant areas of hemorrhage or necrosis.[27]

There are two ways to calculate contrast washout. The first is called absolute percentage washout (APW) and the second is called relative percentage washout (RPW).

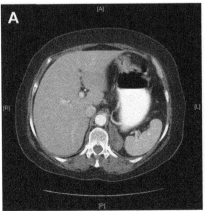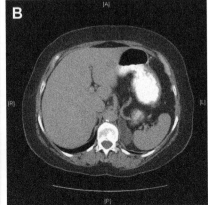

Fig. 4. CT imaging with contrast of a benign adrenal neoplasm (A) immediate and (B) delayed.

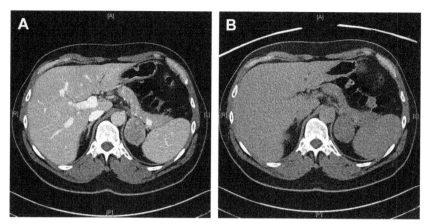

Fig. 5. CT imaging with contrast of an ACC (*A*) immediate and (*B*) delayed.

APW requires a noncontrast HU measurement. APW is calculated using the formula ([enhanced HU−delayed HU]÷[enhanced HU−noncontrast HU]) × 100. Frequently, only contrast and delayed images are performed so an APW cannot be calculated. In these cases, the RPW must be used and is calculated as ([enhanced HU−delayed HU]÷enhanced HU) × 100. Because the APW includes the noncontrast measurement, it is considered more accurate.[14]

Protocols designed for adrenal imaging call for both noncontrast and contrast-enhanced scanning so that the more accurate APW may be calculated. Most centers use 15-minute delayed imaging for calculating washout. To characterize an adrenal neoplasm as benign, the current standard minimum values for washout percentages are an APW of 60% and an RPW of 40% at 15 minutes.[35] In the study by Caoili and colleagues,[35] these cutoffs produced 95% specificity and 89% sensitivity for APW, and 93% specificity and 83% sensitivity for RPW. Dunnick and colleagues[36] reported sensitivity of 96% and specificity of 100% for diagnosing adenoma if RPW is greater than or equal to 40% at 15 minutes.

Some centers have used 10-minute delayed imaging and reported excellent results. Using an APW of greater than or equal to 52%, a sensitivity of 100% and specificity of 98% has been reported.[35] However, in a study of 323 adrenal lesions, using an APW threshold of 60%, the sensitivity was only 38.8% with a specificity of 93.3% for lipid-poor adenomas. Using an RPW threshold of 37.5%, the sensitivity dropped to 30.6%.[37] Because of such findings, most centers continue to use the 15-minute delay.

Another CT technique for adrenal neoplasm characterization is histogram analysis, which obviates immediate and delayed CT contrast imaging and which can be used with enhanced or unenhanced images. However, it is most clinically useful when only a noncontrast scan is available.[27] It relies on an assessment of the lipid content of the mass, calculated by placing a cursor over roughly two-thirds of the lesion, avoiding areas of necrosis. The individual attenuation values are measured for each pixel and the percentage of negative pixels (<0 HU) is determined. Because intralesional fat is proportional to the percentage of negative pixels, thresholds are established to accurately predict adenoma.[38] Unfortunately, studies have reported inconsistent sensitivity and specificity; however, recent literature supports sensitivity of 85% to 91% and specificity of 100% when greater than or equal to 10% of pixels are negative for noncontrast CT. Thus, this tool can possibly increase the sensitivity of a noncontrast CT from 66% to 91% for a benign adenoma.[39,40]

PET SCAN

The most recent and possibly fastest growing segment of adrenal imaging is PET-CT scanning (**Fig. 6**). Using PET with fludeoxyglucose F 18 (^{18}F FDG-PET), studies have shown very high accuracy for detecting adrenal malignancies, with sensitivity as high as 100% and specificity between 87% and 97%.[41,42] The FDG uptake does not significantly differ for lipid-rich versus lipid-poor adenomas, and the sensitivity and specificity for lipid-poor adenomas are 98.5% and 92%, respectively.[43] Only 5% of normal adrenals are seen on PET alone, whereas 68% are seen on PET-CT.[44] Adrenal FDG uptake is compared with that of liver, with most adenomas having lower[45] and most nonadenomas having higher uptake.[27] There is overlap, however, in the moderate uptake range.[45] When quantitative assessment of uptake is made using standardized uptake values (SUVs), accurate distinction markedly improves. Using an SUV cut-off of 2.68 to 3.0 detects malignant adrenal neoplasms with 98.5% sensitivity, 92% specificity, 89.3% positive predictive value, and 98.9% negative predictive value.[43] The problem of false-positives can be ameliorated by using the CT findings because some of these lesions will be revealed by their low CT attenuation coefficients.[27]

The rate of false-positive PET scan for nonfunctioning adrenal incidentalomas is 5% due to inflammatory lesions, such as sarcoid and tuberculosis, or adrenocortical hyperplasia.[46] False-negative PET is rare but can occur if there has been extensive hemorrhage or necrosis,[47,48] or if the adrenal lesion is a metastasis from a primary that is not FDG-avid.

Most studies agree that an adrenal lesion with a visual uptake and SUV less than liver can be confidently diagnosed as benign. However, because of low specificity, the clinician cannot conversely be assured that a lesion with visual and SUV uptake greater than liver is malignant.

IMAGING CHARACTERISTICS OF INDIVIDUAL LESIONS

There are certain benign adrenal neoplasms that are recognized by pathognomonic radiographic findings. These include myelolipoma, cyst, hemorrhage, and lipid-rich adenoma.

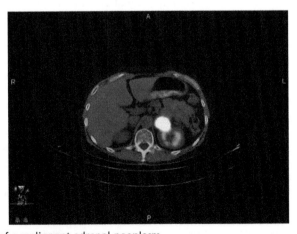

Fig. 6. PET-CT of a malignant adrenal neoplasm.

Myelolipoma

Myelolipomas are common benign adrenal tumors that can grow to more than 20 cm (**Fig. 7**). They are uniformly benign and, fortunately, they have distinctive radiographic characteristics that make their diagnosis reasonably straightforward. They often present as incidentalomas but can present with mass effect. The pathognomonic finding on CT is macroscopic fat. On MRI, the lesions are T1-hyperintense and suppress with "frequency selective fat saturation."[14] Most myelolipomas have at least 50% fat.[49] Calcifications are frequent. There can sometimes be a pseudocapsule of normal adrenal tissue surrounding the tumor.

Studies have shown that macroscopic fat can be found in other types of adrenal neoplasms, including benign adenomas and even ACC, but this is rare. In a review of 41 ACCs, Zhang and colleagues[50] reported a CT finding of macroscopic fat in 10% of their cases. Therefore, the finding of macroscopic fat, although highly suggestive of myelolipoma, needs to be considered along with all the other imaging features before concluding that the neoplasm is indeed a benign myelolipoma.

Cyst

Adrenal cysts are relatively uncommon but, fortunately, reasonably simple to characterize radiographically. They can range from a centimeter to larger than 20 cm (**Fig. 8**). Causes include congenital cysts and those that develop after an adrenal hemorrhage. Congenital cysts usually have thin nonenhancing walls that are often calcified and uniform appearance with HU less than or equal to 20, whereas posthemorrhagic cysts tend to have thicker walls and septations.[14]

Hemorrhage

Adrenal hemorrhage is often an underrecognized diagnosis. Patients may present with acute flank pain, or these may be silent. It is most often associated with trauma, coagulopathy, sepsis, and stress. However, hemorrhage can occur in benign or malignant adrenal neoplasms, as well as pheochromocytomas. CT findings of acute hemorrhage include high HU (50–90) density and periadrenal stranding.[51] Over time, the HU density decreases along with the size of the lesion (**Fig. 9**).

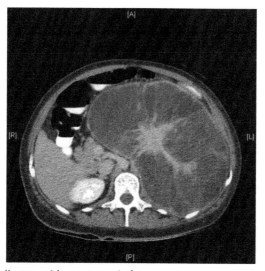

Fig. 7. Large myelolipoma with macroscopic fat.

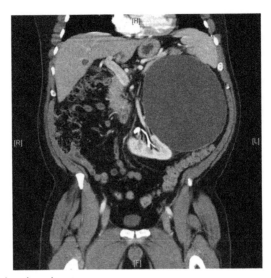

Fig. 8. Large simple adrenal cyst.

On MRI, acute hemorrhage appears isointense on T1 and hypointense on T2. Over time, the hematoma becomes hyperintense on T1 and T2, and is often heterogenous.[14] If hemorrhage is suspected, follow-up imaging with CT or MRI should be performed to document resolution of the periadrenal inflammatory response and shrinkage of the overall lesion.

Lesions that cannot confidently be placed into one of the benign categories are called indeterminate. They include lipid-poor adenomas, adrenal metastases, ACC, and pheochromocytoma.

Adrenocortical Cancer

If there were radiographic features that were 100% sensitive and specific for adrenocortical cancer, many patients would be spared the diagnostic adrenalectomy that is

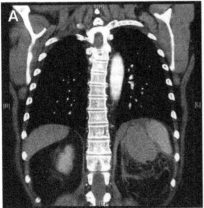
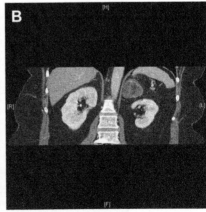

Fig. 9. (A) Acute adrenal hemorrhage with periadrenal stranding. (B) 3-months later with resolution of stranding and lesion shrinkage.

performed for many of the indeterminate nonfunctioning adrenal incidentalomas now being discovered. When evaluating an adrenal neoplasm for its malignant potential, it is important to remember that approximately 30% of ACCs are biochemically active. Size has always been a predictor of malignancy[52] and the traditionally quoted risks based on size are 2% for tumors smaller than or equal to 4 cm, 6% for tumors 4.1 to 6 cm, and 25% for tumors larger than 6 cm.[7] The current standard of care among endocrine surgeons is to recommend laparoscopic adrenalectomy for most nonfunctioning neoplasms larger than 4 cm. However, less than 1% of adrenal incidentalomas prove to be malignant and published risks have been higher due to the bias of surgical series.[13] These traditionally accepted risks need to be reevaluated because they are not applicable to the large population of patients who undergo cross-sectional imaging for unrelated reasons.

Thus, clinicians are often left building a radiographic case for or against adrenocortical cancer when evaluating adrenal incidentalomas. This is a critical process because it ultimately determines whether a patient will undergo adrenalectomy and whether that adrenalectomy will be performed laparoscopically or open. Increased size remains one of the strongest predictors and a lesion diameter larger than or equal to 6 cm, without findings that strongly suggest a benign lesion such as myelolipoma, should continue to raise suspicions of malignancy.

On noncontrast CT, a feature often associated with ACCs includes central necrosis, which can occur as the tumor outstrips its blood supply. Radiographically, this will produce heterogeneity of the attenuation coefficient. Approximately 30% of ACCs contain calcifications. It is rare to see macroscopic fat.[53] On contrast-enhanced CT, there is expected imaging heterogeneity (**Fig. 10**). Usually, the absolute and relative washout is less than it is for benign adenomas; however, there are rare case reports of ACCs with benign washout characteristics.[50,54]

The MRI findings of ACC also include heterogeneity because of necrosis and hemorrhage (**Fig. 11**). On T1 imaging, ACCs are isointense to hypointense to the liver parenchyma, with areas of hemorrhage demonstrating high intensity. CSI typically does not show dropout, due to the lack of fat within malignant lesions. Yet, rare ACCs can contain intracytoplasmic fat, especially the ones that are hormonally active, and may

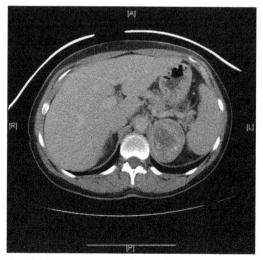

Fig. 10. Heterogeneity of ACC on contrast-enhanced CT.

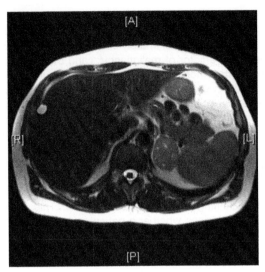

Fig. 11. MRI of ACC.

demonstrate signal loss on opposed-phase imaging.[55,56] Unlike benign adenomas, these lesions tend to be heterogenous.

Any evidence on CT or MRI of retroperitoneal adenopathy, loss of normal periadrenal tissue planes, gross invasion of periadrenal structures, or venous involvement immediately makes the probability of malignancy extremely high.

PET scans have a reported 100% sensitivity and 95% specificity for ACC, with the added potential for identifying additional lesions in 30% of patients.[57]

Patients with a Known Nonadrenal Malignancy

Patients who carry a diagnosis of nonadrenal cancer must be differently evaluated. The prevalence of adrenal neoplasms in these patients is higher, ranging from 9% to 13%.[58,59] The risk of such a neoplasm representing an adrenal metastasis ranges from 26% to 36%.[60] However, that risk rapidly increases for lesions larger than 4 cm and for those that increase in size on follow-up imaging.[61]

Adrenal metastases

In a patient with a previous malignancy, the development of a new adrenal lesion is almost certainly an adrenal metastasis and, in such patients, these lesions are not called incidentalomas. Metastases showing up as incidentalomas are extremely rare.[19] Adrenal metastases usually are heterogenous and exhibit rapid growth (**Fig. 12**). On CT, HU density is greater than 10 and MRI shows lack of dropout on out-of-phase imaging with SI-i greater than 16.5.[14]

PROTOCOL FOR RADIOGRAPHIC WORKUP

When an adrenal incidentaloma is identified, it should always be assessed for cortisol and catecholamine production, even if there are no clinical signs of hormonal secretion, because both subclinical Cushing and pheochromocytoma may not manifest any overt clinical symptoms. This can easily be accomplished with a low-dose overnight dexamethasone suppression test and plasma metanephrines.[2] Once these diagnoses are eliminated, the evaluation of a lesion's malignant potential should commence.

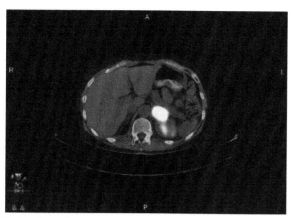

Fig. 12. Fused PET-CT of a pulmonary squamous cell metastasis to left adrenal, not present on scan 3 months earlier.

Although most current guidelines recommend resection for lesions larger than 4 cm,[62,63] this size threshold came about after the successful adoption of laparoscopic adrenalectomy. Before that technique's development, the threshold for resection was 5 to 6 cm.[64–66] After laparoscopic adrenalectomy became widespread, the rates of adrenalectomy doubled while the number of adrenocortical cancers remained unchanged.[67,68] The proven low rates of adrenocortical cancer in lesions smaller than 6 cm and the ever-increasing ability to characterize incidentalomas radiographically should give clinicians pause to reconsider whether resecting most lesions larger than 4 cm is warranted. However, it remains true that risk of adrenocortical malignancy significantly increases for lesions larger than or equal to 6 cm. Unless the radiographic signature is unquestionably benign, such as is the case with myelolipoma and cyst, these lesions still warrant resection.

The clinician should always seek out previous cross-sectional imaging studies because stability of any adrenal lesion over long periods, regardless of size, is highly predictive of a benign process. For lesions smaller than 6 cm, there are several reliable predictors of benignity. First, if the lesion has not grown over 1 year, it is very unlikely to be malignant.[69] Second, if the initial imaging includes a noncontrast CT and the unenhanced HU is less than 10, it is nearly certain that the lesion is benign.[20] Third, if the initial study obtained is an MRI, then CSI should be performed; loss of signal on the out-of-phase images is predictive of a benign lipid-rich adenoma.[70] However, if on CT the HU are greater than 10, the MR does not show signal loss on out-of-phase imaging, or there are other concerning features, an adrenal protocol CT with and without contrast should be performed to calculate the APW. If the APW is greater than 40% and there are no findings that otherwise raise the suspicion for ACC, the lesion can be observed.

FOLLOW-UP

Currently published guidelines for follow-up of nonfunctional adrenal incidentalomas are shown in **Table 2**. These guidelines were developed based on the recent use of a cutoff of 4 cm for resection. Therefore, the presumption exists that most nonfunctioning lesions larger than 4 cm would have undergone laparoscopic resection. Recommendations are for reassessment of hormone production and growth of the

Table 2
Current recommendations for follow-up

Group	Hormonal Tests	Frequency	Duration	Time Interval
Grumbach et al[7]	1 mg DXT, metanephrines, K renin-aldosterone in patients with HTN	Annual	4 y	2 CTs at least 6 mo apart No data to support further imaging if no change in size
Young[6]	1 mg DXT, metanephrines, K renin-aldosterone in patients with HTN	Annual	4 y	CT at 6, 12, and 24 mo
American College of Radiology[72]	—	—	—	No follow-up if lesion has diagnostic features of a benign neoplasm

Abbreviations: DXT, dexamethasone; HTN, hypertension.

neoplasm. Both the NIH guidelines[7] and those of Young[6] recommend multiple follow-up CT scans over the ensuing 2 years. However, recently published guidelines in the radiology literature[69] illustrate a growing confidence in the ability of CT, MRI, and PET to accurately diagnose benign adrenal adenoma. These new guidelines state that no follow-up imaging is required if the initial studies are diagnostic of a benign adenoma. Although it will take time for such an approach to take hold in both endocrine and surgery practices, it will likely be adopted more readily by radiologists, who are on the frontlines of this epidemic.

Reasons to reassess the earlier guidelines include the cost to the patient and the health care system of repeated biochemical and radiographic testing for ongoing surveillance when the chance of developing malignancy is less than 1%.[15] Although it is established that 5% to 20% of adrenal incidentalomas will show slow growth of 1 cm or more over an average of 4 years, these are almost always benign.[71] Also, the advances made in imaging quality and evaluation enable involved clinicians to be more confident in their assessments of the likelihood of benignity for lesions in the 4 to 6 cm range. Therefore, a reasonable approach to lesions smaller than 4 cm that are nonfunctional and clearly meet imaging criteria of a benign lipid-rich adenoma is to not perform further imaging,[72] as well as limit repeat biochemical evaluation to patients who are hypertensive or develop symptoms and signs associated with cortisol, catecholamine, or aldosterone excess. Lesions between 4 and 6 cm that carry slightly higher malignancy rates should be excised if imaging cannot confidently characterize them as benign. However, if imaging suggests a lipid-rich adenoma, a nonoperative approach may be pursued and repeat adrenal imaging may be obtained in 6 to 12 months. Lesions larger than or equal to 6 cm should be resected unless there is unequivocal imaging evidence of a benign nature. If radiographic features are suggestive of possible adrenocortical cancer, strong consideration should be given to open adrenalectomy instead of an open approach.

REFERENCES

1. Kloos RT, Gross MD, Francis IR, et al. Incidentally discovered adrenal masses. Endocr Rev 1995;16(4):460–84.
2. Mazzaglia P, Miner T. Adrenal incidentaloma. In: Cameron JL, editor. Current surgical therapy.
3. Robbins. Robbins pathologic basis of disease. 4th edition.

4. Harrison's principles of internal medicine. 12th edition.
5. Schteingart DE, Doherty GM, Gauger PG, et al. Management of patients with adrenal cancer: recommendations of an international consensus conference. Endocr Relat Cancer 2005;12(3):667–80.
6. Young WF Jr. Clinical practice. The incidentally discovered adrenal mass. N Engl J Med 2007;356(6):601–10.
7. Grumbach MM, Biller BM, Braunstein GD, et al. Management of the clinically inapparent adrenal mass ("incidentaloma"). Ann Intern Med 2003;138(5):424–9.
8. Henneman D, Chang Y, Hodin RA, et al. Effect of laparoscopy on the indications for adrenalectomy. Arch Surg 2009;144(3):255–9 [discussion: 9].
9. Brunt LM, Doherty GM, Norton JA, et al. Laparoscopic adrenalectomy compared to open adrenalectomy for benign adrenal neoplasms. J Am Coll Surg 1996;183(1):1–10.
10. Miccoli P, Raffaelli M, Berti P, et al. Adrenal surgery before and after the introduction of laparoscopic adrenalectomy. Br J Surg 2002;89(6):779–82.
11. Gagner M, Lacroix A, Bolte E. Laparoscopic adrenalectomy in Cushing's syndrome and pheochromocytoma. N Engl J Med 1992;327(14):1033.
12. Heniford BT, Arca MJ, Walsh RM, et al. Laparoscopic adrenalectomy for cancer. Semin Surg Oncol 1999;16(4):293–306.
13. Mazzaglia PJ, Vezeridis MP. Laparoscopic adrenalectomy: balancing the operative indications with the technical advances. J Surg Oncol 2010;101(8):739–44.
14. Taffel M, Haji-Momenian S, Nikolaidis P, et al. Adrenal imaging: a comprehensive review. Radiol Clin North Am 2012;50(2):219–43, v.
15. Cawood TJ, Hunt PJ, O'Shea D, et al. Recommended evaluation of adrenal incidentalomas is costly, has high false-positive rates and confers a risk of fatal cancer that is similar to the risk of the adrenal lesion becoming malignant; time for a rethink? Eur J Endocrinol 2009;161(4):513–27.
16. Angeli A, Osella G, Ali A, et al. Adrenal incidentaloma: an overview of clinical and epidemiological data from the National Italian Study Group. Horm Res 1997;47(4–6):279–83.
17. Young WF Jr. Management approaches to adrenal incidentalomas. A view from Rochester, Minnesota. Endocrinol Metab Clin North Am 2000;29(1):159–85, x.
18. Lee MJ, Hahn PF, Papanicolaou N, et al. Benign and malignant adrenal masses: CT distinction with attenuation coefficients, size, and observer analysis. Radiology 1991;179(2):415–8.
19. Song JH, Chaudhry FS, Mayo-Smith WW. The incidental adrenal mass on CT: prevalence of adrenal disease in 1,049 consecutive adrenal masses in patients with no known malignancy. AJR Am J Roentgenol 2008;190(5):1163–8.
20. Boland GW, Lee MJ, Gazelle GS, et al. Characterization of adrenal masses using unenhanced CT: an analysis of the CT literature. AJR Am J Roentgenol 1998; 171(1):201–4.
21. Blake MA, Kalra MK, Sweeney AT, et al. Distinguishing benign from malignant adrenal masses: multi-detector row CT protocol with 10-minute delay. Radiology 2006;238(2):578–85.
22. Reinig JW, Doppman JL, Dwyer AJ, et al. Adrenal masses differentiated by MR. Radiology 1986;158(1):81–4.
23. Glazer GM, Woolsey EJ, Borrello J, et al. Adrenal tissue characterization using MR imaging. Radiology 1986;158(1):73–9.
24. Inan N, Arslan A, Akansel G, et al. Dynamic contrast enhanced MRI in the differential diagnosis of adrenal adenomas and malignant adrenal masses. Eur J Radiol 2008;65(1):154–62.

25. Semelka RC, Shoenut JP, Lawrence PH, et al. Evaluation of adrenal masses with gadolinium enhancement and fat-suppressed MR imaging. J Magn Reson Imaging 1993;3(2):337–43.

26. Krestin GP, Steinbrich W, Friedmann G. Adrenal masses: evaluation with fast gradient-echo MR imaging and Gd-DTPA-enhanced dynamic studies. Radiology 1989;171(3):675–80.

27. Sahdev A, Willatt J, Francis IR, et al. The indeterminate adrenal lesion. Cancer Imaging 2010;10:102–13.

28. Boland GW, Blake MA, Hahn PF, et al. Incidental adrenal lesions: principles, techniques, and algorithms for imaging characterization. Radiology 2008; 249(3):756–75.

29. Blake MA, Cronin CG, Boland GW. Adrenal imaging. AJR Am J Roentgenol 2010;194(6):1450–60.

30. McNicholas MM, Lee MJ, Mayo-Smith WW, et al. An imaging algorithm for the differential diagnosis of adrenal adenomas and metastases. AJR Am J Roentgenol 1995;165(6):1453–9.

31. Fujiyoshi F, Nakajo M, Fukukura Y, et al. Characterization of adrenal tumors by chemical shift fast low-angle shot MR imaging: comparison of four methods of quantitative evaluation. AJR Am J Roentgenol 2003;180(6):1649–57.

32. Rescinito G, Zandrino F, Cittadini G Jr, et al. Characterization of adrenal adenomas and metastases: correlation between unenhanced computed tomography and chemical shift magnetic resonance imaging. Acta Radiol 2006;47(1):71–6.

33. Haider MA, Ghai S, Jhaveri K, et al. Chemical shift MR imaging of hyperattenuating (>10 HU) adrenal masses: does it still have a role? Radiology 2004;231(3): 711–6.

34. Korobkin M, Brodeur FJ, Francis IR, et al. CT time-attenuation washout curves of adrenal adenomas and nonadenomas. AJR Am J Roentgenol 1998;170(3): 747–52.

35. Caoili EM, Korobkin M, Francis IR, et al. Adrenal masses: characterization with combined unenhanced and delayed enhanced CT. Radiology 2002;222(3): 629–33.

36. Dunnick NR, Korobkin M, Francis I. Adrenal radiology: distinguishing benign from malignant adrenal masses. AJR Am J Roentgenol 1996;167(4):861–7.

37. Sangwaiya MJ, Boland GW, Cronin CG, et al. Incidental adrenal lesions: accuracy of characterization with contrast-enhanced washout multidetector CT–10-minute delayed imaging protocol revisited in a large patient cohort. Radiology 2010;256(2):504–10.

38. Bae KT, Fuangtharnthip P, Prasad SR, et al. Adrenal masses: CT characterization with histogram analysis method. Radiology 2003;228(3):735–42.

39. Halefoglu AM, Bas N, Yasar A, et al. Differentiation of adrenal adenomas from nonadenomas using CT histogram analysis method: a prospective study. Eur J Radiol 2010;73(3):643–51.

40. Ho LM, Paulson EK, Brady MJ, et al. Lipid-poor adenomas on unenhanced CT: does histogram analysis increase sensitivity compared with a mean attenuation threshold? AJR Am J Roentgenol 2008;191(1):234–8.

41. Boland GW, Blake MA, Holalkere NS, et al. PET/CT for the characterization of adrenal masses in patients with cancer: qualitative versus quantitative accuracy in 150 consecutive patients. AJR Am J Roentgenol 2009;192(4):956–62.

42. Groussin L, Bonardel G, Silvera S, et al. 18F-Fluorodeoxyglucose positron emission tomography for the diagnosis of adrenocortical tumors: a prospective study in 77 operated patients. J Clin Endocrinol Metab 2009;94(5):1713–22.

43. Metser U, Miller E, Lerman H, et al. 18F-FDG PET/CT in the evaluation of adrenal masses. J Nucl Med 2006;47(1):32–7.
44. Bagheri B, Maurer AH, Cone L, et al. Characterization of the normal adrenal gland with 18F-FDG PET/CT. J Nucl Med 2004;45(8):1340–3.
45. Blake MA, Slattery JM, Kalra MK, et al. Adrenal lesions: characterization with fused PET/CT image in patients with proved or suspected malignancy—initial experience. Radiology 2006;238(3):970–7.
46. Bakheet SM, Powe J, Ezzat A, et al. F-18-FDG uptake in tuberculosis. Clin Nucl Med 1998;23(11):739–42.
47. Caoili EM, Korobkin M, Brown RK, et al. Differentiating adrenal adenomas from nonadenomas using (18)F-FDG PET/CT: quantitative and qualitative evaluation. Acad Radiol 2007;14(4):468–75.
48. Yun M, Kim W, Alnafisi N, et al. 18F-FDG PET in characterizing adrenal lesions detected on CT or MRI. J Nucl Med 2001;42(12):1795–9.
49. Kenney PJ, Wagner BJ, Rao P, et al. Myelolipoma: CT and pathologic features. Radiology 1998;208(1):87–95.
50. Zhang HM, Perrier ND, Grubbs EG, et al. CT features and quantification of the characteristics of adrenocortical carcinomas on unenhanced and contrast-enhanced studies. Clin Radiol 2012;67(1):38–46.
51. Dunnick NR. Hanson lecture. Adrenal imaging: current status. AJR Am J Roentgenol 1990;154(5):927–36.
52. Hussain S, Belldegrun A, Seltzer SE, et al. Differentiation of malignant from benign adrenal masses: predictive indices on computed tomography. AJR Am J Roentgenol 1985;144(1):61–5.
53. Bharwani N, Rockall AG, Sahdev A, et al. Adrenocortical carcinoma: the range of appearances on CT and MRI. AJR Am J Roentgenol 2011;196(6):W706–14.
54. Simhan J, Canter D, Teper E, et al. Adrenocortical carcinoma masquerading as a benign adenoma on computed tomography washout study. Urology 2012; 79(2):e19–20.
55. Ferrozzi F, Bova D. CT and MR demonstration of fat within an adrenal cortical carcinoma. Abdom Imaging 1995;20(3):272–4.
56. Schlund JF, Kenney PJ, Brown ED, et al. Adrenocortical carcinoma: MR imaging appearance with current techniques. J Magn Reson Imaging 1995;5(2):171–4.
57. Becherer A, Vierhapper H, Potzi C, et al. FDG-PET in adrenocortical carcinoma. Cancer Biother Radiopharm 2001;16(4):289–95.
58. Bovio S, Cataldi A, Reimondo G, et al. Prevalence of adrenal incidentaloma in a contemporary computerized tomography series. J Endocrinol Invest 2006; 29(4):298–302.
59. Glazer HS, Weyman PJ, Sagel SS, et al. Nonfunctioning adrenal masses: incidental discovery on computed tomography. AJR Am J Roentgenol 1982;139(1):81–5.
60. Oliver TW Jr, Bernardino ME, Miller JI, et al. Isolated adrenal masses in nonsmall-cell bronchogenic carcinoma. Radiology 1984;153(1):217–8.
61. Frilling A, Tecklenborg K, Weber F, et al. Importance of adrenal incidentaloma in patients with a history of malignancy. Surgery 2004;136(6):1289–96.
62. Zeiger MA, Thompson GB, Duh QY, et al. American Association of Clinical Endocrinologists and American Association of Endocrine Surgeons Medical Guidelines for the management of adrenal incidentalomas: executive summary of recommendations. Endocr Pract 2009;15(5):450–3.
63. Berland LL. The American College of Radiology strategy for managing incidental findings on abdominal computed tomography. Radiol Clin North Am 2011;49(2):237–43.

64. Prinz RA, Brooks MH, Churchill R, et al. Incidental asymptomatic adrenal masses detected by computed tomographic scanning. Is operation required? JAMA 1982;248(6):701–4.
65. Herrera MF, Grant CS, van Heerden JA, et al. Incidentally discovered adrenal tumors: an institutional perspective. Surgery 1991;110(6):1014–21.
66. Bornstein SR, Stratakis CA, Chrousos GP. Adrenocortical tumors: recent advances in basic concepts and clinical management. Ann Intern Med 1999; 130(9):759–71.
67. Saunders BD, Wainess RM, Dimick JB, et al. Trends in utilization of adrenalectomy in the United States: have indications changed? World J Surg 2004;28(11): 1169–75.
68. Gallagher SF, Wahi M, Haines KL, et al. Trends in adrenalectomy rates, indications, and physician volume: a statewide analysis of 1816 adrenalectomies. Surgery 2007;142(6):1011–21 [discussion: 21].
69. Berland LL, Silverman SG, Gore RM, et al. Managing incidental findings on abdominal CT: white paper of the ACR incidental findings committee. J Am Coll Radiol 2010;7(10):754–73.
70. Mayo-Smith WW, Lee MJ, McNicholas MM, et al. Characterization of adrenal masses (<5 cm) by use of chemical shift MR imaging: observer performance versus quantitative measures. AJR Am J Roentgenol 1995;165(1):91–5.
71. Terzolo M, Stigliano A, Chiodini I, et al. AME position statement on adrenal incidentaloma. Eur J Endocrinol 2011;164(6):851–70.
72. Choyke PL, ACR Committee on Appropriateness Criteria. ACR Appropriateness Criteria on incidentally discovered adrenal mass. J Am Coll Radiol 2006;3(7): 498–504.

Hyperaldosteronism
Diagnosis, Lateralization, and Treatment

Adrian M. Harvey, MD, MEd, MSc, FRCSC

KEYWORDS

- Primary hyperaldosteronism • Secondary hypertension • Aldosterone
- Aldosterone-to-renin ratio • Adrenal venous sampling
- Laparoscopic adrenalectomy

KEY POINTS

- Although initially believed to be rare, less restrictive screening has demonstrated that primary hyperaldosteronism (PA) may be found in more than 10% of hypertensive patients.
- The aldosterone-to-renin ratio is widely accepted as the first-line screening test for PA.
- PA has several underlying pathologic causes. Most patients have either an aldosterone-producing adenoma or bilateral hyperplasia.
- Lateralization of the source of autonomous aldosterone production is critical to the selection of appropriate (medical vs surgical) treatment.
- Patients with unilateral disease who are appropriate surgical candidates should be treated with laparoscopic adrenalectomy.
- Following surgery, cure of hypertension is observed in 30% to 50% of patients with improvement of blood pressure control in most patients.
- Patients with bilateral disease and those who are not appropriate candidates for surgery should be treated with a mineralocorticoid antagonist.

HISTORY AND EPIDEMIOLOGY

Dr Jerome Conn, an endocrinologist from the University of Michigan first described primary hyperaldosteronism (PA) in 1955.[1,2] The initial case he reported was a 34-year-old woman with severe hypertension and hypokalemia. This patient had evidence of increased aldosterone in the urine and she was ultimately found to have a 4 cm solitary adrenal adenoma. Surgical resection resulted in resolution of hypertension and hypokalemia.

The presentation and understanding of PA has evolved significantly in the almost 60 years since its initial description. Dr Conn had originally speculated that PA might

Disclosures: None.
Section of General Surgery and Surgical Oncology, Department of Surgery, Faculty of Medicine, Foothills Medical Center, University of Calgary, 1403 29th Street Northwest, FMC, North Tower, Calgary, Alberta T2N 2T9, Canada
E-mail address: adrian.harvey@albertahealthservices.ca

be found in up to 20% of hypertensive patients. However, early series seemed to indicate that PA was a rare phenomenon, found in less than 1%.[3-6] This initial underrepresentation was largely the result of selective screening restricted to patients with both hypertension and hypokalemia. Broader screening criteria have been adopted with the realization that hypokalemia is not universally present. In fact, most patients are clinically indistinguishable from those with essential hypertension. Mulatero and colleagues[7] (2004) retrospectively reviewed the results of less restrictive screening in clinical centers on five continents. These centers reported hypokalemia in just 9% to 37% of patients with confirmed PA. As screening criteria have adapted to reflect our evolving understanding of PA prevalence, estimates in excess of 10% have been reported in many contemporary series.[5,7-21]

The underlying cause of secondary hypertension in Conn's original patient was autonomous aldosterone production from a solitary adrenal adenoma. However, PA has more than one underlying cause (**Table 1**). Most patients have either an aldosterone-producing adenoma (APA) or bilateral adrenal hyperplasia (BAH).[7,10,22-25] Less common causes include unilateral hyperplasia, adrenal cortical carcinoma, and rare familial forms of PA. The distinction between these underlying pathologic conditions is important clinically because bilateral disease tends to responds poorly to surgical intervention.[22,26-28] Broader patterns of screening have resulted in a shift in the proportion of patients with each underlying cause. In fact, as less restrictive criteria have been adopted, a decline in patients with APA, from between 68% and 89% to approximately 40%, has been observed.[7,29]

PATHOPHYSIOLOGY AND CLINICAL IMPACT

The renin-angiotensin-aldosterone system is an important regulator of fluid volume status and blood pressure. Renin is secreted by the juxtaglomerular cells of the kidney in response to reduced renal vascular perfusion. Renin subsequently cleaves angiotensinogen to angiotensin 1, which is converted to angiotensin 2 by angiotensin-converting enzyme in vascular endothelial cells. Angiotensin 2 and potassium are the major long-term stimulants of aldosterone release. Aldosterone, in turn, induces resorption of sodium and secretion of potassium and hydrogen ions in the cortical collecting duct and distal nephron. The result is an expansion of extracellular fluid volume, which acts in a negative feedback manner to suppress further renin secretion. In PA, production of aldosterone is autonomous, resulting in inappropriate expansion of intravascular volume and hypertension.

The importance of potentially correctable forms of hypertension such as PA cannot be underestimated. Hypertension is a well-established risk factor for cardiac disease, stroke, and renal failure. More importantly, ischemic cardiac disease and stroke

Table 1 Underlying causes and their frequency in PA		
Pathologic State	**Frequency**	**Unilateral (U) or Bilateral (B)**
Aldosterone-producing adenoma	30%–40%	U
Bilateral adrenal hyperplasia	60%–65%	B
Primary adrenal hyperplasia	~2%	U
Adrenal cortical carcinoma	<1%	U
Familial		
FH-I (glucocorticoid remediable)	<1%	B
FH-II	<1%	U

risk can be lowered by even minor reductions in blood pressure.[30] In addition, elevated aldosterone independently induces inflammation and fibrosis, resulting in end-organ damage beyond what would be expected from the extent of hypertension alone. Milliez and colleagues[31] compared cardiovascular complication rates in 124 patients with PA to 465 controls with essential hypertension matched by age, sex, and blood pressure. The investigators observed an increased risk of stroke (odds ratio [OR] = 4.2), nonfatal myocardial infarction (OR = 6.5), and atrial fibrillation (OR = 12.1) in subjects with PA.[31] Thus, there is significant potential clinical benefit from appropriate screening, diagnosis, and treatment.

DIAGNOSIS
Screening

Given the revelation that PA is more prevalent than initially thought and that most patients do not present with hypokalemia, screening has evolved to include a broader subset of the population. The decision of who to screen represents a delicate balance between the benefit of increased sensitivity in case detection with the potential harm of work-up and treatment. Practice guidelines have been recently published by endocrine societies in Japan and the United States.[22,24] Although the Japanese guidelines suggest screening may be appropriate for all hypertensive patients, the US guidelines focus on screening efforts on patient groups with known or suspected high prevalence of PA.

Patients in whom screening for PA is recommended include[22]

- Hypertensive patients with hypokalemia (spontaneous or diuretic-induced)
- Patients with resistant hypertension (systolic blood pressure >140 or diastolic blood pressure >90 despite treatment with ≥3 antihypertensive medications; prevalence 8%–23%)
- Patients with moderate (160–179/100–109 mm Hg; prevalence 8%) or severe (>180/>110 mm Hg; prevalence 13%) hypertension
- Patients with hypertension and an adrenal incidentaloma (prevalence 1%–10%).

The aldosterone-to-renin ratio (ARR) is widely accepted to be the most appropriate screening test for PA.[10,13,16,18,19,22,24,32–37] Given its low prevalence, hypokalemia clearly lacks the sensitivity required. In addition, measurements of aldosterone (low sensitivity) or renin (low specificity) alone have demonstrated inferior performance in screening for PA.[22,34,38,39] Consistent estimates of the sensitivity and specificity of the ARR are elusive in the literature.[16,32–36] This is a consequence of the numerous patient, methodological, and interpretation factors that may affect the results of each assay. However, Yin and colleagues[36] (2012) demonstrated that careful attention to testing protocols, consideration of patient factors, and appropriate selection of cutoff values could result in sensitivity approaching 100% and specificity in the 92% to 97% range.

In preparation for ARR testing, serum potassium should be measured and corrected if low. In addition, the patient should be encouraged not to restrict salt intake. Medications that have a significant effect on the ARR (**Table 2**) should be withdrawn for 4 weeks.[22,35,37] Patients should also eliminate products derived from the licorice root because these can interfere with 11β-hydroxysteroid dehydrogenase, producing a state of apparent mineralocorticoid excess.[40] Additional medications with lesser impact on the ARR may be discontinued if initial testing yields borderline values and hypertension can be adequately controlled with noninterfering agents (see **Table 2**). The blood samples should be drawn in a laboratory experienced with endocrine

Table 2
Medication that may affect the interpretation of the ARR

Medication	ARR
1. Significant effect	
K⁺-sparing diuretic	
Spironolactone or eplerenone	↓
Amiloride or triamterene	↓
K⁺-wasting diuretic	↓
Other (licorice root)	↓ or ← →
2. Lesser effect	
ACE inhibitor	↓
Angiotensin receptor blocker	↓
β-blocker	↑
α-agonist (central)	↑
NSAID	↑
Dihydropyridine CCB	↓
3. Minimal effect	
Verapamil ± hydralazine	← →
Selective α1-blocker (doxazosin, terazosin)	← →

Abbreviations: ACE, angiotensin-converting enzyme; CCB, calcium channel blocker; NSAID, nonsteroidal antiinflammatory drug.

testing procedures using a standardized approach.[22] Blood should be drawn after the patient has been up for at least 2 hours and seated for 5 to 15 minutes. Samples should be transferred for analysis expeditiously and at room temperature. Prolong storage (>24 hours) at low temperature has been shown to result in conversion of prorenin to renin by cryoactivation.[41]

Considerable variability in the interpretation of the ARR exists in the literature. Standard US units express the plasma aldosterone concentration (PAC) in nanograms per deciliter and the plasma renin activity (PRA) in nanograms per milliliters per hour. Cutoff values reported in the literature vary widely; however, most centers that use a seated morning measurement use values between 20 and 40.[10,12,16,22,24,32–37] Laboratories that use the International System of Units or direct renin concentration measurements will naturally use different cutoff ratios. Some centers also require an elevated aldosterone level to reduce false-positives that may result from a very low renin.[22]

Confirmatory Testing

Positive ARR values are typically followed by a confirmatory test to make a definitive diagnosis. Confirmatory tests used in clinical practice include (1) oral sodium loading, (2) saline infusion, (3) fludrocortisone suppression, and (4) captopril challenge.[22,24,33,37,42–46] These tests share a common principle of attempting to suppress aldosterone production either by increasing intravascular volume or medically inhibiting some step in its production. Failure of suppression is interpreted as evidence for autonomous production and considered diagnostic of PA.

During the oral sodium loading test, patients ingest a high sodium diet for 3 days followed by a 24-hour urine measurement of aldosterone. The saline infusion test involves giving patients 2 L of 0.9% normal saline over 4 hours followed by a measurement of PAC. Failure of intravascular volume expansion to suppress aldosterone level through its action on renin indicates autonomous production. Given that these tests may involve acute increases in intravascular volume, they should be used with caution in elderly patients with severe hypertension or heart failure.

The fludrocortisone suppression test uses oral sodium loading in addition to the synthetic mineralocorticoid effect in an attempt to suppress aldosterone. The protocol is complex and the test is somewhat cumbersome, often requiring several days of hospital admission. Patients are given 0.1 mg of fludrocortisone every 6 hours and a high-salt diet for 4 days. On day four, an upright plasma aldosterone is measured. Again, failure of suppression is considered diagnostic. Although some centers consider this the gold standard test for the diagnosis of PA, its widespread use is limited owing to the complexity and expense of the protocol and lack of prospective validation. In addition, Mulatero and colleagues[42] (2006) demonstrated similar performance from the more straightforward saline infusion test. Because this test involves oral sodium loading, it must also be used cautiously with patients with significant cardiovascular comorbidity.

The captopril challenge test attempts to suppress aldosterone production by inhibiting the conversion of angiotensin 1 to angiotensin 2. Patients are given 25 to 50 mg of captopril and have plasma measurements of aldosterone, PRA, and cortisol measured at 0, 1, and 2 hours. Because autonomous production of aldosterone is independent of angiotensin 2, patients with PA will fail to show suppression. Although clearly more straightforward with respect to protocol, some investigators have reported that this test may have an unacceptable false-negative rate.[47]

Currently, US and Japanese guidelines recommend confirmatory testing in the work-up of PA.[22,24] However, obligatory use of confirmatory testing is not without opposition in the literature. Nanba and colleagues[44] (2012) reported that most patients with positive ARR also had positive confirmatory tests. This was particularly true when the ARR was quite high. In addition, Salva and colleagues[45] (2012) pointed to the lack of prospective validation and variable sensitivity to specificity. The investigators concluded that their position in the diagnostic algorithm was "unresolved." Indeed, even the US guidelines report that the recommendation for confirmatory testing is based on low-quality evidence.[22] Proponents of confirmatory testing point to the potential cost and risk associated with proceeding to more invasive lateralization procedures in patients who may not ultimately have the disease.

The author's center stopped performing confirmatory tests after ARR case detection in 2005. The protocol directs patients with elevated ARR who are appropriate surgical candidates and who accept further work-up to have an adrenal protocol CT and adrenal venous sampling (AVS) performed (**Fig. 1**). The ARR is set relatively low (>550 PAC pmol/L: PRA ng/mL/hour) to maximize sensitivity and avoid missing patients with potentially correctable disease. This protocol has not shown an increase in proportion of nonlateralized disease, which would be expected if the false-positive rate of ARR were unacceptably high (Kline and colleagues, unpublished result, 2012). Overall, only 3 of 83 patients undergoing AVS had laboratory tests classified as possible PA in which a false-positive diagnosis would have to be considered.

The adoption of this protocol was predicated on the availability of safe and reliable AVS performed by an experienced radiologist. Our current biochemical success rate for AVS is greater than 95%.[29] In addition, laboratory results are evaluated by a consistent group of dedicated hypertensive specialists and endocrine surgeons. In the absence of these resources, adoption of a protocol such as ours would be problematic.

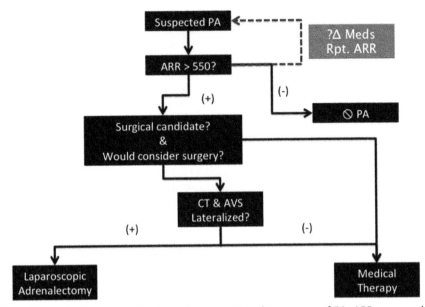

Fig. 1. The author's current algorithm for work-up and treatment of PA. ARR expressed in units (aldosterone, pmol/L; renin, ng/ml/h) and set at 550 to maximize sensitivity.

Lateralization

Following diagnosis, the priority shifts to differentiating between unilateral and bilateral sources of aldosterone excess. Underlying pathologic conditions in PA are listed in **Table 1**.[7,25,48–51] Accurate determination of the underlying subtype is critical to the recommendation of appropriate therapy because bilateral hyperplasia is unlikely to respond to surgery.[22,26–28] Currently, most protocols rely on cross-sectional imaging with CT often in conjunction with AVS.

Anatomic imaging

Adrenal protocol CT provides anatomic information important for surgical planning and may demonstrate a unilateral adenoma (**Fig. 2**). However, CT has some significant limitations when it comes to accurate lateralization.[22,24,25,52–55] CT scanning has limited sensitivity for small adenomas, detecting fewer than 25% less than 1 cm.[22] This is problematic given that APAs tend to be small. In most series, the median size is between 1.5 and 2 cm.[54,56–62] In addition, CT does not provide any functional information. Thus, the presence of an adenoma on CT does not confirm that this is the source of autonomous aldosterone production. Given that the incidence of adrenal incidentalomas on CT scans is reported to be 4% to 5%, the possibility that an apparent adenoma is unrelated to PA must be considered.[63] In addition, small adrenal masses may be part of a bilateral macronodular hyperplasia subtype.

Given the described limitations of cross-sectional, anatomic imaging, the US and Japanese Endocrine Society guidelines recommend against the use of CT scan as a stand-alone lateralization test.[22,24] In a series of 203 patients with PA from the Mayo Clinic, CT scan accurately identified the source of excess aldosterone in just 53%.[54] In this series, the investigators reported that if operative decisions were based on CT alone 24.7% of patients would have had unnecessary surgery and 21.7% would have been excluded from surgical management of potential benefit. However, noting

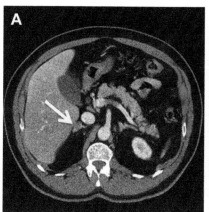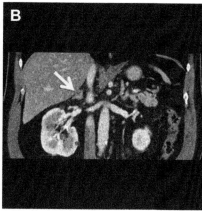

Fig. 2. CT scan showing right adrenal mass lesion on axial (*A*) and coronal (*B*) views in a patient with elevated ARR. AVS showed clear lateralization to the right side and the patient underwent right laparoscopic adrenalectomy. *Arrows* indicate right adrenal adenoma.

that incidentalomas are less common in young patients, the investigators also suggested that patients less than 40 years old with a unilateral adrenal mass greater than 1 cm and a normal contralateral gland could potentially undergo surgery without AVS.[54]

AVS
AVS provides biochemical evidence of laterality in patients with PA. Japanese and US clinical practice guidelines recommend AVS in all patients in whom surgical management is considered.[22,24] Unfortunately, AVS is an invasive and technically demanding test with a broad range of reported success rates. A large review of AVS demonstrated that the overall success rate in 47 reports was just 74%.[37] Before the establishment of our current protocol, AVS procedures at our institution were reviewed. Despite radiological procedure reports almost universally describing successful cannulation of both adrenal veins, the technical success rate, judged by biochemical criteria, was just 44%.[64] Following this review, we made several changes to our AVS protocol including: (1) assignment of a single, experienced interventional radiologist; (2) standardized protocol, including corticotropin infusion; and (3) standardized interpretation by a consistent, dedicated group of specialists. A subsequent review of our institutional experience revealed that our technical success rate increased to 95%.[29] These improvements enabled the establishment of our current protocol in which all patients with PA who are potential surgical candidates undergo AVS. In experienced hands, the complication rate of AVS is low (<2.5%).[54] Potential complications include groin hematoma, adrenal vein dissection, and adrenal hemorrhage.

A dedicated and experienced radiologist performs AVS on all patients referred for further work-up. Catheters are inserted percutaneously into the femoral veins (**Fig. 3**). Blood is drawn from the inferior vena cava (IVC) and both adrenal veins. Baseline samples are taken and then repeated following administration of Cortrosyn (corticotropin, 250 µg bolus and 10 µg/min, infusion over 15 minutes). Corticotropin aids in the interpretation of AVS by reducing stress-induced or spontaneous fluctuations in steroid secretion.[10,22,54,65] This maneuver helps to correctly identify appropriate catheter placement. In addition, APAs may be more responsive to corticotropin, resulting in an exaggerated lateralization ratio in these patients.

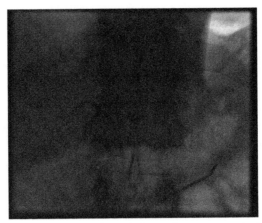

Fig. 3. AVS. Catheters are introduced through femoral puncture and advanced up the inferior vena cava and into both adrenal veins. Samples are taken from the IVC and both adrenal veins before and after corticotropin infusion.

Criteria by which the results are interpreted vary significantly between centers. At the author's center, the same group of specialists using a standard set of guidelines interprets all results. The first priority in interpretation is to determine if the adrenal veins were both successfully cannulated. This is done biochemically because the radiologic report correlates poorly with accepted markers of success.[64] This determination requires comparison of cortisol measurements from the IVC with those taken from the adrenal veins. We use an adrenal vein/IVC ratio of 3:1 at baseline and 5:1 in the corticotropin-stimulated state.[29,65,66] Once technical success is established, results are evaluated for evidence of lateralization. The use of absolute aldosterone levels with a ratio greater than 10:1 has been reported in the literature.[37] However, this method fails to account for periodic changes in steroid secretion and anatomic dilution of the left adrenal vein affluent leading to poor sensitivity. To control for these variables, results are typically expressed as a ratio of aldosterone-to-cortisol (A/C). When A/C values of the affected and unaffected sides are compared, a ratio of 4:1 is used to define lateralization.[29,64–66] Suppression of the A/C ratio on the unaffected side less than the level seen in the IVC provides further evidence. These ratios have been evaluated in the literature and shown to be the most accurate measures in AVS.[67]

At the author's center, samples are also drawn for the measurement of epinephrine. In the case of borderline localization values, these measures are used to clarify the issue of technical success. Due to their expense, the samples are not processed unless deemed necessary to aid interpretation. Recent series have shown that epinephrine results can be useful for determining technical success as well as for lateralization.[68,69]

Additional lateralization tests

Several other tests have been used for lateralization in PA. For the most part these investigations lack the accuracy of CT and AVS in combination. However, they may still be useful in the setting of unsuccessful or unavailable AVS. The postural stimulation test is based on the observation that APAs tend to be relatively unresponsive to angiotensin 2 in comparison with BAH.[22] In addition, measurements of 18-hydroxycorticosterone tend to be higher in APAs.[22,70] Thus, in the setting of an abnormality on CT and unsuccessful AVS these tests might contribute to confirming unilateral disease. Finally, radiolabeled iodocholesterol scintigraphy has been available since the 1970s. Unfortunately, it lacks specificity for smaller adenomas and thus is unlikely to contribute to the subtype classification in patients with equivocal CT.[22]

Genetic testing

Although familial forms are rare, identification may have important implications. In particular, identification of patients with familial hyperaldosteronism (FH) type I (glucocorticoid remediable aldosteronism) will direct appropriate therapy. Genetic testing for FH-I is sensitive and specific. It should be selectively used in patients with an elevated pretest probability of familial disease. As such, the Endocrine Society guidelines recommend considering genetic testing in patients with an early diagnosis of PA (<20 years) and those with a family history of PA or stroke at an early age.[22] FH-II is clinically similar to nonfamilial disease and is treated similarly. Regardless, genetic testing may have implications for screening family members.

TREATMENT
Surgical

Unilateral adrenal disease (APA or unilateral hyperplasia) in a patient who is an appropriate surgical candidate is best treated with adrenalectomy. Usually this is done via a laparoscopic approach (transabdominal or retroperitoneal). Compared with traditional open surgery, laparoscopic adrenalectomy has proven safe and effective with reduced hospital stay, less analgesic requirement, and earlier intake by mouth.[71,72]

Outcomes following adrenalectomy for unilateral PA have been well documented in the literature.[18,29,51,56,57,59–62,72–74] ARRs and hypokalemia normalize in most patients. In addition, 30% to 60% of patients are cured when cure of hypertension is defined as blood pressure lower than 140 over 90 with no antihypertensive medications. Most patients (80%–95%) experience an improvement in blood pressure control. Changes in blood pressure largely occur during the first 6 months postoperatively. Several factors have been proposed as predictors of postoperative blood pressure normalization. These include (1) number of medications, (2) duration of hypertension, (3) response to spironolactone, (4) age, (5) gender, (6) preoperative ARR, (7) family history, and (8) body mass index (BMI). Zarnegar and colleagues[74] (2008) used logistic regression on data from 100 subjects to generate a score predictive of response to surgery. The most accurate scoring system was based on four factors that could predict a high (4 factors, 75%) or low (≤1 factor, 27%) likelihood of blood pressure resolution. The factors found to be most predictive were (1) fewer than or equal to 2 blood pressure medications, (2) duration of hypertension less than or equal to 6 years, (3) female sex, and (4) BMI greater than 25.

Patients with unilateral disease who are not appropriate for surgery should be treated with a mineralocorticoid antagonist.[10,22,24,75] Although patients may require additional antihypertensive medications, long-term blood pressure control has been demonstrated in most patients. Widespread use of medical therapy in unilateral disease is limited due to side effects and cost-effectiveness of therapy. Spironolactone, the most commonly used agent, has significant potential side effects mainly due to its antiandrogenic effects. These include gynecomastia, breast engorgement or tenderness, and reduced libido.[10,76] In addition, Sywak and Pasieka[60] (2002) demonstrated that adrenalectomy was more cost-effective than life-long medical therapy in patients with unilateral disease.

Patients with bilateral hyperplasia respond poorly to surgery. Even with bilateral adrenalectomy, cure rates are less than 20%.[22,26–28] As such, clinical practice guidelines recommend that patients with bilateral disease be treated with mineralocorticoid antagonists with additional antihypertensive medications as required.[22,24] Patients should be carefully monitored for electrolyte abnormalities and adverse side effects of medications. Spironolactone is generally considered first-line therapy. However, patients unable to tolerate this can be treated with eplerenone, a more expensive but selective mineralocorticoid receptor blocker with fewer antiandrogenic effects. In addition, amiloride, a medication that blocks the effects of aldosterone at the epithelial sodium channel in the cortical collecting ducts, is commonly used. Bilateral disease resulting from FH-I is responsive to low-dose glucocorticoid treatment.[22] At the author's center, patients with bilateral disease who continue to have difficult to control hypertension despite appropriate medical therapy may occasionally undergo unilateral adrenalectomy if a subclinical gradient favoring one side is found on AVS.

SUMMARY

PA is a relatively common secondary cause of hypertension. Patients with PA have associated cardiovascular morbidity and mortality greater than would be predicted based on hypertension alone. As such, appropriate screening, diagnosis, and treatment have the potential to positively affect many patients. Following screening and diagnosis, management algorithms should endeavor to lateralize the source of excess aldosterone secretion. Patients who are appropriate surgical candidates and have a documented unilateral source of aldosterone production should be offered laparoscopic adrenalectomy. In contrast, BAH is best treated medically with an antihypertensive regime that includes a mineralocorticoid receptor antagonist.

REFERENCES

1. Conn JW. Presidential address. I. Painting background. II. Primary aldosteronism, a new clinical syndrome. J Lab Clin Med 1955;45:3–17.
2. Conn JW, Louis LH. Primary aldosteronism: a new clinical entity. Trans Assoc Am Physicians 1955;68:215–31 [discussion: 231].
3. Andersen GS, Toftdahl DB, Lund JO, et al. The incidence rate of phaeochromocytoma and Conn's syndrome in Denmark, 1977–1981. J Hum Hypertens 1988; 2:187–9.
4. Berglund G, Andersson O, Wilhelmsen L. Prevalence of primary and secondary hypertension: studies in a random population sample. Br Med J 1976;2:554–6.
5. Kaplan NM. Hypokalemia in the hypertensive patient, with observations on the incidence of primary aldosteronism. Ann Intern Med 1967;66:1079–90.
6. Sinclair AM, Isles CG, Brown I, et al. Secondary hypertension in a blood pressure clinic. Arch Intern Med 1987;147:1289–93.
7. Mulatero P, Stowasser M, Loh KC, et al. Increased diagnosis of primary aldosteronism, including surgically correctable forms, in centers from five continents. J Clin Endocrinol Metab 2004;89:1045–50.
8. Calhoun DA, Nishizaka MK, Zaman MA, et al. Hyperaldosteronism among black and white subjects with resistant hypertension. Hypertension 2002;40:892–6.
9. Calhoun DA, Nishizaka MK, Zaman MA, et al. Aldosterone excretion among subjects with resistant hypertension and symptoms of sleep apnea. Chest 2004;125:112–7.
10. Carey RM. Primary aldosteronism. J Surg Oncol 2012;106:575–9.
11. Douma S, Petidis K, Doumas M, et al. Prevalence of primary hyperaldosteronism in resistant hypertension: a retrospective observational study. Lancet 2008;371: 1921–6.

12. Fogari R, Preti P, Zoppi A, et al. Prevalence of primary aldosteronism among un-selected hypertensive patients: a prospective study based on the use of an aldo-sterone/renin ratio above 25 as a screening test. Hypertens Res 2007;30:111–7.

13. Gordon RD, Stowasser M, Tunny TJ, et al. High incidence of primary aldoste-ronism in 199 patients referred with hypertension. Clin Exp Pharmacol Physiol 1994;21:315–8.

14. Lim PO, Dow E, Brennan G, et al. High prevalence of primary aldosteronism in the Tayside hypertension clinic population. J Hum Hypertens 2000;14:311–5.

15. Loh KC, Koay ES, Khaw MC, et al. Prevalence of primary aldosteronism among Asian hypertensive patients in Singapore. J Clin Endocrinol Metab 2000;85: 2854–9.

16. Mulatero P, Dluhy RG, Giacchetti G, et al. Diagnosis of primary aldosteronism: from screening to subtype differentiation. Trends Endocrinol Metab 2005;16: 114–9.

17. Rossi GP, Bernini G, Caliumi C, et al. A prospective study of the prevalence of primary aldosteronism in 1,125 hypertensive patients. J Am Coll Cardiol 2006; 48:2293–300.

18. Schirpenbach C, Segmiller F, Diederich S, et al. The diagnosis and treatment of primary hyperaldosteronism in Germany: results on 555 patients from the German Conn Registry. Dtsch Arztebl Int 2009;106:305–11.

19. Stowasser M, Gordon RD, Gunasekera TG, et al. High rate of detection of pri-mary aldosteronism, including surgically treatable forms, after 'non-selective' screening of hypertensive patients. J Hypertens 2003;21:2149–57.

20. Strauch B, Zelinka T, Hampf M, et al. Prevalence of primary hyperaldosteronism in moderate to severe hypertension in the Central Europe region. J Hum Hyper-tens 2003;17:349–52.

21. Williams JS, Williams GH, Raji A, et al. Prevalence of primary hyperaldosteron-ism in mild to moderate hypertension without hypokalaemia. J Hum Hypertens 2006;20:129–36.

22. Funder JW, Carey RM, Fardella C, et al. Case detection, diagnosis, and treat-ment of patients with primary aldosteronism: an Endocrine Society clinical prac-tice guideline. J Clin Endocrinol Metab 2008;93:3266–81.

23. Iacobone M, Citton M, Viel G, et al. Unilateral adrenal hyperplasia: a novel cause of surgically correctable primary hyperaldosteronism. Surgery 2012;152: 1248–55.

24. Nishikawa T, Omura M, Satoh F, et al. Guidelines for the diagnosis and treatment of primary aldosteronism—the Japan Endocrine Society 2009. Endocr J 2011; 58:711–21.

25. Rossi GP, Sacchetto A, Chiesura-Corona M, et al. Identification of the etiology of primary aldosteronism with adrenal vein sampling in patients with equivocal computed tomography and magnetic resonance findings: results in 104 consecutive cases. J Clin Endocrinol Metab 2001;86:1083–90.

26. Baer L, Sommers SC, Krakoff LR, et al. Pseudo-primary aldosteronism. An entity distinct from true primary aldosteronism. Circ Res 1970;27:203–20.

27. Priestley JT, Ferris DO, ReMine WH, et al. Primary aldosteronism: surgical man-agement and pathologic findings. Mayo Clin Proc 1968;43:761–75.

28. Rhamy RK, McCoy RM, Scott HW, et al. Primary aldosteronism: experience with current diagnostic criteria and surgical treatment in fourteen patients. Ann Surg 1968;167:718–27.

29. Harvey A, Pasieka JL, Kline G, et al. Modification of the protocol for selective ad-renal venous sampling results in both a significant increase in the accuracy and

necessity of the procedure in the management of patients with primary hyperaldosteronism. Surgery 2012;152:643–9 [discussion: 649].

30. Lewington S, Clarke R, Qizilbash N, et al. Age-specific relevance of usual blood pressure to vascular mortality: a meta-analysis of individual data for one million adults in 61 prospective studies. Lancet 2002;360:1903–13.
31. Milliez P, Girerd X, Plouin PF, et al. Evidence for an increased rate of cardiovascular events in patients with primary aldosteronism. J Am Coll Cardiol 2005;45: 1243–8.
32. Fischer E, Reuschl S, Quinkler M, et al. Assay characteristics influence the aldosterone to renin ratio as a screening tool for primary aldosteronism: results of the German Conn's registry. Horm Metab Res 2013;45:526–31.
33. Giacchetti G, Ronconi V, Lucarelli G, et al. Analysis of screening and confirmatory tests in the diagnosis of primary aldosteronism: need for a standardized protocol. J Hypertens 2006;24:737–45.
34. Montori VM, Young WF. Use of plasma aldosterone concentration-to-plasma renin activity ratio as a screening test for primary aldosteronism. A systematic review of the literature. Endocrinol Metab Clin North Am 2002;31:619–32, xi.
35. Stowasser M, Ahmed AH, Pimenta E, et al. Factors affecting the aldosterone/renin ratio. Horm Metab Res 2012;44:170–6.
36. Yin G, Zhang S, Yan L, et al. Effect of age on aldosterone/renin ratio (ARR) and comparison of screening accuracy of ARR plus elevated serum aldosterone concentration for primary aldosteronism screening in different age groups. Endocrine 2012;42:182–9.
37. Young WF, Klee GG. Primary aldosteronism. Diagnostic evaluation. Endocrinol Metab Clin North Am 1988;17:367–95.
38. Hiramatsu K, Yamada T, Yukimura Y, et al. A screening test to identify aldosterone-producing adenoma by measuring plasma renin activity. Results in hypertensive patients. Arch Intern Med 1981;141:1589–93.
39. McKenna TJ, Sequeira SJ, Heffernan A, et al. Diagnosis under random conditions of all disorders of the renin-angiotensin-aldosterone axis, including primary hyperaldosteronism. J Clin Endocrinol Metab 1991;73:952–7.
40. Farese RV, Biglieri EG, Shackleton CH, et al. Licorice-induced hypermineralocorticoidism. N Engl J Med 1991;325:1223–7.
41. Ulmer PS, Meikle AW. Sample requirements for plasma renin activity and immunoreactive renin. Clin Chem 2000;46:1442–4.
42. Mulatero P, Milan A, Fallo F, et al. Comparison of confirmatory tests for the diagnosis of primary aldosteronism. J Clin Endocrinol Metab 2006;91:2618–23.
43. Mysliwiec J, Zukowski L, Grodzka A, et al. Diagnostics of primary aldosteronism: is obligatory use of confirmatory tests justified? J Renin Angiotensin Aldosterone Syst 2012;13:367–71.
44. Nanba K, Tamanaha T, Nakao K, et al. Confirmatory testing in primary aldosteronism. J Clin Endocrinol Metab 2012;97:1688–94.
45. Salva M, Cicala MV, Mantero F. Primary aldosteronism: the role of confirmatory tests. Horm Metab Res 2012;44:177–80.
46. Solar M, Malirova E, Ballon M, et al. Confirmatory testing in primary aldosteronism: extensive medication switching is not needed in all patients. Eur J Endocrinol 2012;166:679–86.
47. Mulatero P, Bertello C, Garrone C, et al. Captopril test can give misleading results in patients with suspect primary aldosteronism. Hypertension 2007;50:e26–7.
48. Chao CT, Wu VC, Kuo CC, et al. Diagnosis and management of primary aldosteronism: an updated review. Ann Med 2013;45:375–83.

49. Goh BK, Tan YH, Chang KT, et al. Primary hyperaldosteronism secondary to uni-lateral adrenal hyperplasia: an unusual cause of surgically correctable hyper-tension. A review of 30 cases. World J Surg 2007;31:72–9.
50. Rayner B. Primary aldosteronism and aldosterone-associated hypertension. J Clin Pathol 2008;61:825–31.
51. Weisbrod AB, Webb RC, Mathur A, et al. Adrenal histologic findings show no difference in clinical presentation and outcome in primary hyperaldosteronism. Ann Surg Oncol 2013;20:753–8.
52. Hammarstedt L, Muth A, Wangberg B, et al. Adrenal lesion frequency: a pro-spective, cross-sectional CT study in a defined region, including systematic re-evaluation. Acta Radiol 2010;51:1149–56.
53. White ML, Gauger PG, Doherty GM, et al. The role of radiologic studies in the evaluation and management of primary hyperaldosteronism. Surgery 2008; 144:926–33 [discussion: 933].
54. Young WF, Stanson AW, Thompson GB, et al. Role for adrenal venous sampling in primary aldosteronism. Surgery 2004;136:1227–35.
55. Zarnegar R, Bloom AI, Lee J, et al. Is adrenal venous sampling necessary in all patients with hyperaldosteronism before adrenalectomy? J Vasc Interv Radiol 2008;19:66–71.
56. Goh BK, Tan YH, Yip SK, et al. Outcome of patients undergoing laparoscopic adrenalectomy for primary hyperaldosteronism. JSLS 2004;8:320–5.
57. Letavernier E, Peyrard S, Amar L, et al. Blood pressure outcome of adrenalec-tomy in patients with primary hyperaldosteronism with or without unilateral ade-noma. J Hypertens 2008;26:1816–23.
58. Mathur A, Kemp CD, Dutta U, et al. Consequences of adrenal venous sampling in primary hyperaldosteronism and predictors of unilateral adrenal disease. J Am Coll Surg 2010;211:384–90.
59. Meyer A, Brabant G, Behrend M. Long-term follow-up after adrenalectomy for primary aldosteronism. World J Surg 2005;29:155–9.
60. Sywak M, Pasieka JL. Long-term follow-up and cost benefit of adrenalectomy in patients with primary hyperaldosteronism. Br J Surg 2002;89:1587–93.
61. Tresallet C, Salepcioglu H, Godiris-Petit G, et al. Clinical outcome after laparo-scopic adrenalectomy for primary hyperaldosteronism: the role of pathology. Surgery 2010;148:129–34.
62. Waldmann J, Maurer L, Holler J, et al. Outcome of surgery for primary hyperal-dosteronism. World J Surg 2011;35:2422–7.
63. Nieman LK. Approach to the patient with an adrenal incidentaloma. J Clin Endo-crinol Metab 2010;95:4106–13.
64. Harvey A, Kline G, Pasieka JL. Adrenal venous sampling in primary hyperaldosteron-ism: comparison of radiographic with biochemical success and the clinical decision-making with "less than ideal" testing. Surgery 2006;140:847–53 [discussion: 853].
65. Kline GA, So B, Dias VC, et al. Catheterization during adrenal vein sampling for primary aldosteronism: failure to use (1-24) ACTH may increase apparent failure rate. J Clin Hypertens (Greenwich) 2013;15:480–4.
66. Kline GA, Harvey A, Jones C, et al. Adrenal vein sampling may not be a gold-standard diagnostic test in primary aldosteronism: final diagnosis depends upon which interpretation rule is used. Variable interpretation of adrenal vein sampling. Int Urol Nephrol 2008;40:1035–43.
67. Webb R, Mathur A, Chang R, et al. What is the best criterion for the interpretation of adrenal vein sample results in patients with primary hyperaldosteronism? Ann Surg Oncol 2012;19:1881–6.

68. Baba Y, Nakajo M, Hayashi S. Adrenal venous catecholamine concentrations in patients with adrenal masses other than pheochromocytoma. Endocrine 2013; 43:219–24.

69. Baba Y, Hayashi S, Nakajo M. Are catecholamine-derived indexes in adrenal venous sampling useful for judging selectivity and laterality in patients with primary aldosteronism? Endocrine 2013;43:611–7.

70. Mulatero P, di Cella SM, Monticone S, et al. 18-hydroxycorticosterone, 18-hydroxycortisol, and 18-oxocortisol in the diagnosis of primary aldosteronism and its subtypes. J Clin Endocrinol Metab 2012;97:881–9.

71. Jacobsen NE, Campbell JB, Hobart MG. Laparoscopic versus open adrenalectomy for surgical adrenal disease. Can J Urol 2003;10:1995–9.

72. Rossi H, Kim A, Prinz RA. Primary hyperaldosteronism in the era of laparoscopic adrenalectomy. Am Surg 2002;68:253–6 [discussion: 256].

73. Catena C, Colussi G, Lapenna R, et al. Long-term cardiac effects of adrenalectomy or mineralocorticoid antagonists in patients with primary aldosteronism. Hypertension 2007;50:911–8.

74. Zarnegar R, Young WF, Lee J, et al. The aldosteronoma resolution score: predicting complete resolution of hypertension after adrenalectomy for aldosteronoma. Ann Surg 2008;247:511–8.

75. Kline GA, Pasieka JL, Harvey A, et al. Medical or surgical therapy for primary aldosteronism: post-treatment follow-up as a surrogate measure of comparative outcomes. Ann Surg Oncol 2013;20:2274–8.

76. Parthasarathy HK, Menard J, White WB, et al. A double-blind, randomized study comparing the antihypertensive effect of eplerenone and spironolactone in patients with hypertension and evidence of primary aldosteronism. J Hypertens 2011;29:980–90.

Subclinical Cushing Syndrome: A Review

Lee F. Starker, MD, PhD[a], John W. Kunstman, MD[a], Tobias Carling, MD, PhD[a,b],*

KEYWORDS

- Subclinical Cushing syndrome • Adrenal incidentalomas
- Dexamethasone-suppressive testing • Corticotropin

KEY POINTS

- Subclinical Cushing syndrome (SCS) may not be as clinically insignificant as previously postulated.
- Diagnosis of the syndrome is somewhat difficult, but possible.
- As most patients present with adrenal incidentalomas, a thorough biochemical workup by both a dedicated endocrinologist and endocrine surgeon is necessary for optimal outcome.
- Given the low rate of complications, minimally invasive adrenalectomy is recommended for patients with biochemically proven or suspected SCS who are appropriate surgical candidates.

INTRODUCTION

Subclinical Cushing syndrome (SCS) has recently become a topic of controversy and interest. The reasons for this are multifactorial. Adrenal masses known as incidentalomas, identified by radiographic imaging obtained for unrelated reasons, are detected more frequently, especially within our aging population; this is due to a combination of more refined diagnostic imaging technologies with higher resolution, and because cross-sectional imaging is much more widely used. This increase in the number of patients with adrenal masses undergoing biochemical evaluation has led to identification of patients with biochemical abnormalities without florid clinical symptoms. A unique situation has thus arisen for clinical intervention, as those patients without florid Cushing syndrome can be spared the development of significant physiologic derangements by early intervention and surgical resection. However, only a portion of patients with SCS progress to Cushing syndrome.

[a] Department of Surgery, Yale University School of Medicine, 333 Cedar Street, New Haven, CT, USA; [b] Yale Endocrine Neoplasia Laboratory, Yale University School of Medicine, 333 Cedar Street, New Haven, CT, USA
* Corresponding author. Section of Endocrine Surgery, Department of Surgery, Yale University School of Medicine, 333 Cedar Street, FMB130, Box 208062, New Haven, CT 06520.
E-mail address: tobias.carling@yale.edu

Surg Clin N Am 94 (2014) 657–668
http://dx.doi.org/10.1016/j.suc.2014.02.008
0039-6109/14/$ – see front matter © 2014 Elsevier Inc. All rights reserved.

Classic Cushing syndrome is characterized by the signs of hypercortisolism: moon face, buffalo hump, central obesity, easy bruising, proximal muscle wasting, deep purple striae, acne, hirsutism, and glucose intolerance. The syndrome is rare with an overall yearly incidence of 1 in 50,000.[1] Primary adrenal lesions only account for roughly 15% of the cases of Cushing syndrome. About 50% of these lesions are adenomas, with the remaining 50% stemming from functional adrenal cortical carcinomas. Nevertheless, most studies report a prevalence of 5% to 24% for SCS in patients with an adrenal incidentaloma (AI). This broad range can likely be attributed to the differing results in the diagnostic criteria used over time.[2–7]

The concept of SCS was first identified and described in 1973 by Beierwaltes and colleagues[8] and then again in 1981 by Charbonnel and colleagues.[9] SCS was defined as an increase in the overall endogenous secretion of glucocorticoids without clinical manifestations of clinical Cushing syndrome. The overwhelming consensus is that the diagnosis can be made when there is a combination of 2 distinct findings: no overt clinical signs of Cushing syndrome and at least 2 distinct alterations in the hypothalamic-pituitary-adrenal (HPA) axis. Nonetheless, patients with SCS usually have an increased prevalence of obesity, hypertension, and type 2 diabetes. It is imperative to assess all patients with an AI for biochemical production before surgical resection, as the unopposed overproduction of glucocorticoids in this case can suppress the contralateral adrenal gland and lead to postoperative Addisonian crisis, which can be fatal.[10]

DEFINITION

SCS presents in patients with a clinically nonfunctioning adrenal adenoma, likely identified for an unrelated reason on diagnostic imaging. Before the term SCS took hold, the term preclinical Cushing syndrome was used and is still used interchangeably. However, this terminology is misleading because the overwhelming majority of patients with SCS will not progress to clinically apparent Cushing syndrome, as the term implies. Therefore, the terminology of SCS has become the preferred and more accurate modality of description.[1]

To facilitate the definition of the disease, a National Institutes of Health (NIH) State of Science Conference was convened and a better, more easily identifiable term was chosen: subclinical autonomous glucocorticoid hypersecretion.[11] The final consensus was that to concretely make the diagnosis, 2 distinct criteria must be fulfilled. First, the patient must not present with a clear Cushing syndrome phenotype, and none of the physical stigmata of the disease must be present. It is imperative that an experienced clinician examine the patient to be absolutely certain that there is no evidence of classic Cushing syndrome.[7] Second, the patient must have presented with an adrenal mass that was identified in an incidental fashion, meaning that the radiographic imaging was obtained for another reason and this lesion was subsequently identified. The likely culprit of this cortisol hypersecretion is commonly a cortical adenoma, although adrenocortical carcinoma (ACC) must not be overlooked[12,13]; however, given the natural course of ACC one must question whether the terminology of SCS can truly apply.[14]

DIAGNOSIS
Rationale

Diagnosis of hypercortisolism may be laborious, even in cases of overt disease. Because of the subtle nature of the clinical manifestations of SCS as already described, biochemical tests are crucial in establishing a diagnosis. Several additional factors increase the difficulty of biochemical testing in cases of SCS. When assessed on a population basis, cortisol secretion and activation of the HPA axis runs in a continuum from unmistakably hypoactive (ie, adrenal insufficiency) to normal to hyperactive. As a corollary, assigning arbitrary cutoff values for the numerous biochemical tests assessing cortisol secretion and the HPA axis risks neglecting disease when such cutoffs are set too stringently, and overtreatment when too lenient. This conundrum is especially true in patients with AI. Moreover, the circadian nature of cortisol secretion, which persists even in disease states, dampens the reproducibility of certain biochemical test results and increases the effort required by provider, patient, and laboratory in obtaining accurate data. This situation has a particularly notable effect in cases of SCS, where potentially small elevations in cortisol levels and the resulting perturbation of the HPA axis may fall below a given test's threshold for detection. Furthermore, the myriad of tests available makes efficient and accurate diagnosis challenging even for experienced clinicians. A summary of described diagnostic criteria for SCS is given in **Table 1**, and individual tests are described here.

Dexamethasone-Suppression Testing

Dexamethasone-suppression testing (DST) is the test most frequently used to evaluate mild elevations in cortisol secretion, and therefore plays a key role in diagnosis of SCS. Dexamethasone is an endogenous steroid, used because it does not

Table 1
Proposed criteria for diagnosis of subclinical hypercortisolism (SCS)

Authors,[Ref.] Year	Criteria	Dexamethasone Dose, DST Cutoff	SCS Prevalence (%)
Reincke et al,[60] 1992	DST alone	1 mg, 3 µg/dL	12
Osella et al,[29] 1994	DST alone	1 mg, 5 µg/dL	16
Ambrosi et al,[28] 1995	DST plus ≥1 of CRH, CCR, ACTH, UFC	1 mg, 5 µg/dL	12
Tsagarakis et al,[31] 1998	Low-dose DST alone	2.5 µg/dL	25
Terzolo et al,[33] 1998	DST plus UFC	1 mg, 5 µg/dL	6
Mantero & Arnaldi,[4] 2000	≥2 of CRH, CCR, ACTH, UFC, DST	1 mg, 5 µg/dL	9.2
Rossi et al,[47] 2000	Low-dose DST plus ≥1 of CRH, CCR, ACTH, UFC	3.0 µg/dL	18.5
Valli et al,[17] 2001	Unilateral uptake on ^{131}I-norcholesterol scintigraphy	N/A	61.3
Emral et al,[25] 2003	DST and high-dose DST	3 mg, 3 µg/dL	5.7
Chiodini et al,[20] 2009	≥2 of ACTH, UFC, DST	1 mg, 3 µg/dL	29.6
Masserini et al,[21] 2009	≥2 of ACTH, UFC, DST	1 mg, 3 µg/dL	21.4
Eller-Vainicher et al,[15] 2010	≥3 of CCR, ACTH, UFC, DST	1 mg, 3 µg/dL	48.3
Di Dalmazi et al,[66] 2012	DST (5 µg/dL) or DST (1.8 µg/dL) plus UFC or ACTH	1 mg, 1.8 µg/dL or 5 µg/dL	21.3

Abbreviations: ACTH, adrenocorticotropic hormone; CCR, alteration in circadian cortisol rhythm (increased midnight serum or salivary cortisol level); CRH, blunted response to corticotropin-releasing hormone; DST, dexamethasone-suppression test; N/A, no data available; SCS, subclinical Cushing syndrome; UFC, elevated 24-hour urinary free cortisol.

cross-react with either immunologic or chemical assays for cortisol. In individuals with corticotropin (adrenocorticotropic hormone [ACTH])-dependent hypercortisolism (either overt or subclinical), dexamethasone administration suppresses the HPA axis and results in suppression of cortisol secretion. For SCS diagnosis, 1 mg overnight DST is the most commonly performed, owing to its simplicity of administration.[4,15–17] In consensus statements, the NIH and the American Association of Clinical Endocrinologists/American Association of Endocrine Surgeons recommend the standard cutoff of 5 µg/dL as the upper limit of normal for serum cortisol following DST in patients with AI.[11,18] This cutoff results in very few false-positive outcomes, as specificity can exceed 90%.[12,15] However, most normal individuals have cortisol levels suppressed to below 1 µg/dL after overnight DST, and sensitivity for detection of SCS is poor at the 5-µg/dL cutoff. As such, some European groups have recommended that a lower cutoff value for DST be used when assessing for SCS.[6] By lowering the serum cortisol level to a lower cutoff value to ascribe a positive DST result, sensitivity increases dramatically, from 20% to 30% at 5 µg/dL to 70% to 90% at 1.8 µg/dL (**Table 2**); this also results in an inverse decline in specificity. Accordingly a compromise cutoff of 3 µg/dL has been widely assessed and clinically validated, which attempts to minimize false-positive results while maintaining a modestly increased sensitivity in comparison with higher cutoff values.[7,15,19–22]

Several additional methods of DST have been evaluated for SCS diagnosis. The 2-day, 2-mg DST (sometimes referred to as low-dose DST) appears, for unclear reasons to be more accurate in patients with alcoholism, diabetes, or psychiatric disorders, but for most patients has no advantage.[23,24] Higher-dose DST, using 3-mg or 8-mg dexamethasone doses, have been proposed to further increase specificity, but this has not been demonstrated in comparison testing and these doses do not appear to have a role in SCS diagnosis.[24–26]

Corticotropin (Adrenocorticotropic Hormone)

Hypercortisolism can be regarded as ACTH-independent when serum ACTH levels are suppressed to lower than 10 pg/mL, as in cases of most adrenal tumors causing

Table 2
Sensitivity and specificity of 1 mg overnight dexamethasone-suppression test at diagnosing subclinical hypercortisolism using various cutoff values for morning serum cortisol measurement

Authors,[Ref.] Year	5 µg/dL Cutoff (Se/Sp)	3 µg/dL Cutoff (Se/Sp)	1.8 µg/dL Cutoff (Se/Sp)	No. of Patients	Criteria for SCS Diagnosis
Barzon et al,[67] 2001	44/100	—	75/72	83	Scintigraphy
Valli et al,[17] 2001	58/83	63/75	100/67[a]	31	Scintigraphy
Eller-Vainicher et al,[68] 2010	33.3/85.7	59/52.4	79.5/23.8	60	Postsurgical hypocortisolism
Morelli et al,[45] 2010	23.8/93.3	52.4/81.4	71.4/49.5	231	Clinical manifestations[b]
Eller-Vainicher et al,[15] 2010	21.7/96.9	—	91.3/56.3[c]	55	Postresection improvement[d]

Abbreviations: SCS, subclinical Cushing syndrome; Se, sensitivity (%); Sp, specificity (%).
[a] Study utilized 2.2 µg/dL cutoff.
[b] Included presence of hypertension, type 2 diabetes mellitus, or vertebral fractures.
[c] Study utilized 2.0 µg/dL cutoff.
[d] Improvement in at least 2 of: cholesterol level, body weight, hypertension, serum glucose.

overt hypercortisolism. Low ACTH levels are a frequent finding in AI, being present in more than 50% of cases in some studies.[4,15,21,27] As such, the specificity of depressed ACTH levels alone in the context of diagnosing SCS is as low as 38% to 60% in some studies. Furthermore, as ACTH levels can be normal even in ACTH-independent hypercortisolism, ACTH is not regarded as a useful primary tool in SCS diagnosis without additional testing.[26] Similarly, addition of CRH (corticotropin-releasing hormone) stimulation before ACTH testing does not increase sensitivity to screening for SCS.[26,28,29] In patients with known SCS, ACTH testing can help to rule out occult ACTH-dependent hypercortisolism as the cause rather than AI. This scenario should be suspected in cases of AI where ACTH is not suppressed, and is especially useful in cases of bilateral or diffuse adrenal enlargement, either of which can occur in ACTH excess. To exclude the presence of pituitary or ectopic ACTH-dependent hypercortisolism, ACTH should be less than 10 pg/mL. In uncertain cases (ie, ACTH >10 pg/mL but <20 pg/mL), CRH stimulation testing can be performed. ACTH-dependent SCS can be excluded if the ACTH level is lower than 30 pg/mL after CRH stimulation.[23,30]

Dehydroepiandrosterone Sulfate

Dehydroepiandrosterone (DHEA) is the most abundant circulating steroid hormone in humans. Reduction in DHEA sulfate (DHEA-S) levels is a frequent finding in AI.[31,32] Adrenal steroid production is very sensitive to ACTH, so it is possible that the reduced DHEA-S levels indicate very subtle decreases in HPA-axis activity attributable to SCS. However, DHEA-S levels also naturally decline with age. Low DHEA-S serum concentration has not been demonstrated to be a useful diagnostic test for SCS.[26,29,33]

Urinary Free Cortisol

Ordinarily, cortisol secretion adheres to a predictable cycle, with serum levels reaching their nadir at midnight and then peaking approximately 1 hour after waking. Consequently, hypercortisolism can be determined via elevated release over 24 hours, which encompasses a complete circadian cycle. More than 90% of serum cortisol is bound to plasma proteins, such as cortisol-binding globulin. Both urinary and salivary assays for cortisol are reflective of unbound, or free, cortisol in the serum. Measurement of urinary free cortisol (UFC) provides a direct and reliable assessment of cortisol secretion.[34] However, the number of reliable reference laboratories for UFC measurement remains limited, and the test itself can be affected by patient factors such as fluid intake, comorbid disease (such as depression), and obesity.[35–37] Overnight urine sample collection protocols from 10 PM to 8 AM, corrected for creatinine excretion, have also been described,[38,39] but are not in widespread clinical practice. Among patients with AI, a wide variance in the prevalence of UFC elevation have been reported, ranging from less than 5% to more than 20% of adrenal incidentalomas.[15,17,27] The sensitivity of UFC to minimal elevations in cortisol secretion is low.[36,40] As such, UFC alone has limited applicability in SCS screening, and should only be used for SCS diagnosis in concert with another modality.[41]

Midnight Cortisol

Random morning serum or salivary cortisol measurements are widely variable even within a single patient, and have minimal diagnostic value in assessing hypercortisolism. However, elevation in cortisol levels at the time of the usual midnight nadir is reflective of an abnormality in the regular circadian rhythm, and indicates hypercortisolism. Midnight cortisol measurement has been shown to be elevated in SCS by several investigators.[15,17,22,39] Both salivary and serum assays have been evaluated in SCS; midnight serum cortisol (MSeC) measurement is more burdensome as it requires the patient to be present for phlebotomy, unlike midnight salivary cortisol (MSaC). Midnight measurements are not skewed by obesity or depressive disorders, although they are unreliable in patients with erratic sleep schedules or who are employed in night-shift work.[42,43] MSaC has gained in popularity recently for diagnosis of overt hypercortisolism, despite challenges to standardization of laboratory practices and techniques.[44] However, MSaC has been shown to have a low sensitivity in the diagnosis of SCS (22%–77%, depending on threshold level for a positive test).[21,41] MSeC appears to correlate well with some of the clinical manifestations of SCS,[33] but has mainly been used as a confirmatory test owing to its cumbersome nature.

Approach to SCS Diagnosis in Adrenal Incidentaloma

When contemplating biochemical testing to assess for the presence of SCS in a patient with newly discovered AI, several contrasting details should be considered. A testing regimen that is sensitive to SCS is desirous, as evidence continues to accumulate that SCS is a frequent finding in disease states such as osteopenia and diabetes mellitus. Similarly, because the treatment of AI is often surgical, testing should be specific enough to avoid false-positive results; this is especially true because SCS is by definition an asymptomatic condition. Studies evaluating the sensitivity and specificity of multiple tests among SCS patients are limited by the lack of a gold-standard definition for SCS. In the largest study to date examining biochemical testing for SCS, Mantero and Arnaldi[4] evaluated CRH, midnight cortisol testing, UFC, ACTH, and overnight DST with a 5 μg/dL cutoff for a positive test. No single test exceeded 80% in sensitivity, and only DST reached 90% in specificity. However, these results must be interpreted carefully, as a positive result in 2 or more of 5 tests was the gold standard for diagnosing SCS and there was no independent standard for SCS diagnosis. However, similar statistics were found by Morelli and colleagues,[45] who assessed the same tests in SCS patients who had an SCS-related complication such as vertebral fractures, hypertension, or diabetes mellitus. Furthermore, in a seminal study, Eller-Vainicher and colleagues[15] found similar results in 60 patients who underwent surgery for SCS. By using postresection hypercortisolism as the gold standard for SCS diagnosis, the investigators were able to ascribe true positivity to the tests they evaluated. Clearly these data demonstrate that no single test offers adequate accuracy to effectively evaluate for the presence or absence of SCS in AI.

Several investigators during the 1990s suggested that the diagnosis of SCS should rely on 2 or more diagnostic criteria,[13,28,33,46] and most suggested regimens included overnight DST as a component. As described earlier, the widely used overnight 1-mg DST offers excellent sensitivity when using a low cutoff for positivity, but with a significant decline in specificity. Over the past decade, multiple investigators have advocated using a battery of biochemical tests to maximize sensitivity while maintaining specificity.[15,16,19,20,47] A potential criticism of a combination approach is that it is currently not known with certainty which tests best correlate with SCS-related negative outcomes. However, Morelli and colleagues[45] found that a combination of overnight 1-mg DST with a 3 μg/dL cutoff elevated UFC above the normal limit, and serum ACTH of less than 10 pg/mL offered an accuracy of 75.8% for predicted SCS-related complications when abnormalities in at least 2 of the 3 tests was considered diagnostic of SCS. The DST-UFC-ACTH combination has been validated clinically in several studies by Chiodini and colleagues.[19,20,27] Other combinations have also been described, but the DST-UFC-ACTH combination has demonstrated sensitivity and specificity exceeding 60% when correlated with actual clinical end points.[15,45] In practice, the authors use a combination approach when determining the presence of hormonal activity in newly diagnosed cases of AI, including DST, UFC, and ACTH measurements in all patients. A thorough history and physical examination must be performed as well, and correlated with any findings. Of course some patients will have equivocal testing. In these patients, the authors pursue serial measurements at regular intervals and consider adjunctive tests, such as DHEA-S. While these measures are necessary in a minority of patients, the authors make every effort to pursue certainty in these diagnostic dilemmas. Crucially, as there are still no widely accepted standard diagnostic criteria for SCS, treatment recommendations should be approached on an individual basis.

ADRENAL SCINTIGRAPHY

Patients with SCS, as previously stated, have minimal alterations in their biochemical profiles and often require an experienced clinician to accurately evaluate potential SCS on physical examination. Given the difficult nature of diagnosis of SCS, additional testing in the form of adrenal scintigraphy has been used. Utilization of iodocholesterol scintigraphy would reveal uptake within the adenoma and would have absent uptake in the contralateral gland. Several studies were able to correlate this unilateral scintigraphic uptake with hypersecreting cortisol adenomas, and subsequent pituitary suppression of ACTH.[12,48–50] Morioka and colleagues[51] reviewed a total of 7 cases whereby they were able to demonstrate marked accumulation of the marker within the tumors. Other studies have also identified adequate localization of the tumors. Rossi and colleagues[47] identified unilateral uptake in 50% of their patients with SCS, and in all but 1 the lesion was localized to the correct side. Although localization was feasible, there was an apparent discordance with the test's ability to aid in the degree of endocrine dysfunction of the gland or the potential for adrenal insufficiency postoperatively. McLeod and colleagues[10] used contralateral gland suppression on NP-59 scans to more accurately ascertain accurate localization of the hyperfunctioning gland. The NP-59–suppression scan gave valuable information not only in its ability to more accurately localize the offending lesion, but also to address the bigger question of potential inadequate adrenal reserve in the contralateral gland postoperatively.[10] The appearance of unilateral scintigraphic uptake, although potentially beneficial with respect to tumor localization, was also argued to be a misleading piece of information, as uptake of the tracer simply identified a more prominent area of adrenal tissue rather than a truly hyperfunctioning gland.[29,52] For this reason adrenal scintigraphy has not gained general acceptance, and therefore is only offered in a few select institutions worldwide.

INDICATIONS FOR SURGERY IN SCS

In the current era of evidence-based medicine, the long-term complications of incidentally discovered adrenal adenomas remain virtually unknown. Therefore, the overall management of these tumors remains empirical. Given the overall questionable long-term effects of incidentally identified adrenal masses, there are broadly 2 clinical options, surveillance and resection. Several studies have been performed in a prospective fashion to monitor patients with SCS to assess disease progression in an attempt to prove the need for early resection of these lesions. In a cohort of 12 patients, Libè and colleagues[16] followed patients with SCS for a mean period of 25.5 months without surgery. Although none of the patients progressed to overt Cushing syndrome, there was some moderate worsening of biochemical indices of the disease, which suggests mild disease progression. One study was able to prove a progression rate from SCS to overt Cushing syndrome in 12.5% of patients at 1 year of follow-up.[53] To date there have been no large prospective randomized trials, but Toniato and colleagues[54] assessed 23 surgically treated subjects and identified an improvement of hypertension, diabetes, obesity, and dyslipidemia in 67%, 63%, 50%, and 38% of patients, respectively. Several smaller studies have shown improvement of glucose metabolism and body weight after surgical resection.[25,55–57]

Adrenalectomy has been proved to ameliorate the biochemical abnormalities associated with SCS, but its long-term effects have yet to be completely elucidated.[58] Nonetheless, patients with SCS have a higher incidence of hypertension, obesity, decreased bone density, and metabolic syndrome.[59] Of importance is that adrenalectomy has been demonstrated to decrease the cardiovascular risk factors associated with SCS.[7,57,59] Another study identified elevated risk factors for cardiac disease, finding patients with SCS to have increased fasting glucose levels, cholesterol, and triglycerides when compared with matched controls.[59] Multiple studies have identified a positive patient benefit from early adrenalectomy in reversing these potentially devastating systemic comorbidities.[47,51,55,60]

In general, a low threshold for surgical resection in patients with biochemically proven or suspected SCS or those that have an overall size of lesion greater than 4 cm is advised in expert hands, given the low morbidity and mortality associated with either laparoscopic or, more recently, posterior retroperitoneoscopic adrenalectomy (PRA). These 2 operative strategies have proved superior to open adrenalectomy owing to shorter hospital stays, quicker recovery times, and fewer perioperative complications.[61–63] Patients should receive perioperative glucocorticoid supplementation because they do run the risk of acute Addisonian crisis.[11,48] It is imperative to rule out SCS before operative resection, given this potentially life-threatening complication if perioperative glucocorticoid supplementation is not administered.[10,64] Given the subclinical nature of SCS, it remains extremely difficult to accurately determine clinical improvement; nevertheless, patients should be monitored and continued on a short steroid course until they have a proven intact HPA axis according to previously established protocols.[65]

The significant proportion of subjects who experience deterioration in biochemical indices and disease progression, and the unknown impact of chronic hypercortisolemia on health outcomes, contrasted with the high cure and low complication rates after minimally invasive adrenalectomy, render surgery an attractive option in patients with biochemically proven or suspected SCS who are appropriate surgical candidates.

SUMMARY

Owing to its diagnostic challenges, SCS is likely to be highly underdiagnosed and undertreated, and the overall incidence may be as high as 5% to 20% in patients with AIs. The diagnosis can be established by a systematic and thorough biochemical evaluation. SCS has been associated with significant morbidity, which at least partly may be reversed by surgery. Given the low rates of complications and the possibility to reverse the detrimental effects of elevated cortisol secretion, the authors recommend minimally invasive adrenalectomy in patients with biochemically proven or suspected SCS who are appropriate surgical candidates.

REFERENCES

1. Ross NS. Epidemiology of Cushing's syndrome and subclinical disease. Endocrinol Metab Clin North Am 1994;23(3):539–46.

2. Young WF Jr. Clinical practice. The incidentally discovered adrenal mass. N Engl J Med 2007;356(6):601–10.
3. Kloos RT, Korobkin M, Thompson NW, et al. Incidentally discovered adrenal masses. Cancer Treat Res 1997;89:263–92.
4. Mantero F, Arnaldi G. Management approaches to adrenal incidentalomas. A view from Ancona, Italy. Endocrinol Metab Clin North Am 2000;29(1): 107–25, ix.
5. Funder JW, Carey RM, Fardella C, et al. Case detection, diagnosis, and treatment of patients with primary aldosteronism: an Endocrine Society clinical practice guideline. J Clin Endocrinol Metab 2008;93(9):3266–81.
6. Terzolo M, Bovio S, Pia A, et al. Subclinical Cushing's syndrome. Arq Bras Endocrinol Metabol 2007;51(8):1272–9.
7. Reincke M. Subclinical Cushing's syndrome. Endocrinol Metab Clin North Am 2000;29(1):43–56.
8. Beierwaltes WH, Sturman MF, Ryo U, et al. Imaging functional nodules of the adrenal glands with 131-I-19-iodocholesterol. J Nucl Med 1974;15(4):246–51.
9. Charbonnel B, Chatal JF, Ozanne P. Does the corticoadrenal adenoma with "pre-Cushing's syndrome" exist? J Nucl Med 1981;22(12):1059–61.
10. McLeod MK, Thompson NW, Gross MD, et al. Sub-clinical Cushing's syndrome in patients with adrenal gland incidentalomas. Pitfalls in diagnosis and management. Am Surg 1990;56(7):398–403.
11. Grumbach MM, Biller BM, Braunstein GD, et al. Management of the clinically inapparent adrenal mass ("incidentaloma"). Ann Intern Med 2003;138(5):424–9.
12. Barzon L, Scaroni C, Sonino N, et al. Incidentally discovered adrenal tumors: endocrine and scintigraphic correlates. J Clin Endocrinol Metab 1998;83(1): 55–62.
13. Bondanelli M, Campo M, Trasforini G, et al. Evaluation of hormonal function in a series of incidentally discovered adrenal masses. Metabolism 1997;46(1): 107–13.
14. Crucitti F, Bellantone R, Ferrante A, et al. The Italian Registry for Adrenal Cortical Carcinoma: analysis of a multiinstitutional series of 129 patients. The ACC Italian Registry Study Group. Surgery 1996;119(2):161–70.
15. Eller-Vainicher C, Morelli V, Salcuni AS, et al. Accuracy of several parameters of hypothalamic-pituitary-adrenal axis activity in predicting before surgery the metabolic effects of the removal of an adrenal incidentaloma. Eur J Endocrinol 2010;163(6):925–35.
16. Libè R, Dall'Asta C, Barbetta L, et al. Long-term follow-up study of patients with adrenal incidentalomas. Eur J Endocrinol 2002;147(4):489–94.
17. Valli N, Catargi B, Ronci N, et al. Biochemical screening for subclinical cortisol-secreting adenomas amongst adrenal incidentalomas. Eur J Endocrinol 2001; 144(4):401–8.
18. Zeiger MA, Thompson GB, Duh QY, et al. American Association of Clinical Endocrinologists and American Association of Endocrine Surgeons Medical Guidelines for the Management of Adrenal Incidentalomas: executive summary of recommendations. Endocr Pract 2009;15(5):450–3.
19. Chiodini I, Losa M, Pavone G, et al. Pregnancy in Cushing's disease shortly after treatment by gamma-knife radiosurgery. J Endocrinol Invest 2004;27(10):954–6.
20. Chiodini I, Morelli V, Masserini B, et al. Bone mineral density, prevalence of vertebral fractures, and bone quality in patients with adrenal incidentalomas with and without subclinical hypercortisolism: an Italian multicenter study. J Clin Endocrinol Metab 2009;94(9):3207–14.

21. Masserini B, Morelli V, Bergamaschi S, et al. The limited role of midnight salivary cortisol levels in the diagnosis of subclinical hypercortisolism in patients with adrenal incidentaloma. Eur J Endocrinol 2009;160(1):87–92.

22. Tanabe A, Naruse M, Nishikawa T, et al. Autonomy of cortisol secretion in clinically silent adrenal incidentaloma. Horm Metab Res 2001;33(7):444–50.

23. Arnaldi G, Angeli A, Atkinson AB, et al. Diagnosis and complications of Cushing's syndrome: a consensus statement. J Clin Endocrinol Metab 2003;88(12): 5593–602.

24. Nieman LK, Biller BM, Findling JW, et al. The diagnosis of Cushing's syndrome: an Endocrine Society Clinical Practice Guideline. J Clin Endocrinol Metab 2008; 93(5):1526–40.

25. Emral R, Uysal AR, Asik M, et al. Prevalence of subclinical Cushing's syndrome in 70 patients with adrenal incidentaloma: clinical, biochemical and surgical outcomes. Endocr J 2003;50(4):399–408.

26. Tsagarakis S, Vassiliadi D, Thalassinos N. Endogenous subclinical hypercortisolism: diagnostic uncertainties and clinical implications. J Endocrinol Invest 2006;29(5):471–82.

27. Chiodini I. Clinical review: diagnosis and treatment of subclinical hypercortisolism. J Clin Endocrinol Metab 2011;96(5):1223–36.

28. Ambrosi B, Peverelli S, Passini E, et al. Abnormalities of endocrine function in patients with clinically "silent" adrenal masses. Eur J Endocrinol 1995;132(4):422–8.

29. Osella G, Terzolo M, Borretta G, et al. Endocrine evaluation of incidentally discovered adrenal masses (incidentalomas). J Clin Endocrinol Metab 1994; 79(6):1532–9.

30. Raff H, Findling JW. A physiologic approach to diagnosis of the Cushing syndrome. Ann Intern Med 2003;138(12):980–91.

31. Tsagarakis S, Roboti C, Kokkoris P, et al. Elevated post-dexamethasone suppression cortisol concentrations correlate with hormonal alterations of the hypothalamo-pituitary adrenal axis in patients with adrenal incidentalomas. Clin Endocrinol (Oxf) 1998;49(2):165–71.

32. Flecchia D, Mazza E, Carlini M, et al. Reduced serum levels of dehydroepiandrosterone sulphate in adrenal incidentalomas: a marker of adrenocortical tumour. Clin Endocrinol (Oxf) 1995;42(2):129–34.

33. Terzolo M, Osella G, Alì A, et al. Subclinical Cushing's syndrome in adrenal incidentaloma. Clin Endocrinol (Oxf) 1998;48(1):89–97.

34. Mengden T, Hubmann P, Müller J, et al. Urinary free cortisol versus 17-hydroxycorticosteroids: a comparative study of their diagnostic value in Cushing's syndrome. Clin Investig 1992;70(7):545–8.

35. Carroll BJ, Curtis GC, Davies BM, et al. Urinary free cortisol excretion in depression. Psychol Med 1976;6(1):43–50.

36. Duclos M, Corcuff JB, Etcheverry N, et al. Abdominal obesity increases overnight cortisol excretion. J Endocrinol Invest 1999;22(6):465–71.

37. Mericq MV, Cutler GB. High fluid intake increases urine free cortisol excretion in normal subjects. J Clin Endocrinol Metab 1998;83(2):682–4.

38. Corcuff JB, Tabarin A, Rashedi M, et al. Overnight urinary free cortisol determination: a screening test for the diagnosis of Cushing's syndrome. Clin Endocrinol (Oxf) 1998;48(4):503–8.

39. Shiwa T, Oki K, Yamane K, et al. Significantly high level of late-night free cortisol to creatinine ratio in urine specimen in patients with subclinical Cushing's syndrome. Clin Endocrinol (Oxf) 2013;79:617–22.

40. Kidambi S, Raff H, Findling JW. Limitations of nocturnal salivary cortisol and urine free cortisol in the diagnosis of mild Cushing's syndrome. Eur J Endocrinol 2007;157(6):725–31.

41. Nunes ML, Vattaut S, Corcuff JB, et al. Late-night salivary cortisol for diagnosis of overt and subclinical Cushing's syndrome in hospitalized and ambulatory patients. J Clin Endocrinol Metab 2009;94(2):456–62.

42. Fekedulegn D, Burchfiel CM, Violanti JM, et al. Associations of long-term shift work with waking salivary cortisol concentration and patterns among police officers. Ind Health 2012;50(6):476–86.

43. Beko G, Varga I, Glaz E, et al. Cutoff values of midnight salivary cortisol for the diagnosis of overt hypercortisolism are highly influenced by methods. Clin Chim Acta 2010;411(5–6):364–7.

44. Sereg M, Toke J, Patócs A, et al. Diagnostic performance of salivary cortisol and serum osteocalcin measurements in patients with overt and subclinical Cushing's syndrome. Steroids 2011;76(1–2):38–42.

45. Morelli V, Masserini B, Salcuni AS, et al. Subclinical hypercortisolism: correlation between biochemical diagnostic criteria and clinical aspects. Clin Endocrinol (Oxf) 2010;73(2):161–6.

46. Kasperlik-Zeluska AA, Rosłonowska E, Słowinska-Srzednicka J, et al. Incidentally discovered adrenal mass (incidentaloma): investigation and management of 208 patients. Clin Endocrinol (Oxf) 1997;46(1):29–37.

47. Rossi R, Tauchmanova L, Luciano A, et al. Subclinical Cushing's syndrome in patients with adrenal incidentaloma: clinical and biochemical features. J Clin Endocrinol Metab 2000;85(4):1440–8.

48. Kloos RT, Gross MD, Francis IR, et al. Incidentally discovered adrenal masses. Endocr Rev 1995;16(4):460–84.

49. Bardet S, Rohmer V, Murat A, et al. [131]I-6 beta-iodomethylnorcholesterol scintigraphy: an assessment of its role in the investigation of adrenocortical incidentalomas. Clin Endocrinol (Oxf) 1996;44(5):587–96.

50. Francis IR, Gross MD, Shapiro B, et al. Integrated imaging of adrenal disease. Radiology 1992;184(1):1–13.

51. Morioka M, Fujii T, Matsuki T, et al. Preclinical Cushing's syndrome: report of seven cases and a review of the literature. Int J Urol 2000;7(4):126–32.

52. Rizza RA, Wahner HW, Spelsberg TC, et al. Visualization of nonfunctioning adrenal adenomas with iodocholesterol: possible relationship to subcellular distribution of tracer. J Nucl Med 1978;19(5):458–63.

53. Barzon L, Fallo F, Sonino N, et al. Development of overt Cushing's syndrome in patients with adrenal incidentaloma. Eur J Endocrinol 2002;146(1):61–6.

54. Toniato A, Merante-Boschin I, Opocher G, et al. Surgical versus conservative management for subclinical Cushing syndrome in adrenal incidentalomas: a prospective randomized study. Ann Surg 2009;249(3):388–91.

55. Bernini G, Moretti A, Iacconi P, et al. Anthropometric, haemodynamic, humoral and hormonal evaluation in patients with incidental adrenocortical adenomas before and after surgery. Eur J Endocrinol 2003;148(2):213–9.

56. Mitchell IC, Auchus RJ, Juneja K, et al. Subclinical Cushing's syndrome is not subclinical: improvement after adrenalectomy in 9 patients. Surgery 2007;142(6):900–5 [discussion: 905.e1].

57. Midorikawa S, Sanada H, Hashimoto S, et al. The improvement of insulin resistance in patients with adrenal incidentaloma by surgical resection. Clin Endocrinol (Oxf) 2001;54(6):797–804.

58. Aron DC. The adrenal incidentaloma: disease of modern technology and public health problem. Rev Endocr Metab Disord 2001;2(3):335–42.

59. Tauchmanovà L, Rossi R, Biondi B, et al. Patients with subclinical Cushing's syndrome due to adrenal adenoma have increased cardiovascular risk. J Clin Endocrinol Metab 2002;87(11):4872–8.

60. Reincke M, Nieke J, Krestin GP, et al. Preclinical Cushing's syndrome in adrenal "incidentalomas": comparison with adrenal Cushing's syndrome. J Clin Endocrinol Metab 1992;75(3):826–32.

61. Thompson GB, Grant CS, van Heerden JA, et al. Laparoscopic versus open posterior adrenalectomy: a case-control study of 100 patients. Surgery 1997; 122(6):1132–6.

62. Korman JE, Ho T, Hiatt JR, et al. Comparison of laparoscopic and open adrenalectomy. Am Surg 1997;63(10):908–12.

63. Constantinides VA, Christakis I, Touska P, et al. Systematic review and meta-analysis of retroperitoneoscopic versus laparoscopic adrenalectomy. Br J Surg 2012;99(12):1639–48.

64. Huiras CM, Pehling GB, Caplan RH. Adrenal insufficiency after operative removal of apparently nonfunctioning adrenal adenomas. JAMA 1989;261(6): 894–8.

65. Arlt W, Allolio B. Adrenal insufficiency. Lancet 2003;361(9372):1881–93.

66. Di Dalmazi G, Vicennati V, Rinaldi E, et al. Progressively increased patterns of subclinical cortisol hypersecretion in adrenal incidentalomas differently predict major metabolic and cardiovascular outcomes: a large cross-sectional study. Eur J Endocrinol 2012;166(4):669–77.

67. Barzon L, Fallo F, Sonino N, et al. Overnight dexamethasone suppression of cortisol is associated with radiocholesterol uptake patterns in adrenal incidentalomas. Eur J Endocrinol 2001;145(2):223–4.

68. Eller-Vainicher C, Morelli V, Salcuni AS, et al. Post-surgical hypocortisolism after removal of an adrenal incidentaloma: is it predictable by an accurate endocrinological work-up before surgery? Eur J Endocrinol 2010;162(1):91–9.

Adrenocortical Cancer Update

Ryaz Chagpar, MD, MSc, Allan E. Siperstein, MD, Eren Berber, MD*

KEYWORDS

- Adrenocortical cancer • Endocrinopathy • Adrenal imaging • Adrenalectomy
- Mitotane

KEY POINTS

- Adrenocortical cancer is a rare neoplasm with a poor prognosis. Patients can present with a nonfunctional or functional adrenal mass, either sporadically or as part of a hereditary endocrinopathy.
- Preoperative suspicion of malignancy based on clinical, biochemical, and radiologic criteria is essential in guiding an appropriate approach to surgical management.
- En bloc surgical resection with microscopically negative margins is the standard of care for locoregional disease, given the paramount prognostic importance of margin status.
- The high locoregional and systemic recurrence rates after initial resection have led to the development of a variety of adjuvant therapies, including surgical reintervention, mitotane-based combination chemotherapy, radioablative techniques, and targeted systemic agents.

INTRODUCTION

Adrenocortical carcinoma (ACC) is a rare neoplasm, with an annual incidence of approximately 1–2/million people worldwide.[1] Although the clinical and biochemical features as well as the stage at initial presentation of these cancers can vary based on their functionality and association with various hereditary endocrinopathies, prognosis has remained unchanged over the past 20 years, with a median survival of 2 years for all patients and an unadjusted 5-year overall survival of approximately 40% for those individuals with surgically resectable disease.[2,3] Despite these unfavorable outcomes, recent strides have been made in terms of our understanding of the pathogenesis of this aggressive cancer, resulting in the introduction of novel multimodality therapies, as well as refinements to surgical techniques, which may lead to improved outcomes for these patients.

Section of Endocrine Surgery, Endocrinology and Metabolism Institute, Cleveland Clinic Foundation, 9500 Euclid Avenue, Cleveland, OH 44195, USA
* Corresponding author.
E-mail address: berbere@ccf.org

Surg Clin N Am 94 (2014) 669–687
http://dx.doi.org/10.1016/j.suc.2014.02.009   surgical.theclinics.com
0039-6109/14/$ – see front matter © 2014 Elsevier Inc. All rights reserved.

CLINICAL PRESENTATION

Most ACC's present in the fifth and sixth decades of life, with a median age of ~55 years, although there is a bimodal age distribution, with a second peak in incidence at less than 5 years of age, which is likely representative of ACCs associated with underlying germline mutations.[3,4] Although most ACCs are sporadic, there is increasing evidence of an association with various hereditary syndromes, including, Li-Fraumeni, Beckwith-Wideman, multiple endocrine neoplasia type 1, congenital adrenal hyperplasia, familial adenomatous polyposis, Lynch syndrome, and Carney complex.[5–7] In children from southern Brazil, for example, the incidence of ACC is ~10 to 15 times higher than that observed worldwide, given the increased prevalence of a germline p53 mutation.[8,9]

Whether sporadic or familial, ACCs can present either as a functional endocrinopathy, or as a nonfunctional adrenal mass, with the latter usually being incidentally discovered on cross-sectional imaging. Approximately 60% of patients present with functional tumors, with more than half of these manifesting as a non-ACTH dependent Cushing syndrome.[10] Virilizing symptoms in females secondary to androgen-only secreting tumors, and feminizing symptoms in males secondary to estrogen-only secretion, are observed in approximately 20% and 10% of functional ACCs, respectively. Isolated hyperaldosteronism is more uncommon, comprising only ~5% of functional ACCs. Up to 10% of functional ACCs show multihormone hypersecretion (eg, corticosteroids and androgens). Although these endocrinopathies can also be associated with benign adrenocortical adenomas, there are several clinical and biochemical factors on presentation that should raise the suspicion of malignancy, including the presence of constitutional symptoms, young age, feminization or virilization, increased urinary 17-ketosteroids, or evidence of multihormonal secretion. More novel biochemical profiling using a panel of urinary adrenal steroids may also be of benefit in assessing risk of malignancy. Using a metabolomics approach, Arlt and colleagues[11] identified a profile of 8 urinary steroids that could distinguish between an adrenocortical adenoma and an ACC, with both a sensitivity and specificity of 88%.

A complete hormonal workup is therefore required for all suspected ACCs, not only to rule out the presence of cortical hyperfunctionality in the form of subclinical Cushing syndrome, hyperaldosteronism, or hyperandrogenism but also to exclude evidence of catecholamine excess, which may suggest the presence of a pheochromocytoma or extra-adrenal paraganglioma.

IMAGING EVALUATION
Computed Tomography

Most patients with ACCs present with large adrenal masses (mean size of 11.5 cm) and evidence of extra-adrenal extension on cross-sectional imaging.[2,3] Although large tumor size has traditionally been one of the diagnostic hallmarks of ACC, this feature is not perfectly sensitive or specific, with approximately 5% to 10% of ACCs being smaller than 4 cm, and only 25% of adrenal incidentalomas greater than 6 cm harboring malignancy.[3,12–14] Various attempts to define an ideal cutoff size have been made, with variable results. In 1 retrospective study of 210 incidentalomas, a cutoff size of 5 cm yielded a sensitivity of 93% and a specificity of 64% for determining malignancy.[15] Hence, in addition to an absolute tumor size greater than 4 to 6 cm, any increase in tumor growth over a 6-month period should also raise the suspicion of malignancy.[16]

Additional morphologic features on computed tomography (CT) that suggest malignancy include tumor heterogeneity, regions of internal hemorrhage or necrosis, a low-attenuation central stellate scar, and ill-defined borders. Those ACCs without ill-defined margins often show a thin enhancing rim.[12] Besides these morphologic features, traditional densitometry and enhancement washout ratios that have been used to distinguish adrenal adenomas from nonadenomas can also be used to aid in the preoperative diagnosis of an ACC. An unenhanced tumor density greater than 10 HU has been shown to have a sensitivity of 71% and specificity of 98% for the detection of malignancy, whereas an absolute percent enhancement washout greater than 60% and a relative percent wash out of more than 50% on delayed postcontrast CT is consistent with a benign adenoma, having a reported sensitivity of 56% to 100% and specificity 98% to 100%.[17–19] Consistent with these findings, Zhang and colleagues,[12] in a recent descriptive analysis of 41 patients with histopathologically proved ACCs evaluated for contrast-enhanced CT characteristics at presentation, found an absolute enhancement washout of 60% or less in 71% of ACCs, whereas 82% of these malignancies had a relative enhancement washout of 40% or less.

Evidence of extra-adrenal disease is also evident in approximately 56% of CT scans obtained at patient presentation. Intracaval tumor thrombus is relatively common, being observed in approximately 14% to 17% of CT scans, although it has been reported to occur in up to 25% of patients with ACC.[12,20–22] Thrombus within the inferior vena cava (IVC) is more common in the setting of right-sided ACCs, likely given the shorter length of the right adrenal vein and its direct drainage into the IVC. Extension of venous thrombus into the right atrium from an intracaval thrombus or into the left gonadal and azygous veins from the left renal vein has also been described. The presence and extent of venous tumor thrombus are therefore a critical consideration in preoperative surgical planning (**Fig. 1**).[23,24]

Suspected regional node involvement, on the other hand, has been variably reported on both imaging and pathologic specimens, given that formal lymphadenectomy is not universally adopted as standard practice during adrenalectomy for ACC.[22] Hence, there is considerable variance in reported rates of regional nodal positivity, which range from 10% to 26%, when based on findings from preoperative CT or surgical pathology specimens, to as high as 68%, when observed at autopsy.[2,12,25,26]

Distant metastases are radiologically evident in 15% to 39% of patients on presentation, with the most common sites including lung, liver, and bone.[10,12,27]

Magnetic Resonance Imaging

Both magnetic resonance imaging (MRI) and CT are comparable modalities in their ability to identify ACC, with MRI having a sensitivity of 81% to 89% and a specificity of 92% to 99% at distinguishing benign versus malignant adrenal masses.[1,28,29]

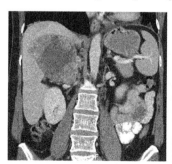 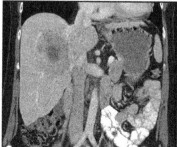

Fig. 1. CT scan of an approximately 10-cm ACC with invasion of the retrohepatic IVC. The patient received an en bloc resection, which included a right hepatectomy and caval tumor thrombectomy.

However, MRI may be better suited for the detection of intracaval tumor thrombus and defining the extent of locoregional disease. ACCs show enhancement after administration of gadolinium, followed by a delayed washout, as well as lower signal intensity on T1-weighted and higher intensity on T2-weighted images when compared with liver. Areas of hemorrhage and necrosis often show hyperintensity on both T1-weighted and T2-weighted images.

Fluorodeoxyglucose Positron Emission Tomography

Given that most ACCs also show uptake of fluorodeoxyglucose (FDG), positron emission tomography (PET) has become an additional diagnostic tool; its usefulness seems most appropriate in the setting of CT suspicious or indeterminate primary lesions, or to provide a more complete clinical staging of known ACC.[30–32] In a prospective study of 77 patients with surgically managed histopathologically diagnosed ACC, Groussin and colleagues[33] reported a sensitivity of 100% and specificity of 88% in the ability of FDG-PET to differentiate between adrenal adenomas and ACC using an adrenal/liver maximum standardized uptake value ratio of 1.45 as a cutoff value. In addition, FDG-PET was able to accurately diagnose 13 of 15 histopathologically benign adrenocortical adenomas that were deemed suspicious for malignancy based on CT densitometric and enhancement washout features.

Metomidate-Based Imaging

Metomidate, radiolabeled with either ^{11}C for PET-based techniques or with ^{123}I for single-photon emission CT (SPECT)-based techniques, is becoming a highly specific functional marker for imaging ACC and other adrenocortical tumors, because both metomidate and iodometomidate (IMTO) are taken up by cortical cells via targeted binding to both 11β-hydroxylase and aldosterone synthase.[34] In a study of 75 histopathologically diagnosed adrenal neoplasms,[35] [^{11}C]metomidate PET had a sensitivity of 89% and specificity of 96% in distinguishing cortical from noncortical lesions. Similarly, functional imaging with IMTO also has the potential to become a powerful tool for accurate staging of ACC. In a recent prospective study of 58 patients with histologically confirmed ENSAT (European Network for the Study of Adrenal Tumours) stage IV ACC, Kreissl and colleagues[36] reported the ability of IMTO SPECT/CT to detect both primary ACC and distant disease with a specificity of 100%, although with only an overall sensitivity of 38% in this preliminary study.

PATHOLOGIC EVALUATION, PROGNOSTIC FACTORS, AND STAGING
Pathologic Evaluation

Although pathologic diagnosis of ACC is still the gold standard, unlike most other solid tumors, the histopathologic diagnosis of carcinoma is frequently not definitive and not perfectly sensitive or specific in predicting clinical behavior. For approximately the past 30 years, the pathologic diagnosis of ACC has been based on the subjective identification of at least 3 of the 9 morphologic features on light microscopy that comprise the Weiss criteria (**Box 1**).[37] Although several components of the Weiss criteria have been shown to be significant independent predictors of prognosis in retrospective studies, the subjectivity in their assessment has resulted in both intraobserver and interobserver variability, which potentially decreases diagnostic reproducibility and accuracy in predicting subsequent recurrence or metastases.[38,39] In addition, for pediatric, oncocytic, myxoid, and sarcomatoid variants of ACC, the Weiss criteria do not show a comparably high diagnostic performance as when used for conventional ACCs.

> **Box 1**
> **Weiss criteria. The presence of 3 or more of these histologic features has traditionally been associated with malignancy**
>
> *Weiss criteria*
>
> 1. High nuclear grade (grade 3 or 4)
>
> 2. Mitosis 6/50 hpf or higher
>
> 3. Atypical mitosis
>
> 4. Clear cells 25% or less
>
> 5. Diffuse architecture 33% surface or more
>
> 6. Confluent necrosis
>
> 7. Venous invasion
>
> 8. Sinusoidal invasion
>
> 9. Capsular infiltration

In an attempt to decrease this variability and increase accuracy, pathologic algorithms incorporating certain Weiss criteria with additional specific and possibly less subjective markers of malignancy, such as reticulin staining and SF-1 immunohistochemistry, have recently been developed, with promising initial results at increasing interrater reliability.[38,40]

Prognostic Factors

Although prognosis is certainly dependent on an accurate diagnosis, whether based on pathologic criteria, or on preoperative clinical, biochemical, and imaging characteristics, survival of patients with ACC is also associated with both intraoperative findings and surgical technique.

The single most important prognostic factor is margin status.[2,41] In an observational study of almost 4000 patients with ACC, an R0 resection was associated with a 5-year relative survival (RS) of approximately 50%, whereas patients who underwent resection in which margins were either microscopically (R1) or grossly (R2) positive had only a 23% and 11% 5-year RS, respectively.[2] After adjustment for age, grade, tumor size, nodal status, presence of distant metastases, laterality, type of resection, and administration of adjuvant chemotherapy or radiotherapy, margin status was still independently associated with survival in a multivariable analysis (R2 vs R0, hazard ratio 2.06, 95% confidence interval 1.74–2.43, $P<.0001$).[2]

Not surprisingly, evidence of nodal or distant metastases or need of a multivisceral resection is also independently associated with poor prognosis, with reported 5-year RS of 14%, 12%, and 35%, respectively. However, tumor size has been inconsistently reported to be associated with outcome in histopathologically diagnosed ACC, although is still used in both the American Joint Committee on Cancer (AJCC)/Union for International Cancer Control and ENSAT/Lee staging systems.[2,42]

The first AJCC staging system for ACC was proposed in 2004, incorporating tumor size, presence of nodal disease, invasion into surrounding fat, tissue, or organs, and the presence of distant metastases. A study attempting to validate this system using the German ACC registry[42] simultaneously proposed an alternative ENSAT staging system, which reported both improved discrimination between stages II and III and increased overall prognostic accuracy in terms of disease-specific survival (DSS). Patients with ENSAT T4 tumors were now classified as those having either tumor extension into surrounding organs or tumor thrombus within the IVC or renal vein, whereas patients with stage IV disease were restricted to those with evidence of distant metastases (**Table 1**). The reported unadjusted 5-year DSS for patients with ENSAT stages I to IV was 82%, 61%, 50%, and 13%, respectively.[42]

In addition to the clinicopathologic criteria mentioned earlier, several other factors have been reported to adversely influence outcome, including increasing age, hormonal hypersecretion, and tumors with evidence of dedifferentiation or high mitotic index/Ki67 expression.[43–45] Moreover, for the up to 85% of patients who suffer a recurrence, a time to first recurrence of more than 12 months and an R0 resection at the time of second surgery are also independently associated with improved progression-free and overall survival.[46]

SURGICAL MANAGEMENT OF LOCOREGIONAL AND LOCALLY ADVANCED DISEASE

Surgical resection with microscopically negative margins is the standard of care for locoregional disease, leading to both an abatement of symptoms for patients with functional ACCs, as well as an increased disease-free and overall survival. Maintaining

Table 1
Comparison of AJCC and ENSAT staging systems for ACC. ENSAT stage III includes all tumors with evidence of nodal metastasis, those with invasion of periadrenal tissue or adjacent organs, and those with evidence of venous tumor thrombus. Only tumors with evidence of distant metastasis are categorized as ENSAT stage IV

TNM Staging of ACC		
Primary Tumor (T)		
Tx: primary tumor cannot be assessed		
T0: no evidence of primary tumor		
T1: tumor ≤5 cm in greatest dimension, no extra-adrenal invasion		
T2: tumor >5 cm in greatest dimension, no extra-adrenal invasion		
T3: tumor of any size with local invasion, but no invasion of adjacent organs		
T4: tumor of any size with invasion of adjacent organs (kidney, great vessels, diaphragm, pancreas, spleen, liver)		
Regional Lymph Nodes (N)		
Nx: regional lymph nodes cannot be assessed		
N0: no regional lymph node metastasis		
N1: metastasis in regional lymph node(s)		
Distant Metastasis (M)		
M0: no distant metastasis		
M1: distant metastasis		
Staging	**AJCC (7th Edition)**	**ENSAT**
I	T1 N0 M0	T1 N0 M0
II	T2 N0 M0	T2 N0 M0
III	T1-2 N1 M0 T3 N0 M0	T1-2 N1 M0 T3-4 N0-1 M0
IV	T3 N1 M0 T4 N0-1 M0 Any T, any N, M1	Any T, any N, M1

Adapted from Edge SB, Byrd DR, Compton CC, et al, editors. AJCC cancer staging manual. 7th edition. New York: Springer; 2010. p. 516–7.

capsule integrity and preventing tumor spillage through en bloc resection of involved periadrenal tissues or viscera is therefore one of the cornerstone principles of surgery for ACC.

Role of Lymphadenectomy

Unlike most other solid organ cancers, regional lymphadenectomy has not traditionally been a standard component of surgical resection for ACC, despite the integration of nodal status within current staging systems.[22,42] However, given the high postoperative recurrence rates, reported as being up to 85% in some series, and the current potential for understaging node-positive disease, there has been recent debate on the indications for and required extent of regional lymphadenectomy.

Lymph node positivity rates have been variably reported in the literature given this heterogeneity in surgical management. Recent retrospective studies using data from the National Cancer Data Base (NCDB) and the German ACC registry report nodal positivity rates of approximately 26% in pathologic specimens obtained after resection from histopathologically diagnosed ACC, although rates as high as 68% have been obtained from autopsy specimens.[2,26,47] Although the greater predominance of lymph node positivity at autopsy relative to the time of surgical resection may be secondary to the aggressive natural history of ACC, it might also suggest a potential understaging of stage III cancers resulting from inadequate lymphadenectomy.

In large observational studies from both the United States and Germany,[2,47] only 17% to 18% of patients with ACC underwent some form of lymphadenectomy at resection. Moreover, the extent of lymphadenectomy obtained in these surgical specimens with respect to nodal count and station is not clear, and therefore a true point estimate for nodal positivity at the time of resection cannot be derived from these data. However, that up to 60% of recurrences are locoregional, and often in the form of bulky nodal disease, suggests that inadequate local control at the initial surgery may be a contributing factor to the frequently short-lived disease-free interval, even with preliminary R0 resection.[48,49]

That the most frequently involved lymph node basins at the time of recurrence include ipsilateral aortocaval nodes, in addition to the more commonly envisioned renal hilar nodes, also shows a potential source of nodal disease, which may not be addressed at the time of initial resection.[48–50] Hence, based on these observations, and our current anatomic understanding of lymphatic drainage from the adrenals, Gaujoux and Brennan[22] recently suggested that regional lymphadenectomy at the time of initial resection should encompass perirenal, celiac, and ipsilateral aortocaval nodes extending from the aortic hiatus to the renal vein. These investigators proposed that celiac lymphadenopathy be classified as locoregional rather than distant disease, given its status as a first-tier station in the lymphatic drainage of the adrenal glands.

However, independent of station, lymph node positivity does seem to be associated with poorer outcome, with reported 5-year RS from the NCDB of 42% and 14% for patients who were node negative relative to those with a positive nodal ratio, respectively.[2]

Moreover, in a retrospective study of 283 patients from the German ACC registry, Reibetanz and colleagues[47] reported improved disease-specific and recurrence-free survival for individuals who received at least a 5-node lymphadenectomy versus those who did not, after controlling for age, ENSAT stage, multivisceral resection, adjuvant treatment, and preoperative image-based lymph node status (median follow-up 40 months). Although this study is subject to several limitations, including its retrospective nature and arbitrary definition of what constitutes a lymphadenectomy, as well as potential variability in the extent and type of both pathologic examination and surgical approach, the suggestion that routine regional lymphadenectomy for patients with ACC may lead to both increased locoregional control and more complete staging is compelling. The current undersampling of regional lymph nodes may be 1 potential explanation for the broad range in survival attributed to patients with stage II ACC. In addition to refining prognostication, more accurate staging may also come to influence decision making on the current and future use of adjuvant treatments such as mitotane-based combination chemotherapy.

Based on studies to date, routine regional lymphadenectomy should be considered for all patients with ACC.

Role of Nephrectomy

Although direct invasion of the kidney by ACC is uncommon, ipsilateral nephrectomy has historically been advocated by some as a means to increase locoregional control and to facilitate a more complete lymphadenectomy.[51,52]

Studies directly examining the role of nephrectomy in the surgical management of ACC are limited. However, in a relatively large observational study of patients with ACC from Italy,[53] the addition of an ipsilateral nephrectomy, which was performed in 16% of individuals receiving standard adrenalectomy, was not associated with an increased disease-free survival on univariate analysis. Caution must be exercised in drawing any conclusions from this study, because the indications for nephrectomy were not explicitly stated, and no adjusted survival data controlling for stage of disease or receipt of adjuvant therapy were reported. Despite the paucity of data on this issue, the current standard of surgical care for ACC does not include nephrectomy if there is no direct involvement of the ipsilateral kidney, given both the potential morbidity involved and lack of evidence supporting any change in outcome.

Although direct invasion of the kidney is unusual, tumor thrombus within the ipsilateral adrenal vein or IVC is more common, with the latter occurring in up to 25% of cases.[12,20,22,23] Local vascular invasion in the absence of distant metastases comprises a subset of ENSAT stage III ACC and carries a relatively poor prognosis, with an approximately 30% 3-year OS.[21,42] The principles of surgical resection vary, depending on both the location and the extent of tumor thrombus. Intracaval tumor thrombus, more commonly observed in the setting of right-sided ACC, given the shorter right adrenal vein and its drainage directly into the IVC, should be extirpated with thrombectomy or vein resection, followed by either primary closure of the cavotomy or graft reconstruction, and with a perennial understanding of the associated morbidity involved.[20,24,54] Delineating the extent of caval thrombus preoperatively is essential for surgical planning and aids in both the determination of the operative approach and method for achieving complete venous control, whether through simple cross-clamping, hepatic vascular exclusion, or even cardiopulmonary bypass, as has been used successfully in the setting of a more extensive suprahepatic caval thrombus.[20,24,54] In the context of an isolated right adrenal vein tumor thrombus, a small segment of IVC is usually taken, with subsequent primary closure of the venotomy. Conversely, if the left adrenal vein contains tumor thrombus, concomitant nephrectomy may be necessary, unless there is sparing of the gonadal or azygous veins, in which case, resection of the left renal vein can be undertaken, still preserving viability and drainage of the left kidney.[22]

Laparoscopic Versus Open Adrenalectomy

Laparoscopic adrenalectomy has been well established as safe for benign functional and nonfunctional tumors and is associated with decreased perioperative pain, length of hospitalization, and perioperative morbidity.[55–57]

However, its use in the setting of ACC has been highly controversial, with concerns over inadequate resection and resulting suboptimal patient outcomes. Early descriptive and more recent multi-institutional studies have suggested potential increased rates of tumor fragmentation, margin positivity, and peritoneal carcinomatosis after laparoscopic adrenalectomy relative to a traditional open approach for patients with histopathologically diagnosed ACC.[58–63]

In a recent single-institution study of 156 patients with stage I to III ACC from the University of Michigan, of whom 46 underwent laparoscopic adrenalectomy, a decreased margin positivity rate, as well as increased time to recurrence and overall survival, were observed in patients with stage II disease after receiving an open versus laparoscopic adrenalectomy (median follow-up 26.5 months).[62]

Similarly, in a multi-institutional study from MD Anderson Cancer Center of 302 patients with ENSAT stage I to III ACC, an increased risk of multifocal peritoneal carcinomatosis was observed in the 46 patients who received laparoscopic adrenalectomy at an outside institution relative to those receiving conventional open adrenalectomy at either an outside or the index institution, despite having a smaller tumor size overall. Moreover, open surgical resection was independently associated with increased recurrence-free and overall survival in a multivariate analysis adjusted for tumor stage.[64]

Conversely, an observational study using the German ACC registry[65] suggested no difference in disease-specific or recurrence-free survival between laparoscopic and open adrenalectomy for patients with stage I to III ACCs that were smaller than 10 cm in a Cox model adjusted for stage, tumor size, adjuvant therapy, and presence of glucocorticoid excess (median follow-up = 39.3 months). Further support of these findings comes from a multi-institutional Italian study of 156 patients with stage I and II ACC,[66] of whom 30 underwent laparoscopic adrenalectomy. On univariate Kaplan-Meier analysis, no difference in 5-year disease-free or overall survival was observed when comparing a minimally invasive versus conventional open technique (median follow-up = 42 months). Although the patient cohorts in this study were reported to be similar in terms of age, sex, and ENSAT stage, no formal statistical method was used to control for these confounders.

The controversy surrounding the surgical approach to ACC has also led to variations in published guidelines. Given the German and Italian studies, a recent position statement from the European Society of Endocrine Surgeons suggested that laparoscopic adrenalectomy may be performed for stage I and II ACCs that are 10 cm or smaller.[67] However, the Society of American Gastrointestinal and Endoscopic Surgeons, although also acknowledging the need for an appropriate oncologic resection, conceded that an open approach may be best.

We agree that a surgical approach in which en bloc resection of the tumor, regional lymphadenectomy, and removal of contiguously involved organs can be effectively performed is the most oncologically sound (**Fig. 2**). Although a highly select group of

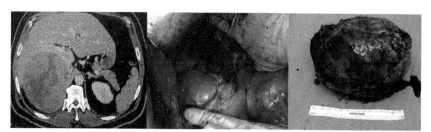

Fig. 2. An ACC larger than 15 cm with associated hepatic, diaphragmatic, and caval compression. This patient underwent an initial open approach with en bloc resection based on preoperative CT scan.

patients with larger, well-circumscribed masses and a low likelihood of ACC based on other preoperative imaging criteria may be suitable candidates for an initial laparoscopic approach, there should be a very low threshold to convert to an open operation based on intraoperative findings of locoregional disease, and before significant dissection is carried out. Moreover, we advocate that any resection for a suspected ACC is best performed in the hands of a skilled adrenal surgeon at a high-volume, specialized center.[68]

SURGICAL MANAGEMENT OF SYSTEMIC AND RECURRENT DISEASE

Approximately 30% to 40% of patients with ACC initially present with distant disease.[39,44] Moreover, of the 40% of patients who suffer a recurrence within the first 2 years of an R0 resection, 40% to 65% have evidence of metastases.[69] These patients have an almost universally poor prognosis, with a 5-year DSS of approximately 15%.[2,42,70,71] Given these guarded outcomes, consideration of multimodality therapy performed at high-volume centers should be the norm. Several surgical modalities have now come to be included in the widening medical armamentarium available for the treatment of patients with stage IV disease.

Recent retrospective studies evaluating the role of pulmonary or hepatic metastasectomy for patients with primary ACC have reported long-term survival, especially in the setting of isolated or oligometastatic disease.[72-76] In a study of 116 metastasectomies from either lung, liver, or alternative sites, Datrice and colleagues[72] reported a 5-year overall survival of 41% from the time to first metastasectomy. In this retrospective study, a disease-free interval of greater than 12 months was also associated with a prolonged median survival on univariate analysis. Similar outcomes for resection of either isolated pulmonary or hepatic metastases have been reported, with some suggestions that repeat metastasectomy may also be associated with improved survival.[73-76] In a retrospective study from Memorial Sloan Kettering Cancer Center of 28 patients who received resection of ACC-related liver metastases,[73] surgical treatment of recurrence, which most often required a repeat metastasectomy, was independently associated with survival in a multivariate model that also adjusted for functional status of the primary tumor, side of the primary lesion, and whether a major hepatectomy was performed.

A recent study using the German ACC registry[46] specifically examined prognostic factors for patients receiving surgical treatment of recurrent disease. Of the 154 patients enrolled, approximately 27% had local recurrence, whereas the remaining 73% suffered from either metastatic disease or a combination of local recurrence and metastatic disease. In a multivariate analysis, only a time to first recurrence of greater than 12 months and receipt of an R0 resection for recurrent tumors was independently associated with improved progression-free and overall survival, after additional adjustment for age, sex, number of affected sites, resection status, and receipt of additional therapy.

These studies suggested that metastasectomy is safe and may lead to prolonged survival in select patients. Moreover, given that disease-free interval seems to be a key prognostic factor, attempts to surgically control recurrence should be entertained in patients with a time to first recurrence of at least 6 to 12 months, and in those in whom an R0 resection is feasible. Although the role of surgical debulking has not been definitively established, it may be considered for symptomatic control in the setting of hormonal excess that is refractory to medical treatment with mitotane or other steroidogenesis inhibitors.[77]

ADJUVANT THERAPY

There is an expanding array of adjuvant therapies for ACC, although given the rarity of the disease, the true efficacy of these treatment modalities has been difficult to discern. Current therapeutic modalities include mitotane-based chemotherapeutic regimens, local and targeted radioablation techniques, and various novel targeted systemic therapies.

Mitotane

Mitotane is a derivative of the pesticide dichlorodiphenyltrichloroethane and has potent adrenocorticolytic activity. Although part of the medical armamentarium for more than the last 50 years, its usefulness in the adjuvant treatment of ACC, whether alone or in combination with other chemotherapeutics, is continuing to be established. Mitotane has a narrow therapeutic window and a host of clinically relevant adverse effects, including gastrointestinal, cardiovascular, and bone marrow toxicity. Moreover, its potent adrenocorticolytic activity necessitates glucocorticoid replacement, often with mineralocorticoid and androgen supplementation. These effects have a significant negative effect on patient quality of life, and therefore, defining a patient cohort that would derive the most benefit from this drug is of ongoing interest.[78,79]

Patients with low-risk to intermediate-risk ACC

There is inconsistency from current retrospective studies with respect to the reported benefit of adjuvant mitotane after R0 resection for ACC.[41,44,70,80] In a European multi-institutional study of 177 patients with stage I to III ACC who received a macroscopically complete resection,[41,81] receipt of adjuvant mitotane was associated with increased recurrence-free survival (42 months vs 10 months for Italian control group vs 25 months for German control group), after adjusting for age, sex, tumor stage, and treatment group in a multivariate analysis. However, this study has been interpreted with caution, given obvious selection bias and potential confounding with respect to type and adequacy of resection.

Consequently, at a 2008 international consensus panel on ACC, it was unanimously agreed that patients with potential residual disease and those at high risk for recurrence, including those who received an R1/Rx resection or tumors with a Ki67 level greater than 10%, should receive a recommendation for adjuvant mitotane. For patients with low-risk to intermediate-risk ACC, including those with ENSAT stage I/II tumors that have been resected with microscopically negative (R0) margins and show a Ki67 expression of 10% or less, recommendations for adjuvant mitotane were not considered mandatory.[82]

Given this controversy, the international ADIUVO (Efficacy of Adjuvant Mitotane Treatment) randomized controlled trial is accruing patients to determine if patients with low-risk to intermediate-risk characteristics benefit from adjuvant mitotane, with disease-free and overall survival as primary and secondary outcomes, respectively.[83]

Patients with locally advanced or metastatic disease

Mitotane, either as monotherapy or part of combination chemotherapy with cytotoxic agents such as streptozocin (Sz) or etoposide, doxorubicin, and cisplatin (EDP), has traditionally been suggested as treatment of patients with unresectable locally advanced or systemic disease. Response rates for monotherapy have been reported in the range of 19% to 33%, with minimal benefits in terms of recurrence-free or overall survival, whereas phase II trials of mitotane as part of combination chemotherapy with Sz or EDP have reported response rates of 36% to 53%.[84–87]

Recently, results of the landmark FIRM-ACT (First International Randomized Trial in Locally Advanced and Metastatic Adrenocortical Cancer Treatment) trial were published.[78] This study randomized 304 patients with advanced ACC to receive either Sz + mitotane or EDP + mitotane as initial first-line therapy, with a primary end point of overall survival. Secondary end points included progression-free survival, tumor response, and quality of life. A higher response rate was observed in the EDP-mitotane group relative to the Sz + mitotane group (23% vs 9%), with a corresponding increase in median progression-free survival (5 months vs 2 months) and no statistically significant difference in quality of life. Although response rates were poor, and no difference was observed in the primary end point of overall survival, these results, as well as the lack of more effective therapeutic regimes, suggest that EDP + mitotane be considered as first-line therapy for patients with unresectable or metastatic ACC.[4]

Radiotherapy

The role of external beam radiotherapy has also been controversial, given reports of the relative radioinsensitivity of ACC, as well as the potential for bystander radiotoxicity to adjacent structures, including small bowel, liver, kidney, and spinal cord.[77,87,88]

However, in a study from the German ACC registry of 28 patients with nonmetastatic ACC who underwent resection with macroscopically negative margins,[48] a substantial decrease in local recurrence was observed on univariate analysis in patients who received adjuvant radiotherapy relative to those who did not (79% vs 12%). Conversely, in a recent study of 48 patients with ACC who underwent resection with variable margin status,[89] no significant difference in 5-year local recurrence was observed between patients who received adjuvant radiotherapy within 3 months of resection versus those who received surgery alone.

Despite this controversy, practice recommendations proposed by Polat and colleagues[50] suggest that adjuvant radiotherapy be considered within 3 months of surgery for all patients who receive an R1/Rx resection, for those with ENSAT stage III disease, and for those whose tumors are either greater than 8 cm, show microvascular invasion, or have a Ki67 level greater than 10%.[4]

In contrast to its role in the adjuvant setting, radiotherapy has a more defined role in the context of symptomatic bone or cerebral metastases, as well as in the setting of superior vena cava or IVC obstruction, when effective palliation has been achieved.[50,90]

Local and Targeted Ablative Therapies

Given the persistently high recurrence rates for patients with ACC, local and targeted radioablative techniques have been used in attempts to gain additional locoregional and systemic control.

Percutaneous radiofrequency ablation (RFA) has been used primarily in the setting of unresectable or metastatic disease, either as a primary form of therapy, or as an adjunct to surgical resection. Ablation of primary ACCs or metastatic deposits seems to be most effective for tumors smaller than 3 to 5 cm in maximal dimension.[72,91] With a carefully selected patient population, RFA has also been used as a potential substitute for surgical resection in advanced disease. In a recent retrospective study of 27 patients with chemotherapy refractory ACC-related liver metastases, similar overall survival was reported on univariate analysis for patients receiving either RFA or hepatic resection.[75]

Transcatheter arterial radioembolization or chemoembolization, which is commonly used in the setting of unresectable hepatocellular cancer either alone or in combination with RFA, has also been applied to the treatment of ACC-related liver metastases, with reported response rates of approximately 21%.[92,93]

More recently, ^{131}I-IMTO has been suggested as a potential targeted radiotherapeutic agent for patients with unresectable advanced ACC that show uptake on ^{123}I-IMTO SPECT/CT.[94]

Targeted Cytotoxic Therapies

At a molecular level, ACCs have been shown to have dysregulation of multiple signaling cascades, including those downstream of the epidermal growth factor receptor (EGFR) and insulinlike growth factor 1 receptor (IGF1R) tyrosine kinases.[95]

Both EGFR and the IGF1R ligand, IGF2, are overexpressed in patients with ACC, with the latter occurring in approximately 90% of all patients.[96–99] Directly targeting these signaling molecules, or the cell-survival and proliferative pathways that they activate, is therefore of ongoing interest (**Fig. 3**).

However, the use of tyrosine kinase inhibitors (TKIs) such as imatinib or erlotinib, as salvage therapy has produced poor response rates, although a phase II trial evaluating the multikinase inhibitor sunitinib in refractory ACC has resulted in moderate tumor response rates, with some patients achieving stable disease.[100–102]

Targeting IGF signaling specifically, such as with the IGF1R TKI, OSI-906 (linsitinib), or with IGF1R monoclonal antibodies, including figitumumab or cixutumumab, seems to have had more success in terms of generating tumor response rates and achieving stable disease in patients with metastatic refractory ACC.[103–105] The phase III, placebo-controlled GALACCTIC (a study of OSI-906 in patients with locally advanced or metastatic adrenocortical carcinoma) trial,[106] evaluating the effect of OSI-906 in patients with locally advanced and metastatic ACC is currently accruing patients, with overall and disease-free survival as primary and secondary outcomes.

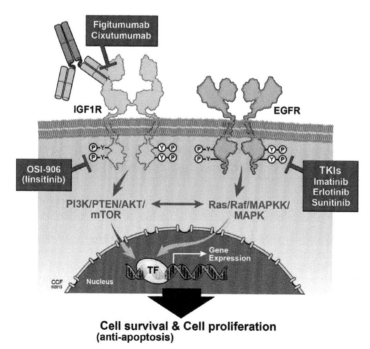

Fig. 3. Targeted therapies being evaluated for ACC.

SUMMARY

ACC is a rare neoplasm with a poor, and historically unchanged, prognosis. Although preoperative clinical, biochemical, and radiologic features can aid in the diagnosis of these cancers, there often remains a degree of uncertainty that is not commonly observed in other solid organ tumors, which are routinely amenable to preoperative pathologic diagnosis. This diagnostic ambiguity and the subsequent potential for an inadequate surgical resection have likely contributed to the currently dismal disease-free survival, although unsettlingly high rates of locoregional recurrences still persist, even in the setting of a supposedly R0 resection. Refinements in both diagnostic criteria and surgical techniques, as well as the increasing use and study of novel multimodality therapies for ACC, such as mitotane-based combination chemotherapy, have provided advances in the treatment of these patients and renewed hope that continued diligence and future breakthroughs may bring about meaningful improvements in patient outcomes.

REFERENCES

1. Fassnacht M, Libe R, Kroiss M, et al. Adrenocortical carcinoma: a clinician's update. Nat Rev Endocrinol 2011;7(6):323–35.
2. Bilimoria KY, Shen WT, Elaraj D, et al. Adrenocortical carcinoma in the United States: treatment utilization and prognostic factors. Cancer 2008;113(11): 3130–6.
3. Kutikov A, Mallin K, Canter D, et al. Effects of increased cross-sectional imaging on the diagnosis and prognosis of adrenocortical carcinoma: analysis of the National Cancer Database. J Urol 2011;186(3):805–10.
4. Berruti A, Baudin E, Gelderblom H, et al. Adrenal cancer: ESMO clinical practice guidelines for diagnosis, treatment and follow-up. Ann Oncol 2012;23(Suppl 7): vii131–8.
5. Else T. Association of adrenocortical carcinoma with familial cancer susceptibility syndromes. Mol Cell Endocrinol 2012;351(1):66–70.
6. Mazzuco TL, Durand J, Chapman A, et al. Genetic aspects of adrenocortical tumours and hyperplasias. Clin Endocrinol 2012;77(1):1–10.
7. Raymond VM, Everett JN, Furtado LV, et al. Adrenocortical carcinoma is a Lynch syndrome-associated cancer. J Clin Oncol 2013;31:3012–8.
8. Custodio G, Parise GA, Kiesel Filho N, et al. Impact of neonatal screening and surveillance for the TP53 R337H mutation on early detection of childhood adrenocortical tumors. J Clin Oncol 2013;31(20):2619–26.
9. Ribeiro RC, Sandrini F, Figueiredo B, et al. An inherited p53 mutation that contributes in a tissue-specific manner to pediatric adrenal cortical carcinoma. Proc Natl Acad Sci U S A 2001;98(16):9330–5.
10. Lafemina J, Brennan MF. Adrenocortical carcinoma: past, present, and future. J Surg Oncol 2012;106(5):586–94.
11. Arlt W, Biehl M, Taylor AE, et al. Urine steroid metabolomics as a biomarker tool for detecting malignancy in adrenal tumors. J Clin Endocrinol Metab 2011; 96(12):3775–84.
12. Zhang HM, Perrier ND, Grubbs EG, et al. CT features and quantification of the characteristics of adrenocortical carcinomas on unenhanced and contrast-enhanced studies. Clin Radiol 2012;67(1):38–46.
13. Mantero F, Terzolo M, Arnaldi G, et al. A survey on adrenal incidentaloma in Italy. Study group on adrenal tumors of the Italian Society of Endocrinology. J Clin Endocrinol Metab 2000;85(2):637–44.

14. Angeli A, Osella G, Ali A, et al. Adrenal incidentaloma: an overview of clinical and epidemiological data from the National Italian Study Group. Horm Res 1997;47(4–6):279–83.
15. Terzolo M, Ali A, Osella G, et al. Prevalence of adrenal carcinoma among incidentally discovered adrenal masses. A retrospective study from 1989 to 1994. Gruppo Piemontese Incidentalomi Surrenalici. Arch Surg 1997;132(8):914–9.
16. Blake MA, Holalkere NS, Boland GW. Imaging techniques for adrenal lesion characterization. Radiol Clin North Am 2008;46(1):65–78, vi.
17. Boland GW, Lee MJ, Gazelle GS, et al. Characterization of adrenal masses using unenhanced CT: an analysis of the CT literature. AJR Am J Roentgenol 1998; 171(1):201–4.
18. Blake MA, Kalra MK, Sweeney AT, et al. Distinguishing benign from malignant adrenal masses: multi-detector row CT protocol with 10-minute delay. Radiology 2006;238(2):578–85.
19. Sangwaiya MJ, Boland GW, Cronin CG, et al. Incidental adrenal lesions: accuracy of characterization with contrast-enhanced washout multidetector CT–10-minute delayed imaging protocol revisited in a large patient cohort. Radiology 2010;256(2):504–10.
20. Chiche L, Dousset B, Kieffer E, et al. Adrenocortical carcinoma extending into the inferior vena cava: presentation of a 15-patient series and review of the literature. Surgery 2006;139(1):15–27.
21. Turbendian HK, Strong VE, Hsu M, et al. Adrenocortical carcinoma: the influence of large vessel extension. Surgery 2010;148(6):1057–64 [discussion: 1064].
22. Gaujoux S, Brennan MF. Recommendation for standardized surgical management of primary adrenocortical carcinoma. Surgery 2012;152(1):123–32.
23. Hedican SP, Marshall FF. Adrenocortical carcinoma with intracaval extension. J Urol 1997;158(6):2056–61.
24. Mihai R, Iacobone M, Makay O, et al. Outcome of operation in patients with adrenocortical cancer invading the inferior vena cava–a European Society of Endocrine Surgeons (ESES) survey. Langenbecks Arch Surg 2012;397(2): 225–31.
25. Fishman EK, Deutch BM, Hartman DS, et al. Primary adrenocortical carcinoma: CT evaluation with clinical correlation. AJR Am J Roentgenol 1987;148(3):531–5.
26. Didolkar MS, Bescher RA, Elias EG, et al. Natural history of adrenal cortical carcinoma: a clinicopathologic study of 42 patients. Cancer 1981;47(9):2153–61.
27. Rodgers SE, Evans DB, Lee JE, et al. Adrenocortical carcinoma. Surg Oncol Clin N Am 2006;15(3):535–53.
28. Young WF Jr. Conventional imaging in adrenocortical carcinoma: update and perspectives. Horm Cancer 2011;2(6):341–7.
29. Honigschnabl S, Gallo S, Niederle B, et al. How accurate is MR imaging in characterisation of adrenal masses: update of a long-term study. Eur J Radiol 2002; 41(2):113–22.
30. Boland GW, Dwamena BA, Jagtiani Sangwaiya M, et al. Characterization of adrenal masses by using FDG PET: a systematic review and meta-analysis of diagnostic test performance. Radiology 2011;259(1):117–26.
31. Gust L, Taieb D, Beliard A, et al. Preoperative 18F-FDG uptake is strongly correlated with malignancy, Weiss score, and molecular markers of aggressiveness in adrenal cortical tumors. World J Surg 2012;36(6):1406–10.
32. Deandreis D, Leboulleux S, Caramella C, et al. FDG PET in the management of patients with adrenal masses and adrenocortical carcinoma. Horm Cancer 2011;2(6):354–62.

33. Groussin L, Bonardel G, Silvera S, et al. 18F-Fluorodeoxyglucose positron emission tomography for the diagnosis of adrenocortical tumors: a prospective study in 77 operated patients. J Clin Endocrinol Metab 2009;94(5):1713–22.
34. Hahner S, Sundin A. Metomidate-based imaging of adrenal masses. Horm Cancer 2011;2(6):348–53.
35. Hennings J, Lindhe O, Bergstrom M, et al. [11C]metomidate positron emission tomography of adrenocortical tumors in correlation with histopathological findings. J Clin Endocrinol Metab 2006;91(4):1410–4.
36. Kreissl MC, Schirbel A, Fassnacht M, et al. [123I]Iodometomidate imaging in adrenocortical carcinoma. J Clin Endocrinol Metab 2013;98(7):2755–64.
37. Lau SK, Weiss LM. The Weiss system for evaluating adrenocortical neoplasms: 25 years later. Hum Pathol 2009;40(6):757–68.
38. Papotti M, Libe R, Duregon E, et al. The Weiss score and beyond–histopathology for adrenocortical carcinoma. Horm Cancer 2011;2(6):333–40.
39. Stojadinovic A, Ghossein RA, Hoos A, et al. Adrenocortical carcinoma: clinical, morphologic, and molecular characterization. J Clin Oncol 2002;20(4):941–50.
40. Duregon E, Fassina A, Volante M, et al. The reticulin algorithm for adrenocortical tumor diagnosis: a multicentric validation study on 245 unpublished cases. Am J Surg Pathol 2013;37:1433–40.
41. Grubbs EG, Callender GG, Xing Y, et al. Recurrence of adrenal cortical carcinoma following resection: surgery alone can achieve results equal to surgery plus mitotane. Ann Surg Oncol 2010;17(1):263–70.
42. Fassnacht M, Johanssen S, Quinkler M, et al. Limited prognostic value of the 2004 International Union Against Cancer staging classification for adrenocortical carcinoma: proposal for a revised TNM classification. Cancer 2009; 115(2):243–50.
43. Morimoto R, Satoh F, Murakami O, et al. Immunohistochemistry of a proliferation marker Ki67/MIB1 in adrenocortical carcinomas: Ki67/MIB1 labeling index is a predictor for recurrence of adrenocortical carcinomas. Endocr J 2008;55(1):49–55.
44. Schulick RD, Brennan MF. Long-term survival after complete resection and repeat resection in patients with adrenocortical carcinoma. Ann Surg Oncol 1999;6(8):719–26.
45. Abiven G, Coste J, Groussin L, et al. Clinical and biological features in the prognosis of adrenocortical cancer: poor outcome of cortisol-secreting tumors in a series of 202 consecutive patients. J Clin Endocrinol Metab 2006;91(7):2650–5.
46. Erdogan I, Deutschbein T, Jurowich C, et al. The role of surgery in the management of recurrent adrenocortical carcinoma. J Clin Endocrinol Metab 2013; 98(1):181–91.
47. Reibetanz J, Jurowich C, Erdogan I, et al. Impact of lymphadenectomy on the oncologic outcome of patients with adrenocortical carcinoma. Ann Surg 2012; 255(2):363–9.
48. Fassnacht M, Hahner S, Polat B, et al. Efficacy of adjuvant radiotherapy of the tumor bed on local recurrence of adrenocortical carcinoma. J Clin Endocrinol Metab 2006;91(11):4501–4.
49. Kendrick ML, Lloyd R, Erickson L, et al. Adrenocortical carcinoma: surgical progress or status quo? Arch Surg 2001;136(5):543–9.
50. Polat B, Fassnacht M, Pfreundner L, et al. Radiotherapy in adrenocortical carcinoma. Cancer 2009;115(13):2816–23.
51. Icard P, Chapuis Y, Andreassian B, et al. Adrenocortical carcinoma in surgically treated patients: a retrospective study on 156 cases by the French Association of Endocrine Surgery. Surgery 1992;112(6):972–9 [discussion: 979–80].

52. Icard P, Louvel A, Chapuis Y. Survival rates and prognostic factors in adrenocortical carcinoma. World J Surg 1992;16(4):753–8.
53. Bellantone R, Ferrante A, Boscherini M, et al. Role of reoperation in recurrence of adrenal cortical carcinoma: results from 188 cases collected in the Italian National Registry for Adrenal Cortical Carcinoma. Surgery 1997;122(6):1212–8.
54. Meniconi RL, Caronna R, Schiratti M, et al. Adrenocortical carcinoma extending into the inferior vena cava in a patient with right kidney agenesis: surgical approach and review of literature. Int J Surg Case Rep 2012;3(7):302–4.
55. Thompson GB, Grant CS, van Heerden JA, et al. Laparoscopic versus open posterior adrenalectomy: a case-control study of 100 patients. Surgery 1997; 122(6):1132–6.
56. Prinz RA. A comparison of laparoscopic and open adrenalectomies. Arch Surg 1995;130(5):489–92 [discussion: 492–4].
57. Lee J, El-Tamer M, Schifftner T, et al. Open and laparoscopic adrenalectomy: analysis of the National Surgical Quality Improvement Program. J Am Coll Surg 2008;206(5):953–9 [discussion: 959–61].
58. Jurowich C, Fassnacht M, Kroiss M, et al. Is there a role for laparoscopic adrenalectomy in patients with suspected adrenocortical carcinoma? A critical appraisal of the literature. Horm Metab Res 2013;45(2):130–6.
59. Porpiglia F, Miller BS, Manfredi M, et al. A debate on laparoscopic versus open adrenalectomy for adrenocortical carcinoma. Horm Cancer 2011;2(6):372–7.
60. Deckers S, Derdelinckx L, Col V, et al. Peritoneal carcinomatosis following laparoscopic resection of an adrenocortical tumor causing primary hyperaldosteronism. Horm Res 1999;52(2):97–100.
61. Gonzalez RJ, Shapiro S, Sarlis N, et al. Laparoscopic resection of adrenal cortical carcinoma: a cautionary note. Surgery 2005;138(6):1078–85 [discussion: 1085–6].
62. Miller BS, Ammori JB, Gauger PG, et al. Laparoscopic resection is inappropriate in patients with known or suspected adrenocortical carcinoma. World J Surg 2010;34(6):1380–5.
63. Suzuki K, Ushiyama T, Ihara H, et al. Complications of laparoscopic adrenalectomy in 75 patients treated by the same surgeon. Eur Urol 1999;36(1):40–7.
64. Cooper AB, Habra MA, Grubbs EG, et al. Does laparoscopic adrenalectomy jeopardize oncologic outcomes for patients with adrenocortical carcinoma? Surg Endosc 2013;27:4026–32.
65. Brix D, Allolio B, Fenske W, et al. Laparoscopic versus open adrenalectomy for adrenocortical carcinoma: surgical and oncologic outcome in 152 patients. Eur Urol 2010;58(4):609–15.
66. Lombardi CP, Raffaelli M, De Crea C, et al. Open versus endoscopic adrenalectomy in the treatment of localized (stage I/II) adrenocortical carcinoma: results of a multiinstitutional Italian survey. Surgery 2012;152(6):1158–64.
67. Henry JF, Peix JL, Kraimps JL. Positional statement of the European Society of Endocrine Surgeons (ESES) on malignant adrenal tumors. Langenbecks Arch Surg 2012;397(2):145–6.
68. Lombardi CP, Raffaelli M, Boniardi M, et al. Adrenocortical carcinoma: effect of hospital volume on patient outcome. Langenbecks Arch Surg 2012;397(2): 201–7.
69. Glover AR, Ip JC, Zhao JT, et al. Current management options for recurrent adrenocortical carcinoma. Onco Targets Ther 2013;6:635–43.
70. Terzolo M, Angeli A, Fassnacht M, et al. Adjuvant mitotane treatment for adrenocortical carcinoma. N Engl J Med 2007;356(23):2372–80.

71. Crucitti F, Bellantone R, Ferrante A, et al. The Italian Registry for Adrenal Cortical Carcinoma: analysis of a multiinstitutional series of 129 patients. The ACC Italian Registry Study Group. Surgery 1996;119(2):161–70.

72. Datrice NM, Langan RC, Ripley RT, et al. Operative management for recurrent and metastatic adrenocortical carcinoma. J Surg Oncol 2012;105(7): 709–13.

73. Gaujoux S, Al-Ahmadie H, Allen PJ, et al. Resection of adrenocortical carcinoma liver metastasis: is it justified? Ann Surg Oncol 2012;19(8):2643–51.

74. Kemp CD, Ripley RT, Mathur A, et al. Pulmonary resection for metastatic adrenocortical carcinoma: the National Cancer Institute experience. Ann Thorac Surg 2011;92(4):1195–200.

75. Ripley RT, Kemp CD, Davis JL, et al. Liver resection and ablation for metastatic adrenocortical carcinoma. Ann Surg Oncol 2011;18(7):1972–9.

76. op den Winkel J, Pfannschmidt J, Muley T, et al. Metastatic adrenocortical carcinoma: results of 56 pulmonary metastasectomies in 24 patients. Ann Thorac Surg 2011;92(6):1965–70.

77. Schteingart DE, Doherty GM, Gauger PG, et al. Management of patients with adrenal cancer: recommendations of an international consensus conference. Endocr Relat Cancer 2005;12(3):667–80.

78. Fassnacht M, Terzolo M, Allolio B, et al. Combination chemotherapy in advanced adrenocortical carcinoma. N Engl J Med 2012;366(23):2189–97.

79. Chortis V, Taylor AE, Schneider P, et al. Mitotane therapy in adrenocortical cancer induces CYP3A4 and inhibits 5alpha-reductase, explaining the need for personalized glucocorticoid and androgen replacement. J Clin Endocrinol Metab 2013;98(1):161–71.

80. Fassnacht M, Johanssen S, Fenske W, et al. Improved survival in patients with stage II adrenocortical carcinoma followed up prospectively by specialized centers. J Clin Endocrinol Metab 2010;95(11):4925–32.

81. Huang H, Fojo T. Adjuvant mitotane for adrenocortical cancer–a recurring controversy. J Clin Endocrinol Metab 2008;93(10):3730–2.

82. Berruti A, Fassnacht M, Baudin E, et al. Adjuvant therapy in patients with adrenocortical carcinoma: a position of an international panel. J Clin Oncol 2010; 28(23):e401–2 [author reply: e403].

83. Efficacy of adjuvant mitotane treatment (ADIUVO). ClinicalTrials.gov (NCT00777244).

84. Berruti A, Terzolo M, Sperone P, et al. Etoposide, doxorubicin and cisplatin plus mitotane in the treatment of advanced adrenocortical carcinoma: a large prospective phase II trial. Endocr Relat Cancer 2005;12(3):657–66.

85. Gonzalez RJ, Tamm EP, Ng C, et al. Response to mitotane predicts outcome in patients with recurrent adrenal cortical carcinoma. Surgery 2007;142(6):867–75 [discussion: 867–75].

86. Khan TS, Imam H, Juhlin C, et al. Streptozocin and o,p'DDD in the treatment of adrenocortical cancer patients: long-term survival in its adjuvant use. Ann Oncol 2000;11(10):1281–7.

87. Lebastchi AH, Kunstman JW, Carling T. Adrenocortical carcinoma: current therapeutic state-of-the-art. J Oncol 2012;2012:234726.

88. Pommier RF, Brennan MF. An eleven-year experience with adrenocortical carcinoma. Surgery 1992;112(6):963–70 [discussion: 970–1].

89. Habra MA, Ejaz S, Feng L, et al. A retrospective cohort analysis of the efficacy of adjuvant radiotherapy after primary surgical resection in patients with adrenocortical carcinoma. J Clin Endocrinol Metab 2013;98(1):192–7.

90. Milgrom SA, Goodman KA. The role of radiation therapy in the management of adrenal carcinoma and adrenal metastases. J Surg Oncol 2012;106(5):647–50.

91. Wood BJ, Abraham J, Hvizda JL, et al. Radiofrequency ablation of adrenal tumors and adrenocortical carcinoma metastases. Cancer 2003;97(3):554–60.

92. Soga H, Takenaka A, Ooba T, et al. A twelve-year experience with adrenal cortical carcinoma in a single institution: long-term survival after surgical treatment and transcatheter arterial embolization. Urol Int 2009;82(2):222–6.

93. Cazejust J, De Baere T, Auperin A, et al. Transcatheter arterial chemoembolization for liver metastases in patients with adrenocortical carcinoma. J Vasc Interv Radiol 2010;21(10):1527–32.

94. Hahner S, Kreissl MC, Fassnacht M, et al. [131I]iodometomidate for targeted radionuclide therapy of advanced adrenocortical carcinoma. J Clin Endocrinol Metab 2012;97(3):914–22.

95. Szabo PM, Tamasi V, Molnar V, et al. Meta-analysis of adrenocortical tumour genomics data: novel pathogenic pathways revealed. Oncogene 2010;29(21): 3163–72.

96. Fernandez-Ranvier GG, Weng J, Yeh RF, et al. Identification of biomarkers of adrenocortical carcinoma using genomewide gene expression profiling. Arch Surg 2008;143(9):841–6 [discussion: 846].

97. Giordano TJ, Thomas DG, Kuick R, et al. Distinct transcriptional profiles of adrenocortical tumors uncovered by DNA microarray analysis. Am J Pathol 2003; 162(2):521–31.

98. Gicquel C, Bertagna X, Gaston V, et al. Molecular markers and long-term recurrences in a large cohort of patients with sporadic adrenocortical tumors. Cancer Res 2001;61(18):6762–7.

99. de Fraipont F, El Atifi M, Cherradi N, et al. Gene expression profiling of human adrenocortical tumors using complementary deoxyribonucleic acid microarrays identifies several candidate genes as markers of malignancy. J Clin Endocrinol Metab 2005;90(3):1819–29.

100. Gross DJ, Munter G, Bitan M, et al. The role of imatinib mesylate (Glivec) for treatment of patients with malignant endocrine tumors positive for c-kit or PDGF-R. Endocr Relat Cancer 2006;13(2):535–40.

101. Quinkler M, Hahner S, Wortmann S, et al. Treatment of advanced adrenocortical carcinoma with erlotinib plus gemcitabine. J Clin Endocrinol Metab 2008;93(6): 2057–62.

102. Kroiss M, Quinkler M, Johanssen S, et al. Sunitinib in refractory adrenocortical carcinoma: a phase II, single-arm, open-label trial. J Clin Endocrinol Metab 2012;97(10):3495–503.

103. Haluska P, Worden F, Olmos D, et al. Safety, tolerability, and pharmacokinetics of the anti-IGF-1R monoclonal antibody figitumumab in patients with refractory adrenocortical carcinoma. Cancer Chemother Pharmacol 2010;65(4):765–73.

104. Demeure MJ, Bussey KJ, Kirschner LS. Targeted therapies for adrenocortical carcinoma: IGF and beyond. Horm Cancer 2011;2(6):385–92.

105. Naing A, Lorusso P, Fu S, et al. Insulin growth factor receptor (IGF-1R) antibody cixutumumab combined with the mTOR inhibitor temsirolimus in patients with metastatic adrenocortical carcinoma. Br J Cancer 2013;108(4):826–30.

106. A study of OSI-906 in patients with locally advanced or metastatic adrenocortical carcinoma (GALACCTIC). ClinicalTrials.gov (NCT00924989).

Nonfunctional Pancreatic Neuroendocrine Tumors

Jennifer H. Kuo, MD[a], James A. Lee, MD[b],*, John A. Chabot, MD[a]

KEYWORDS

- Pancreas • Neuroendocrine • Nonfunctional • Neuroendocrine liver metastases
- PanNET

KEY POINTS

- Pancreatic neuroendocrine tumors are rare, heterogeneous tumors that compose 3% of all pancreatic neoplasms and 7% of all neuroendocrine tumors.
- The incidence of pancreatic neuroendocrine tumors has been increasing over the past 20 years because of the increased diagnosis of pancreatic incidentalomas.
- Ninety percent of pancreatic neuroendocrine tumors are nonfunctional tumors that are often malignant and present with symptoms of mass effect or metastatic disease.
- Formal surgical resection is the treatment of choice for most locoregional disease; however, surgical decision making must include many variables.
- Hepatic metastasis is common, and resection is recommended in the absence of extrahepatic disease.
- Interventional liver-directed therapies and targeted systemic therapies offer promising alternatives for patients with advanced disease, improving morbidity and increasing progression-free survival.

INTRODUCTION

Neuroendocrine tumors (NETs) are a group of rare, diverse neoplasms, which can be found throughout the body. They are most commonly located in the gastrointestinal tract and lung but are also found in the pancreas.[1] Historically known as islet cell tumors, they are now classified as pancreatic NETs (PanNETs) by the World Health Organization (WHO). When compared with adenocarcinomas, PanNETs account for a relatively small percentage of pancreatic neoplasms,[2,3] but their incidence has been increasing over the past 20 years. Based on the Surveillance, Epidemiology, and End Results (SEER) database, the incidence of NETs in the United States increased

[a] Division of GI/Endocrine Surgery, Columbia University, 161 Fort Washington Avenue, 8th Floor, New York, NY 10032, USA; [b] COACH Education, Endocrine Surgery, Adrenal Center, New York Thyroid/Parathyroid Center, Simulation Center, Columbia University, 161 Fort Washington Avenue, 8th Floor, New York, NY 10032, USA
* Corresponding author.
E-mail address: jal74@columbia.edu

Surg Clin N Am 94 (2014) 689–708
http://dx.doi.org/10.1016/j.suc.2014.02.010
0039-6109/14/$ – see front matter © 2014 Elsevier Inc. All rights reserved.
surgical.theclinics.com

nearly 5-fold over the past 3 decades and was 5.25 per 100,000 in 2004.[4] PanNETs account for 7% of all NETs[5] and have an incidence of 0.43 per 100,000 people in 2007,[5] a greater than 2-fold increase in the incidence of PanNETs since the 1980s. The increased frequency of abdominal imaging, specifically computed tomography (CT) and ultrasound, has increased the incidence of abnormal pancreatic findings detected in asymptomatic patients. Of these patients, 17% will ultimately undergo pancreatectomy.[6] This increase in pancreatic incidentalomas may reflect a historical underestimation of the prevalence of this disease; autopsy studies suggest that the prevalence of PanNETs may be higher than we expect, with prevalence rates of 3% to 10%.[7–9]

RELEVANT ANATOMY/PATHOPHYSIOLOGY

Traditionally, PanNETs have been thought to arise from the islets of Langerhans that perform the endocrine function of the pancreas. More recent investigation, however, has demonstrated that these neoplasms originate from pluripotent cells in the pancreatic ductal/acinar system.[10] All PanNETs express neuroendocrine markers, such as synaptophysin, neuron-specific enolase, and chromogranin A (CgA) (present in 88%–100% of patients with PanNETs). A multitude of cellular and molecular alterations have been implicated in the pathogenesis of PanNETs, involving at least 14 different types of cells and genetic alterations in the MEN-1 gene, the p16/MTS1 tumor-suppressor gene, the DPC4/Smad 4 gene, amplification of the Her-2/neu proto-oncogene, and alterations in transcription factors Hox C6, growth factors, and their receptor expressions.[11] Several of these genetic alterations have been shown to correlate with tumor aggressiveness and may have prognostic significance.[12] This molecular heterogeneity translates to heterogeneity in the clinical presentation, including both the multiple syndromes of overproduction and hypersecretion of hormones that have traditionally characterized these tumors as well as hormonally silent tumors. Thus, PanNETs are often classified as functional or nonfunctional based on the presence or absence of a particular clinical syndrome associated with hormone hypersecretion. According to the SEER database, from 1973 to 2000, most PanNETs diagnosed were nonfunctional tumors (90.8%); the remaining 9% included malignant functional tumors, such as gastrinomas (4.2%), insulinomas (2.5%), glucagonomas (1.6%), and VIPomas (0.9%).[13,14] In addition to variability in the production of pancreatic endocrine hormones, PanNETs exhibit a broad range of growth rates, malignant potential, and overall prognosis. Although commonly perceived to be indolent tumors because they have a far better prognosis than pancreatic adenocarcinoma, most patients with PanNETs (60%–70%) present with metastatic disease.[4,13,14] Even when they are resectable, many patients ultimately succumb to the disease. Following surgical resection of PanNETs, the 5-year survival for PanNETs other than insulinomas is roughly 65%, with a 10-year survival of 45%.[14]

In 2000, the WHO introduced a classification system based on clinical and histopathologic features that divides PanNETs into well-differentiated endocrine tumors with either benign or uncertain behavior, well-differentiated endocrine carcinomas, or poorly differentiated endocrine carcinomas.[15] More recent classification systems have acknowledged the increasing importance of a proliferative index, specifically expression of the nuclear antigen Ki-67, and evidence of its prognostic value for PanNET.[15–17] In 2010, the WHO revised the classification of PanNETs to reflect a proliferation-based grading system in conjunction with the traditional histopathologic diagnostic criteria (**Table 1**). They delineated a 3-tier grading system of PanNETs designating tumors as well-differentiated NETs versus poorly differentiated

Table 1		
WHO classification of PanNETs		
Grade	Ki-67 Index (%)	Mitotic Count/10 HPF
G1	≤2	<2
G2	3–20	2–20
G3	>20	>20
TNM	Size (cm)	Muscularis Propria Invasion
T1a	<1	−
T1b	1–2	−
T2	>2	+

In the World Health Organization (WHO) 2010, the higher grade is assumed if the Ki-67 index and mitotic count differ; in the WHO 2010 TNM, the tumor is classified as T2 if it is larger than 2 cm in diameter or if it invades the muscularis propria. T3 and T4 tumors are locally aggressive tumors (data not shown in the table).

Abbreviation: HPF, high-power field.

Data from Bosman F, Carneiro F, Hruban R, editors. WHO classification of tumors of the digestive system. Lyon (France): IARC Press; 2010.

neuroendocrine carcinomas. The well-differentiated NETs were further divided into grade 1 (Ki-67 <2%) and grade 2 (Ki-67 of 2%–20%). The poorly differentiated tumors are considered grade 3 (Ki-67 >20). Mitotic rate or Ki-67 should be assessed on all PanNETs. When both mitotic rate and Ki-67 are obtained, the higher grade is assigned. If the biopsy specimen is inadequate, a repeat biopsy is recommended.[18]

The European Neuroendocrine Tumor Society (ENETS) and the American Joint Committee on Cancer (AJCC) describe alternative classification systems for Pan-NETs. The ENETS' classification[19] for PanNETs combines a staging TNM classification including the tumor diameter along with a grading system based on the mitotic rate and Ki-67.[20] The AJCC's TNM classification is based on a staging system for exocrine pancreatic adenocarcinomas, differentiating tumors based on the extent of disease rather than the tumor grade to determine tumor resectability.[20] Although both systems emphasize different tumor characteristics, both classification systems have been demonstrated to be prognostic for relapse-free survival.[20] It is important to note that histopathology is not always predictive of malignancy, and the only true measures of whether a PanNET is benign or malignant include evidence of local invasion, metastases, and/or recurrent disease.

CLINICAL PRESENTATION

Most PanNETs are sporadic and tend to affect older individuals. Men have a slightly increased risk of developing PanNETs than women (55.2% vs 44.8%), and there is a Caucasian predominance in the United States (84.1% Caucasian vs 15.9% other background).[13] Functional tumors present with symptoms that result from the specific hormone being elaborated. The most common functional PanNETs are insulinomas composing 30% to 45% of functioning PanNETs[2,21] and gastrinomas composing 16% to 30%.[21] Glucagonoma, VIPomas, and somatostatinomas are rarer PanNETs, and other rare functional PanNETs also exist.[22] The presentation of these tumors is summarized in **Table 2** but is not discussed in further detail in this article.

Patients with nonfunctional tumors typically present with symptoms related to local mass effect or metastatic disease, indicating a more advanced stage of disease.[9]

Table 2
Summary of functional NETs

Tumor Type	Number[a]	Secretory Hormone	Clinical Features	Laboratory Tests	Symptomatic Treatment
Insulinoma	40%–60%	Insulin	Hypoglycemia; symptoms of catecholamine excess; 90% benign	Insulin level, C-reactive protein; 72-h inpatient fasting with monitoring of glucose and insulin levels	Dietary modifications; octreotide; diazoxide
Gastrinoma	20%–50%	Gastrin	Peptic ulcer disease; GERD; secretory diarrhea; most common PanNET in MEN-1; 60%–90% malignant	Fasting serum gastrin; gastric pH analysis, gastrin provocation testing (calcium or secretin challenge)	Proton pump inhibitor; octreotide
Glucagonoma	Rare	Glucagon	Glucose intolerance; migratory necrolytic erythema; weight loss; anemia; 90% malignant	Serum glucagon	Octreotide; insulin; zinc supplement (rash); TPN (malnutrition)
Somatostatinoma	Rare	Somatostatin	Diabetes; gallstones; secretory diarrhea	Clinical and pathologic diagnoses; increased somatostatinlike immunoreactivity in resected tumor	Octreotide
VIPoma	Rare	Vasoactive intestinal peptide	Choleralike, secretory diarrhea; hypokalemia; hypochlorhydria	Serum VIP	Octreotide

Abbreviations: GERD, gastroesophageal reflux disease; MEN-1, multiple endocrine neoplasia type 1; TPN, total parenteral nutrition; VIP, vasoactive intestinal polypeptide.
[a] Percentage among PanNETs.

Nonfunctioning tumors either do not produce any hormone, produce very small amounts of hormones that are insufficient to produce symptoms, or produce hormones that do not generate specific symptoms (pancreatic polypeptide, human chorionic gonadotropin subunits, calcitonin, or neurotensin).[23,24] Most nonfunctional tumors occur in the head of the pancreas and often produce symptoms of mass effect that mimic those of pancreatic adenocarcinoma, including jaundice, abdominal pain, weight loss, abdominal mass, nausea and vomiting, backache, and pancreatitis.[22,25,26] As previously mentioned, the number of pancreatic tumors discovered incidentally before any onset of symptoms is dramatically increasing because of the widespread use of abdominal imaging.[6,9,23] Bruzoni and colleagues[27] found that 19% of these pancreatic incidentalomas were NETs on the final pathology.

Although most PanNETs occur sporadically, nearly 10% are associated with predisposing genetic syndromes. These hereditary syndromes include multiple endocrine neoplasia type 1 (MEN-1 syndrome), von Hippel-Lindau disease (VHL), von Recklinghausen disease or neurofibromatosis type 1 (NF-1), and tuberous sclerosis complex (TSC).[2,9,14,21] These patients are generally diagnosed at a younger age, have multiple synchronous lesions throughout the pancreas, and have a family history of endocrine disorders or their associated cancers.[9,21] The most recognized of these hereditary syndromes is MEN-1.[2,9,14,21] Most patients with MEN-1 (80%–100%) develop nonfunctioning PanNETs, 50% to 60% develop gastrinomas, 20% insulinomas, and 3% to 5% VIPomas or glucagonomas.[2,9,14,21] Nonfunctional PanNETs, cystic pancreatic lesions, and mixed serous-NETs can be seen in 20% of patients with VHL.[2,14,21] In contrast to MEN-1 and VHL, PanNETs are relatively uncommon in patients with NF-1 and TSC (<10%).[2,14,21]

The evaluation of patients with PanNETs should include a comprehensive history assessing for signs or symptoms of tumor mass effect, metastatic disease, or specific functioning tumors. Eliciting a family history or genetic testing can determine whether the tumor is sporadic or associated with a genetic syndrome and can have a significant impact on preoperative planning. For example, patients with MEN-1 are more likely to have multiple tumors throughout the pancreas necessitating altered surgical planning.

DIAGNOSIS

When a tumor of neuroendocrine origin is suspected, a complete biochemical evaluation looking for the most commonly secreted pancreatic hormones should be performed to determine functionality. Levels of NET markers can be very helpful for diagnosis and determining the prognosis of nonfunctional PanNETs.[2,11] Serum chromogranin A, a 49-kd protein contained in the neurosecretory vesicles of the NET cells, is the most widely used as it reflects tumor burden. It is most helpful for well-differentiated NETs. Elevated plasma chromogranin A levels have been associated with a poor overall prognosis, and early decreases may be associated with favorable treatment outcomes. It can be helpful in screening for persistent, recurrent, or metastatic disease[11]; the recent North American Neuroendocrine Tumor Society's management guidelines recommend following chromogranin A levels in patients with advanced disease and in patients who have elevated CgA levels at diagnosis and to consider following levels in those who have undergone resection.[18] Elevated CgA levels can also be caused by renal or liver failure and the use of proton-pump inhibitors.

The PP cells of the islets of Langerhans secrete pancreatic polypeptide. It is found to be elevated in 63% of PanNETs[28] but has not been widely used because of its low sensitivity. However, high pancreatic polypeptide levels at baseline may be useful in identifying false-negative CgA determinations in the diagnosis of PanNETs and has a high specificity for follow-up in predicting controlled disease (84%).[29] When there is concordance of CgA and PP levels in follow-up, the ability to predict an increase in tumor burden is increased (from 51%–54% independently to 81% together).[29] The diagnostic accuracy of CgA and PP may be lower in the MEN-1 patient population.[30]

Pancreastatin, a posttranslational fragment of CgA, has shown diagnostic value in monitoring carcinoid tumors. Its levels are not influenced by decreased acid production and, thus, may lead to fewer false-positive determinations. Recent studies have shown some promise in using pancreastatin as a diagnostic and prognostic tumor marker for NETs.[31]

Neuron-specific enolase (NSE) is another tumor marker that is found to be elevated in 50% of NETs, most commonly in pulmonary NETs. High levels of NSE have been associated with poorly differentiated NETs.[32] Synaptophysin, glucagon, progastrin-releasing peptide, and cytokeratin fragments have all been evaluated as potential tumor markers but have low sensitivity for detecting NETs.[33]

Screening for MEN-1 with measurement of parathyroid hormone and calcium levels is also recommended given the high prevalence of PanNETs (80%–100%) in this patient population.[2,23]

DIAGNOSTIC PROCEDURES

The diagnosis of PanNETs centers on biopsy and staging of the disease. Cross-sectional imaging studies with either a multiphasic CT scan or magnetic resonance imaging (MRI) dedicated to the evaluation of the pancreas play a key role.

CT

- It is recommended for the initial evaluation of PanNETs.
- PanNETs are well circumscribed, hypervascular lesions (**Fig. 1**).
- It has a sensitivity of 80% to 100% (decreased in tumors smaller than 2 cm, but most symptomatic nonfunctioning tumors are >3 cm).

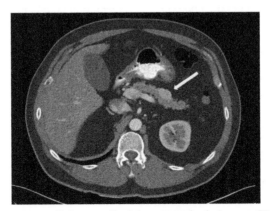

Fig. 1. PanNETs appear as well-circumscribed, hypervascular lesions on CT imaging. CT has a high sensitivity for detecting PanNETs greater than 2 cm in size and offers excellent anatomic and spatial detail. *Arrow* points to neuroendocrine tumor.

- The sensitivity of contrast-enhanced CT approaches 100% (imaging study of choice).
- Dual-phase (arterial and portal) imaging detects pancreatic neoplasms and delineates local vascular anatomy.
- Oral contrast allows optimum visualization of the duodenum, improving the detection of duodenal gastrinomas.

MRI

- PanNETs are typically characterized by low signal intensity on T1-weighted images and high signal intensity on T2-weighted images. (Tumors <1 cm are not detected by MRI with gadolinium; 50% of tumors between 1 and 2 cm are identified.)[34]
- Larger tumors can be visualized without contrast.
- It has a greater sensitivity for liver metastases than CT or somatostatin receptor scintingraphy.[35]

Endoscopic Ultrasonography

- Able to detect small tumors as small as 2 to 3 mm in diameter
- Sensitivity of 79% to 82%, specificity of 95%[36,37]
- Enables histologic analysis with endoscopic ultrasonography (EUS)-guided fine-needle aspiration[38]
- Useful in MEN-1 detecting 55% to 100% of nonfunctional PanNETs in asymptomatic patients[39]
- Operator dependent

Somatostatin Receptor Scintigraphy (Indium In Pentetreotide [Octreoscan])

- Uses indium- 111-labeled somatostatin analogue resulting in high-resolution imaging of the pancreas
- Effective for visualizing gastrinomas (100%), glucagonomas, and nonfunctioning pancreatic tumors
- Not sensitive for detection of insulinomas and poorly differentiated NETs
- Additional advantage of whole-body scanning allowing for detection of metastatic disease outside of the abdomen (**Fig. 2**)
- Provides functional information on level of somatostatin receptor expression, which may be used to guide somatostatin-based therapies in patients with advanced disease
- Does not provide information on tumor size or surgical resectability
- Accuracy improved with fusion of somatostatin analogues to positron emission tomography isotopes in single-photon emission CT; allows differentiation between areas of pathologic and physiologic uptake in the abdomen

Fig. 3 provides a simple algorithm summarizing the diagnostic tests for PanNETs. Other diagnostic procedures, including visceral arteriography and selective intra-arterial stimulation, are used to localize occult functional tumors.

SURGICAL MANAGEMENT

Surgical resection is the only curative therapy for functional and nonfunctional PanNETs and is the cornerstone of the treatment of patients with PanNETs without evidence of metastatic disease or significant comorbidities. There is a significant survival benefit in patients with localized, regional, and metastatic disease who undergo resection (average overall survival 114 months vs 35 months) when compared with those

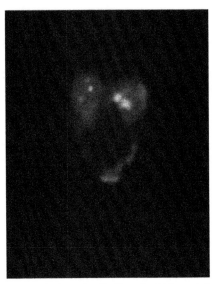

Fig. 2. Somatostatin receptor scintigraphy (indium In 111 pentetreotide [Octreoscan]) allows whole-body imaging and is sensitive for detecting metastatic disease, especially outside of the abdomen. It also allows assessment of somatostatin receptor expression levels that can be used to guide systemic therapy.

who did not undergo surgery.[40] Thus, surgical therapy should be considered if most (approximately 90%) of the gross disease can be resected safely. The primary exception to this rule is PanNETs associated with MEN-1 and Zollinger-Ellison syndrome whereby tumors tend to be multiple and nonfunctional and may warrant close surveillance and/or symptom management.

Given the variable biology and behavior of PanNETs, deciding on the appropriate surgical therapy requires taking into account a myriad of factors, including risk of malignancy, presence/absence of metastases, as well as the patients' overall health and wishes. **Fig. 4** summarizes an algorithm that provides guidance on the surgical treatment of patients with solitary PanNETs. In general, nonfunctional PanNETs should undergo resection. However, evidence is emerging that with more accurate pathologic analysis of biopsy material, there are situations when small lesions can be observed. Most nonfunctional PanNETs are malignant as manifested by local invasion, lymph node involvement, and/or liver metastases. Patients without evidence of metastatic disease should be treated with formal resection and lymphadenectomy. Patients with low-grade metastatic disease should be treated with surgical resection (including resection of metastatic sites) in conjunction with adjuvant therapies, such as ablation, embolization, hormonal therapy, and chemotherapy. Patients with high-grade metastatic disease should receive medical therapy, often including cytotoxic chemotherapy.

All nonfunctional PanNETs greater than 3 cm should be resected if possible. Controversy exists as to whether enucleation is sufficient resection for nonfunctional PanNETs smaller than 3 cm. In a retrospective review of 318 patients with sporadic, nonfunctional, nonsyndromic PanNETs resected at a single institution, 9% to 37% of tumors less than 3 cm in size were associated with lymph node metastases. They also found on multivariate analysis that the presence of positive lymph nodes conferred a poorer survival.[41] Therefore, formal resection is preferred over enucleation

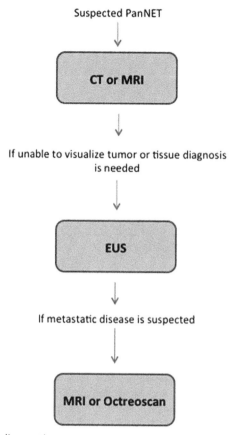

Fig. 3. Algorithm for diagnostic tests.

for nonfunctional PanNETs smaller than 3 cm in size. However, enucleation may be appropriate in elderly patients or those with significant comorbidities, a tumor with a low proliferative index, and patients who do not wish to have a formal resection.[42] Central pancreatectomy is another parenchyma-sparing procedure that can be considered for small benign lesions.[43]

For even smaller tumors less than 2 cm, surgical resection may not necessarily be mandated. The ENETS' guidelines state "no data exist with respect to a positive effect of surgery on overall survival in small (<2 cm), possibly benign or intermediate-risk pancreatic endocrine tumors" and advocate careful balancing of surgical risk before proceeding to resection over observation.[44] Lee and colleagues[45] described a cohort of 67 patients with small (median size 1 cm), incidentally found nonfunctional PanNETs who were observed for a median of 45 months. There were no cases of disease progression over this observation period. Therefore, for small tumors less than 2 cm with a low proliferative index (Ki-67), observation may be an appropriate option. **Table 3** summarizes the surgical options for management of PanNETs.

There have been descriptions and small series of minimally invasive approaches to most of the types of pancreatic resections. These approaches include laparoscopic and robotic techniques for both traditional, formal resections like pancreaticoduodenectomy to parenchyma-sparing operations like enucleations and central

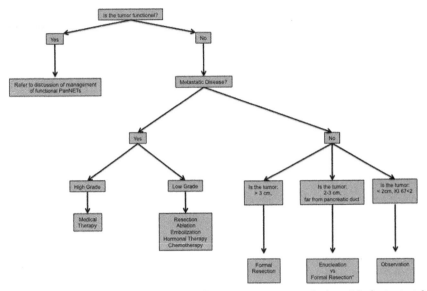

Fig. 4. Decision tree for surgical resection of PanNET. PD, pancreatic duct. * Refer to text for discussion of enucleation versus formal resection.

pancreatectomies. The most commonly performed minimally invasive pancreatic operations are laparoscopic enucleations and laparoscopic distal pancreatectomy. Gagner and colleagues[46] first described their approach to the laparoscopic distal pancreatectomy with spleen preservation for insulinoma in 1996. It has become the gold standard for small, benign lesions or low-grade malignancies. In 2012, a meta-analysis showed that laparoscopic distal pancreatectomy resulted in decreased morbidity (39.3% vs 44.2%), with decreased estimated blood loss by approximately 350 mL and a decreased length of hospital stay by 4 days.[47] They found no difference in operative time, margin positivity, incidence of postoperative pancreatic fistula, and mortality.

Although laparoscopic pancreaticoduodenectomy was described before laparoscopic distal pancreatectomy in 1994,[48] the technique has been slow to gain popularity because of the complex technique and long operative times. However, a recent meta-analysis showed statistically significant differences with respect to less blood loss, lower transfusion rates, lower wound infection rates, lower morbidity rates, and shorter hospital stays. The laparoscopic approach is significantly longer compared with the open approach for pancreaticoduodenectomy.[49] There was no significant difference in oncological outcomes between laparoscopic pancreatectomy and the open technique.[49] Although there is often a learning curve involved, laparoscopic operations can be performed safely and offer a good alternative to formal open operations in the appropriate patients.

Robotic surgery has quickly evolved over the last decade, and several case series describing robotic approaches to distal pancreatectomy and pancreaticoduodenectomy have been published. Cirocchi and colleagues[50,51] reviewed these studies and concluded that although the operative times were longer for robotic distal pancreatectomy and pancreaticoduodenectomy, the robotic technique is feasible with similar morbidity and mortality to the laparoscopic and open techniques and is associated with a decreased length of hospital stay with distal pancreatectomies.[50] They

Table 3
Summary of operative management options for PaNETs

Procedure	Approach	Indications	Contraindications	Outcomes
Traditional resections				
Pancreaticoduodenectomy	Most commonly open Laparoscopic approach gaining popularity Robotic approach being investigated	Large tumors of the pancreatic head, uncinate, or neck	Involvement of the superior mesenteric artery Exclusion based on portal vein involvement may vary by institution	Significant survival benefit in patients who undergo resection[9]
Distal pancreatectomy	Open Laparoscopic	Large tumors of the pancreatic body or tail	Splenic preservation contraindicated for patients with suspected malignancy	Laparoscopic approach affords better postoperative pain, shorter hospital stay, shorter recovery, and better cosmesis[40]
Parenchyma-sparing resections				
Enucleation	Open Laparoscopic	Tumors ≤3 cm in size	Large tumors Nodal or metastatic disease Lesions in close proximity to the pancreatic duct	Similar morbidity and 5-y survival as traditional resections[53] Increased rate of pancreatic fistulas but less severe Decreased blood loss, operative time, and length of hospital stay
Central pancreatectomy	Open Laparoscopic	Small, benign, or low-grade tumors of the neck or proximal body of the pancreas	High-grade and/or advanced tumors	Better preservation of pancreas function with similar morbidity and mortality[43]

concluded that randomized trials were needed to compare oncologic outcomes and the cost-effectiveness of these procedures.

MANAGEMENT OF HEPATIC METASTASES

The liver is the predominant site of extranodal metastatic disease in PanNETs and is the predominant cause of mortality in many patients. Resection of hepatic metastases has been shown to improve outcomes in more than 90% of cases.[11,52–54] Survival rates of approximately 60% are reported at 5 years after hepatic metastasectomy compared with 30% in patients with untreated liver metastases,[54,55] with a median survival of 24 to 128 months. In patients without (or mild nonclinically significant) extrahepatic disease, resection should be considered for treatment. Asymptomatic patients who have resectable disease should also be considered for surgical debulking. **Table 4** summarizes the interventional treatment options for hepatic metastases in patients who are not candidates for surgical resection. In general, the use of these treatments either alone or in conjunction with surgical resection is recommended for locoregional control and symptom relief.[56–58] Liver transplantation is a viable option for symptomatic, well-differentiated gastrointestinal NETs when standard surgical resection is not an option or for disease that has not responded to other treatment options. The 5-year survival rate is 45%.[59] However, a primary PanNET was found to be a negative prognostic factor[60]; therefore, liver transplantation is not recommended in the treatment of NETs arising from the pancreas.

SYSTEMIC THERAPY

Patients with high-grade metastatic disease not amenable to surgical resection or liver-directed therapies can be treated with multiple medical therapeutic approaches. The goal of treatment is to improve quality of life and to extend progression-free survival as well as overall survival. Medical treatment can control the associated symptoms and signs of the specific tumors and shrink tumor mass.

Somatostatin Analogues

Octreotide is the prototypical somatostatin analogue used to treat patients with advanced PanNETs. Nearly 80% of NETs express somatostatin receptors as evidenced by radiotracer uptake on Octreoscans, providing an effective means of delivering cytotoxic treatments to neoplastic cells.[61] Radiolabeled somatostatin analogues bind to the somatostatin receptor, and a fraction of the ligand-receptor complex is internalized, delivering targeted radiotherapy to PanNETs.[62] The most frequently used radionuclides for therapy in PanNETs are indium, yttrium, and lutetium, which differ from one another in terms of emitted particles, particle energy, and tissue penetration.[63] Overall, tumor response rates have been reported between 30% and 50%; stable disease following treatment has been reported in up to 70%.[64,65] In the PROMID study, the use of octreotide-LAR (octreotide acetate long-acting injectable solution) increased the time to progression (14.3 months) as compared with placebo (6 months).[66] Stable disease was achieved in 66.7% and 37.2% of patients with octreotide-LAR and placebo, respectively. It was found to be effective in both functioning and nonfunctioning tumors. The duration of the therapy response is reported to be greater than 30 months; when kidney protective agents are used, the side effects of this therapy are few and mild.[65] Ongoing clinical trials are evaluating the efficacy of novel somatostatin analogues (SOM230 or pasireotide) that have 30 to 40 times higher binding affinity to somatostatin receptors than octreotide and lanreotide.[67]

Table 4
Summary of interventional liver-directed therapies for metastatic PaNETs

Treatment	Indications	Contraindications	Approach	Outcomes
Hepatic artery embolization	Palliation of patients who are not candidates for surgical resection Metastasis limited to the liver	Prior pancreaticoduodenectomy Significant hepatic insufficiency Portal vein thrombosis Poor performance status	Bland embolization: infusion of absorbable gelatin sponge (Gelfoam) powder Chemoembolization (TACE): infusion of cytotoxic drugs (doxorubicin, cisplatin, and streptozocin) or use of drug-eluting beads Radioembolization: use of radioactive isotopes (eg, yttrium-90)	Response rates generally exceed 50%[58-60]
Radiofrequency ablation, microwave ablation, and cryoablation	Patients with <10 lesions, each lesion <4 cm in size Small tumors deep in hepatic parenchyma	Large tumors	Used alone or in combination with surgical resection Percutaneous or laparoscopic approach	Morbidity benefit when compared with hepatic arterial embolization Recurrences common, but multiple treatments may be given with good tolerance
Infusional chemotherapy	Uncommon technique Used in conjunction with radiotherapy	Diffuse disease	Percutaneous infusion of 5-FU or melphalan with extraction of the drug from hepatic veins Multiple treatments possible	Good locoregional control with tumor response seen in 80% of patients when combined with radiotherapy[58]

Abbreviations: TACE, trans-arterial chemoembolization; 5-FU, 5-fluorouracil.

Peptide receptor radionucleotide therapy is a newer treatment option that couples cytotoxic drugs to somatostatin analogues to target PanNETs. Initially octreotide was used, but this has been largely replaced by yttrium-90 or lutetium-177 coupled analogues. This treatment has been shown to be effective for both symptom relief and tumor remission. Adverse effects are typically mild and limited primarily to toxicity to the bone marrow and kidneys.[68]

Cytotoxic Chemotherapy

Historically, well-differentiated PanNETs have been resistant to standard chemotherapy, with reported response rates varying from 8% to 45%.[69] Because of the limited efficacy of these agents, they were often started when patients demonstrated progressive disease despite somatostatin analogues. More recently, a randomized trial comparing the combination of streptozocin with doxorubicin versus streptozocin with fluorouracil demonstrated a mortality benefit as well as radiological and biochemical regression of disease in 69% of patients.[70] Therapy with streptozocin is limited by its toxicity and cumbersome administration schedule. Oral temozolomide (an alkylating agent) is better tolerated and has been shown to have comparable efficacy.[70] An 18-month median progression-free survival in patients with metastatic PanNETs was demonstrated in patients who received temozolomide and capecitabine.[62] Cytotoxic therapies should be considered in the palliation of patients with advanced PanNETs and symptoms related to tumor bulk.

Targeted Therapy

NETs have been shown to express a multitude of growth factors and their corresponding receptors leading to the development of targeted therapeutic agents. Recent phase III studies have shown tremendous promise for 2 drugs designed for targeted therapy in the treatment of PanNETs, everolimus and sunitinib. Both drugs are recommended for patients with progressive metastatic PanNETs.

Everolimus

mTOR (mammalian target of rapamycin) is a serine/threonine kinase involved in the regulation of cell growth and death through apoptosis. It is also capable of impacting multiple downstream pathways, including vascular endothelial growth factor (VEG-F) and other growth factors. There is a relationship between the TSC and the phosphatase and tensin homolog (PTEN), NF-1, and VHL genes that contribute to the development of neuroendocrine tumors. Downregulation of TSC2 and PTEN have been shown to be a poor prognostic factor in PanNETs, supporting an important role for the PI3K/Akt/mTOR pathway and its inhibition in the treatment of PanNETs.[69,71,72] Everolimus (RAD001), an oral mTOR inhibitor, has been shown to have antitumor activity in many solid tumors, including PanNETs. The RAD001 in Advanced Neuroendocrine Tumors-3 (RADIANT-3) study by Yao and colleagues[73] is a randomized phase 3 study evaluating the efficacy of everolimus in advanced PanNETs. In this international multisite study, 410 patients with low- or intermediate-grade, progressive, advanced PanNETs were randomized to receive everolimus, 10 mg oral daily, or placebo. The response rate was 5% in the everolimus arm compared with 2% in the placebo arm, with a median progression-free survival of 11.0 months with everolimus compared with 4.6 months with placebo (hazard ratio, 0.35; 95% confidence interval, 0.27–0.45; $P<.001$). The median overall survival has not been reached. The Food and Drug Administration (FDA) has approved everolimus for advanced PanNETs. Adverse events associated with everolimus are rare and most commonly include stomatitis, rash, diarrhea, fatigue, infections, and pneumonitis.

Sunitinib

PanNETs express an abundance of VEG-F and platelet-derived growth factor (PDGF) receptors. Three tyrosine kinase inhibitors have shown activity against VEG-F receptor: pazopanib, sorafenib, and sunitinib. Sunitinib is an oral, small-molecule, multi-targeted tyrosine kinase inhibitor with activity against VEG-F and PDGF. A phase II trial demonstrated a response rate of 17% with a stable disease rate of 68%.[74] In a multinational randomized controlled trial of 171 patients with advanced, well-differentiated, and progressive pancreatic neuroendocrine carcinomas, patients were randomized to receive sunitinib, 37.5 mg orally daily, or placebo. Sunitinib increased progression-free survival (11.4 months) versus placebo (5.5 months, $P<.0001$).[75] This study was terminated early because of more serious adverse events and deaths in the placebo group (25%) compared with the group receiving sunitinib; thus, the benefit in overall survival could not be determined. It can also be safely combined with somatostatin analogues without affecting the quality of life. Adverse events associated with sunitinib include diarrhea, nausea, asthenia, vomiting, fatigue, and hypothyroidism. The FDA and European Medicines Agency have approved sunitinib for the treatment of unresectable or metastatic, well-differentiated PanNETs with disease progression in adults.

Bevacizumab

Bevacizumab is a humanized monoclonal antibody that inhibits VEG-F and has recently been tested in combination with capecitabine and oxaliplatin for patients with advanced neuroendocrine tumors.[76] In patients with PanNETs, 30% exhibited partial responses with a median progression-free survival of 13.7 months. Prospective, randomized phase III studies combining bevacizumab with octreotide, temozolomide, CAPOX (oxaliplatin and capecitabine), FOLFOX (oxaliplatin and fluorouracil), and everolimus are still ongoing.[77,78]

SUMMARY

PanNETs are a heterogeneous group of tumors that pose a significant challenge because of the heterogeneous clinical presentations and varying degree of aggressiveness. The incidence of PanNETs is increasing, in part, because of the increased use of cross-sectional imaging and increased incidence of pancreatic incidentalomas. Most PanNETs are nonfunctional tumors, and most are malignant in nature. Surgery remains the only curative modality for PanNETs; resection of the primary tumor in localized, regional, and even metastatic disease can improve patient survival. Selecting an operative approach for PanNETs is a complex decision that must consider a myriad of factors, including functional status, benign or malignant nature, involvement with contiguous structures, presence of metastatic disease, proliferative index, and whether the tumor is sporadic or associated with a genetic syndrome. Indications for surgery in patients with nonfunctional PanNETs include local compressive symptoms caused by mass effect and prevention of malignant transformation or dissemination. In general, nonfunctional PanNETs, even those smaller than 3 cm, are best treated with formal resection and appropriate lymphadenectomy because a significant percentage of even small nonfunctional PanNETs will have lymph node metastases. However, in certain clinical scenarios (eg, low Ki-67, patient with significant comorbidities, patient who does not want an extensive resection, and so forth), nonfunctional PanNETs that are 3 cm or less in size that do not impinge on the common bile or pancreatic ducts can be enucleated. There is evidence to suggest observation is appropriate for selected patients with tumors smaller than 2 cm and a low proliferation index. PanNETs greater than 3 cm should be resected with an appropriate oncologic operation based on the location within the pancreas. For lesions located in the head, uncinate, or neck of the pancreas, pancreaticoduodenectomy can be performed. For lesions located in the body or tail of the pancreas, distal pancreatectomy can be performed. For lesions in the neck and proximal body, either an extended pancreatico-duodenectomy or extended distal pancreatectomy may be performed depending on the specific anatomy. For select lesions in the neck and proximal body of the pancreas, central pancreatectomy may be performed. Patients with evidence of metastatic hepatic disease should be considered for metastasectomy if possible. In those patients who are not surgical candidates, early, aggressive treatment of unresectable liver metastases using interventional techniques may improve symptom relief and quality of life and should be considered for palliation of disease. For patients with advanced, metastatic disease not amenable to surgical resection, somatostatin analogues and targeted therapies offer promising therapeutic alternatives for decreasing morbidity and increasing progression-free survival.

REFERENCES

1. Yao JC, Phan AT, Chang DZ, et al. Efficacy of RAD001 (everolimus) and octreotide LAR in advanced low- to intermediate-grade neuroendocrine tumors: results of a phase II study. J Clin Oncol 2008;26(26):4311.
2. Metz DC, Jensen RT. Gastrointestinal neuroendocrine tumors: pancreatic endocrine tumors. Gastroenterology 2008;135(5):1469.
3. Carriaga MT, Henson DE. Liver, gallbladder, extrahepatic bile ducts, and pancreas. Cancer 1995;75(Suppl 1):171.
4. Yao JC, Hassan M, Phan A, et al. One hundred years after "carcinoid": epidemiology of and prognostic factors for neuroendocrine tumors in 35,825 cases in the United States. J Clin Oncol 2008;26(18):3063.
5. Lawrence B, Gustafsson BI, Chan A, et al. The epidemiology of gastroenteropancreatic neuroendocrine tumors. Endocrinol Metab Clin North Am 2011;40(1):1.
6. Lahat G, Ben Haim M, Nachmany I, et al. Pancreatic incidentalomas: high rate of potentially malignant tumors. J Am Coll Surg 2009;209(3):313.
7. Grimelius L, Hultquist GT, Stenkvist B. Cytological differentiation of asymptomatic pancreatic islet cell tumours in autopsy material. Virchows Arch A Pathol Anat Histol 1975;365(4):275.
8. Kimura W, Jimi A, Miyasaka K, et al. Immunohistochemical study of the distribution of pancreastatin in endocrine tumors of the pancreas and in normal pancreatic tissue: analysis of autopsy cases. Pancreas 1991;6(6):688.
9. Burns WR, Edil BH. Neuroendocrine pancreatic tumors: guidelines for management and update. Curr Treat Options Oncol 2012;13(1):24.
10. Vortmeyer AO, Huang S, Lubensky I, et al. Non-islet origin of pancreatic islet cell tumors. J Clin Endocrinol Metab 2004;89(4):1934.
11. Muniraj T, Vignesh S, Shetty S, et al. Pancreatic neuroendocrine tumors. Dis Mon 2013;59(1):5.
12. Duerr EM, Chung DC. Molecular genetics of neuroendocrine tumors. Best Pract Res Clin Endocrinol Metab 2007;21(1):1.
13. Halfdanarson TR, Rabe KG, Rubin J, et al. Pancreatic neuroendocrine tumors (PNETs): incidence, prognosis and recent trend toward improved survival. Ann Oncol 2008;19(10):1727.
14. de Wilde RF, Edil BH, Hruban RH, et al. Well-differentiated pancreatic neuroendocrine tumors: from genetics to therapy. Nat Rev Gastroenterol Hepatol 2012; 9(4):199.

15. Kloppel G, Perren A, Heitz PU. The gastroenteropancreatic neuroendocrine cell system and its tumors: the WHO classification. Ann N Y Acad Sci 2004;1014:13.
16. Panzuto F, Campana D, Fazio N, et al. Risk factors for disease progression in advanced jejunoileal neuroendocrine tumors. Neuroendocrinology 2012;96(1):32.
17. Boninsegna L, Panzuto F, Partelli S, et al. Malignant pancreatic neuroendocrine tumour: lymph node ratio and Ki-67 are predictors of recurrence after curative resections. Eur J Cancer 2012;48(11):1608.
18. Kunz PL, Reidy-Lagunes D, Anthony LB, et al. Consensus guidelines for the management and treatment of neuroendocrine tumors. Pancreas 2013;42(4):557.
19. Rindi G, de Herder WW, O'Toole D, et al. Consensus guidelines for the management of patients with digestive neuroendocrine tumors: why such guidelines and how we went about it. Neuroendocrinology 2006;84(3):155.
20. Strosberg JR, Cheema A, Weber JM, et al. Relapse-free survival in patients with nonmetastatic, surgically resected pancreatic neuroendocrine tumors: an analysis of the AJCC and ENETS staging classifications. Ann Surg 2012;256(2):321.
21. Sadaria MR, Hruban RH, Edil BH. Advancements in pancreatic neuroendocrine tumors. Expert Rev Gastroenterol Hepatol 2013;7(5):477.
22. Li J, Luo G, Fu D, et al. Preoperative diagnosis of nonfunctioning pancreatic neuroendocrine tumors. Med Oncol 2011;28(4):1027.
23. Zarate X, Williams N, Herrera MF. Pancreatic incidentalomas. Best Pract Res Clin Endocrinol Metab 2012;26(1):97.
24. O'Toole D, Saveanu A, Couvelard A, et al. The analysis of quantitative expression of somatostatin and dopamine receptors in gastro-entero-pancreatic tumours opens new therapeutic strategies. Eur J Endocrinol 2006;155(6):849.
25. O'Grady HL, Conlon KC. Pancreatic neuroendocrine tumours. Eur J Surg Oncol 2008;34(3):324.
26. Nissen NN, Kim AS, Yu R, et al. Pancreatic neuroendocrine tumors: presentation, management, and outcomes. Am Surg 2009;75(10):1025.
27. Bruzoni M, Johnston E, Sasson AR. Pancreatic incidentalomas: clinical and pathologic spectrum. Am J Surg 2008;195(3):329.
28. Panzuto F, Severi C, Cannizzaro R, et al. Utility of combined use of plasma levels of chromogranin A and pancreatic polypeptide in the diagnosis of gastrointestinal and pancreatic endocrine tumors. J Endocrinol Invest 2004;27(1):6.
29. Walter T, Chardon L, Chopin-laly X, et al. Is the combination of chromogranin A and pancreatic polypeptide serum determinations of interest in the diagnosis and follow-up of gastro-entero-pancreatic neuroendocrine tumours? Eur J Cancer 2012;48(12):1766.
30. de Laat JM, Pieterman CR, Weijmans M, et al. Low accuracy of tumor markers for diagnosing pancreatic neuroendocrine tumors in multiple endocrine neoplasia type 1 patients. J Clin Endocrinol Metab 2013;98(10):4143.
31. Rustagi S, Warner RR, Divino CM. Serum pancreastatin: the next predictive neuroendocrine tumor marker. J Surg Oncol 2013;108(2):126–8.
32. Baudin E, Gigliotti A, Ducreux M, et al. Neuron-specific enolase and chromogranin A as markers of neuroendocrine tumours. Br J Cancer 1998;78(8):1102.
33. Korse CM, Taal BG, Vincent A, et al. Choice of tumour markers in patients with neuroendocrine tumours is dependent on the histological grade. A marker study of chromogranin A, neuron specific enolase, progastrin-releasing peptide and cytokeratin fragments. Eur J Cancer 2012;48(5):662.

34. Boukhman MP, Karam JH, Shaver J, et al. Insulinoma–experience from 1950 to 1995. West J Med 1998;169(2):98.
35. Dromain C, Baudin E. Endocrine pancreas. J Radiol 2005;86(6 Pt 2):797 [in French].
36. Rosch T, Lightdale CJ, Botet JF, et al. Localization of pancreatic endocrine tumors by endoscopic ultrasonography. N Engl J Med 1992;326(26):1721.
37. Bernstein J, Ustun B, Alomari A, et al. Performance of endoscopic ultrasound-guided fine needle aspiration in diagnosing pancreatic neuroendocrine tumors. Cytojournal 2013;10:10.
38. Chatzipantelis P, Salla C, Konstantinou P, et al. Endoscopic ultrasound-guided fine-needle aspiration cytology of pancreatic neuroendocrine tumors: a study of 48 cases. Cancer 2008;114(4):255.
39. Konda VJ, Aslanian HR, Wallace MB, et al. First assessment of needle-based confocal laser endomicroscopy during EUS-FNA procedures of the pancreas (with videos). Gastrointest Endosc 2011;74(5):1049.
40. Hill JS, McPhee JT, McDade TP, et al. Pancreatic neuroendocrine tumors: the impact of surgical resection on survival. Cancer 2009;115(4):741.
41. Ellison TA, Olino K, Cameron JL, et al. Tumor size correlates with lymph node metastasis in primary pancreatic endocrine neoplasms. New Orleans (LA): The Society for Surgery of the Alimentary Tract; 2010.
42. Pitt SC, Pitt HA, Baker MS, et al. Small pancreatic and periampullary neuroendocrine tumors: resect or enucleate? J Gastrointest Surg 2009;13(9):1692.
43. DiNorcia J, Ahmed L, Lee MK, et al. Better preservation of endocrine function after central versus distal pancreatectomy for mid-gland lesions. Surgery 2010;148(6):1247.
44. Falconi M, Bettini R, Boninsegna L, et al. Surgical strategy in the treatment of pancreatic neuroendocrine tumors. J Pancreas 2006;7(1):150.
45. Lee LC, Grant CS, Salomao DR, et al. Small, nonfunctioning, asymptomatic pancreatic neuroendocrine tumors (PNETs): role for nonoperative management. Surgery 2012;152(6):965.
46. Gagner M, Pomp A, Herrera MF. Early experience with laparoscopic resections of islet cell tumors. Surgery 1996;120(6):1051.
47. Venkat R, Edil BH, Schulick RD, et al. Laparoscopic distal pancreatectomy is associated with significantly less overall morbidity compared to the open technique: a systematic review and meta-analysis. Ann Surg 2012;255(6):1048.
48. Gagner M, Pomp A. Laparoscopic pylorus-preserving pancreatoduodenectomy. Surg Endosc 1994;8(5):408.
49. Nakamura M, Nakashima H. Laparoscopic distal pancreatectomy and pancreatoduodenectomy: is it worthwhile? A meta-analysis of laparoscopic pancreatectomy. J Hepatobiliary Pancreat Sci 2013;20(4):421.
50. Cirocchi R, Partelli S, Coratti A, et al. Current status of robotic distal pancreatectomy: a systematic review. Surg Oncol 2013;22(3):201.
51. Cirocchi R, Partelli S, Trastulli S, et al. A systematic review on robotic pancreaticoduodenectomy. Surg Oncol 2013;22(4):238–46.
52. Kulke MH, Benson AB 3rd, Bergsland E, et al. Neuroendocrine tumors. J Natl Compr Canc Netw 2012;10(6):724.
53. Sarmiento JM, Que FG. Hepatic surgery for metastases from neuroendocrine tumors. Surg Oncol Clin N Am 2003;12(1):231.
54. Touzios JG, Kiely JM, Pitt SC, et al. Neuroendocrine hepatic metastases: does aggressive management improve survival? Ann Surg 2005;241(5):776.

55. Chamberlain RS, Canes D, Brown KT, et al. Hepatic neuroendocrine metastases: does intervention alter outcomes? J Am Coll Surg 2000;190(4):432.
56. Halperin DM, Kulke MH. Management of pancreatic neuroendocrine tumors. Gastroenterol Clin North Am 2012;41(1):119.
57. Minter RM, Simeone DM. Contemporary management of nonfunctioning pancreatic neuroendocrine tumors. J Gastrointest Surg 2012;16(2):435.
58. Toumpanakis C, Meyer T, Caplin ME. Cytotoxic treatment including embolization/chemoembolization for neuroendocrine tumours. Best Pract Res Clin Endocrinol Metab 2007;21(1):131.
59. Le Treut YP, Gregoire E, Belghiti J, et al. Predictors of long-term survival after liver transplantation for metastatic endocrine tumors: an 85-case French multicentric report. Am J Transplant 2008;8(6):1205.
60. Gregoire E, Le Treut YP. Liver transplantation for primary or secondary endocrine tumors. Transpl Int 2010;23(7):704.
61. Wang C, Xu H, Chen H, et al. Somatostatin stimulates intestinal NHE8 expression via p38 MAPK pathway. Am J Physiol Cell Physiol 2011;300(2): C375.
62. Strosberg JR, Cheema A, Kvols LK. A review of systemic and liver-directed therapies for metastatic neuroendocrine tumors of the gastroenteropancreatic tract. Cancer Control 2011;18(2):127.
63. Teunissen JJ, Kwekkeboom DJ, de Jong M, et al. Endocrine tumours of the gastrointestinal tract. Peptide receptor radionuclide therapy. Best Pract Res Clin Gastroenterol 2005;19(4):595.
64. Waldherr C, Pless M, Maecke HR, et al. Tumor response and clinical benefit in neuroendocrine tumors after 7.4 GBq (90)Y-DOTATOC. J Nucl Med 2002;43(5): 610.
65. Kwekkeboom DJ, de Herder WW, Krenning EP. Somatostatin receptor-targeted radionuclide therapy in patients with gastroenteropancreatic neuroendocrine tumors. Endocrinol Metab Clin North Am 2011;40(1):173.
66. Rinke A, Muller HH, Schade-Brittinger C, et al. Placebo-controlled, double-blind, prospective, randomized study on the effect of octreotide LAR in the control of tumor growth in patients with metastatic neuroendocrine midgut tumors: a report from the PROMID Study Group. J Clin Oncol 2009;27(28): 4656.
67. Demirkan BH, Eriksson B. Systemic treatment of neuroendocrine tumors with hepatic metastases. Turk J Gastroenterol 2012;23(5):427.
68. Forrer F, Valkema R, Kwekkeboom DJ, et al. Neuroendocrine tumors. Peptide receptor radionuclide therapy. Best Pract Res Clin Endocrinol Metab 2007;21(1): 111.
69. Chan JA, Kulke MH. New treatment options for patients with advanced neuroendocrine tumors. Curr Treat Options Oncol 2011;12(2):136.
70. Moertel CG, Kvols LK, O'Connell MJ, et al. Treatment of neuroendocrine carcinomas with combined etoposide and cisplatin. Evidence of major therapeutic activity in the anaplastic variants of these neoplasms. Cancer 1991;68(2): 227.
71. Wang L, Ignat A, Axiotis CA. Differential expression of the PTEN tumor suppressor protein in fetal and adult neuroendocrine tissues and tumors: progressive loss of PTEN expression in poorly differentiated neuroendocrine neoplasms. Appl Immunohistochem Mol Morphol 2002;10(2):139.
72. Kulke MH. Gastrointestinal neuroendocrine tumors: a role for targeted therapies? Endocr Relat Cancer 2007;14(2):207.

73. Yao JC, Shah MH, Ito T, et al. Everolimus for advanced pancreatic neuroendocrine tumors. N Engl J Med 2011;364(6):514.
74. Kulke MH, Lenz HJ, Meropol NJ, et al. Activity of sunitinib in patients with advanced neuroendocrine tumors. J Clin Oncol 2008;26(20):3403.
75. Raymond E, Dahan L, Raoul JL, et al. Sunitinib malate for the treatment of pancreatic neuroendocrine tumors. N Engl J Med 2011;364(6):501.
76. Kunz PL, Fisher GA. Advances in the treatment of gastroenteropancreatic neuroendocrine tumors. Clin Exp Gastroenterol 2010;3:79–86.
77. Terris B, Scoazec JY, Rubbia L, et al. Expression of vascular endothelial growth factor in digestive neuroendocrine tumours. Histopathology 1998;32(2):133.
78. Yao JC, Phan A, Hoff PM, et al. Targeting vascular endothelial growth factor in advanced carcinoid tumor: a random assignment phase II study of depot octreotide with bevacizumab and pegylated interferon alpha-2b. J Clin Oncol 2008;26(8):1316.

Index

Note: Page numbers of article titles are in **boldface** type.

Surg Clin N Am 94 (2014) 709–719
http://dx.doi.org/10.1016/S0039-6109(14)00060-7
0039-6109/14/$ – see front matter © 2014 Elsevier Inc. All rights reserved.

surgical.theclinics.com

Moving?

Make sure your subscription moves with you!

To notify us of your new address, find your **Clinics Account Number** (located on your mailing label above your name), and contact customer service at:

Email: journalscustomerservice-usa@elsevier.com

800-654-2452 (subscribers in the U.S. & Canada)
314-447-8871 (subscribers outside of the U.S. & Canada)

Fax number: 314-447-8029

Elsevier Health Sciences Division
Subscription Customer Service
3251 Riverport Lane
Maryland Heights, MO 63043

*To ensure uninterrupted delivery of your subscription, please notify us at least 4 weeks in advance of move.

Printed and bound by CPI Group (UK) Ltd, Croydon, CR0 4YY

03/10/2024

01040497-0005